Trigeminal Nerve Pain

Alaa Abd-Elsayed

Editor

Trigeminal Nerve Pain

A Guide to Clinical Management

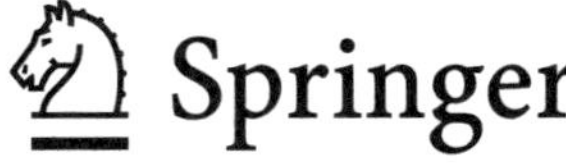 Springer

Editor
Alaa Abd-Elsayed
Department of Anesthesiology
University of Wisconsin School of Medicine and Public Health
Madison, WI
USA

ISBN 978-3-030-60689-3   ISBN 978-3-030-60687-9   (eBook)
https://doi.org/10.1007/978-3-030-60687-9

This Springer imprint is published by the registered company Springer Nature Switzerland AG
The registered company address is: Gewerbestrasse 11, 6330 Cham, Switzerland

To my parents, my wife, and my two beautiful kids Maro and George

Preface

Trigeminal nerve pain and related headache conditions impact millions of people in the USA and across the world. Affected persons can suffer with debilitating pain leading to a deterioration of overall quality of life and psychological well-being. Unfortunately, the diagnosis and treatment of these syndromes can be challenging given a lack of strong training in managing these conditions.

This book discusses the different painful trigeminal nerve conditions with a special focus on trigeminal neuralgia which is the most common trigeminal pain condition. Authors fully and comprehensively discuss these syndromes, including the epidemiology, anatomy, diagnosis, and the different available treatment strategies including non-pharmacological, pharmacological, interventional, and surgical modalities.

This book provides excellent information that will be useful for all practitioners who deal with trigeminal nerve conditions in any setting. It is important to recognize that treating trigeminal nerve conditions requires a multidisciplinary collaboration among pain physicians, neurologists, surgeons, primary care providers, and psychiatrists. Consequently, this book discusses the different approaches taken by and expertise provided from these varying physicians.

I hope that this book will facilitate your understanding of trigeminal nerve conditions and help you utilize the available modalities for treating them. I also hope that this knowledge will help provide comfort in approaching patients with these conditions.

I would like to thank all the authors who contributed to this book and Springer for sponsoring this book for publication.

Madison, WI   Alaa Abd-Elsayed, MD, MPH

Contents

History

1

Hemant Kalia, Jay Karri, and Alaa Abd-Elsayed

Introduction

Trigeminal Neuralgia (TN), also known as *tic douloureux*, has been a topic of great debate and discussion since the sixteenth century. Some of the early work by Galen and Avicenna reference this clinical entity but the first accurate clinical descriptions were provided by Drs. Johannes Michael Fehr and Elias Schmidt, secretaries of the Imperial Leopoldina Academy of the Natural Sciences, and famous philosopher John Locke [1].

In 1756, Nicholas Andre coined the term *tic douloureux,* as he believed that the condition stems from a nerve being in distress and considered it to be a convulsive disorder. The term was used to describe facial contortions and grimaces associated with intermittent sharp, stabbing, and often unbearable pain [2]. The name was accepted despite lack of facial tics in all the patients suffering from this entity.

In 1773, an English physician, Dr. John Fothergill published his experience with 14 patients and attributed TN to be a manifestation of some type of cancer instead of a convulsive disorder thus coining the term *Fothergill's disorder*. In his own words, he stated "The affection seems to be peculiar to persons advancing in years, and to women more than to men. The pain comes suddenly and is excruciating; it lasts but a short time, perhaps a quarter or half a minute, and then goes off; it returns at irregular intervals, sometimes in half an hour, sometimes there are two or three

H. Kalia
Rochester Regional Health System, Rochester, NY, USA

J. Karri
Physical Medicine and Rehabilitation, Baylor College of Medicine, Houston, TX, USA

A. Abd-Elsayed (✉)
Department of Anesthesiology, University of Wisconsin School of Medicine and Public Health, Madison, WI, USA
e-mail: abdelsayed@wisc.edu

A. Abd-Elsayed (ed.), *Trigeminal Nerve Pain*,
https://doi.org/10.1007/978-3-030-60687-9_1

repetitions in a few minutes. Eating will bring it on some persons. Talking, or the least motion of the muscles of the face affects the others; the gentlest touch of a hand-kerchief will sometimes bring on the pain, while a strong pressure on the part has no effect." [3].

In 1820, Dr. Charles Bell was the first physician to localize this syndrome to trigeminal ganglion. TN continued to be a major neurosurgical concern ever since the field emerged as a distinct specialty in the early twentieth century.

Although the etiology of TN continued to be an enigma for quite some time, initial common pathophysiological basis of the disease revolved around the concepts of segmental demyelination at dorsal root entry zone of trigeminal complex, some of the evolved concepts ranged from vascular compression, a compressive mass lesion, postinfectious, multiple sclerosis, trigeminal deafferentation syndrome to even somatoform pain disorder. Historically, TN has also been named as "suicide disease" by Harvey Cushing due to its recalcitrant nature and its psychological effect [4].

Traditionally, treatment of choice was medical management, however, recalcitrant cases were referred for neurosurgical interventions, which later on led to development of specific approaches to target trigeminal ganglion with varying success rates.

Medical Therapies

Early eighteenth and nineteenth centuries saw the use of various compounds like quinine [3], mercury, opium, arsenic [5], and powder of gelsenium as some of the treatments for TN [3]. Sodium diphenylhydantoin was the first antiepileptic medication described in the literature to be used by Bergouignan in 1942 [6].

In current clinical context, carbamazepine is the primary drug of choice, with oxcarbazepine also utilized given this relatively more favorable side effect profile. These medications have rates of efficacy above 90% with a more tolerable risk–benefit ratio. Phenytoin is the second-line drug of choice in TN [7].

Percutaneous Approaches

In 1904, Schloesser and his colleagues described a percutaneous approach for chemoneurolysis of trigeminal ganglion using alcohol; however, this technique fell out of favor due to significant side effects namely weakness of the muscles of mastication, transient dysesthesias, and higher rates of recurrence [1].

In 1913, Rethi first attempted and described electrocoagulation of the trigeminal ganglion [1]. In 1931, a stereotactic approach to insert insulated electrodes through the foramen ovale for electrocoagulation of trigeminal ganglion using monopolar cautery was described by Kirschner [8]. Since initial description of percutaneous approach to trigeminal ganglion, there have been considerable modifications to the approach and electrode types as well. Of all the percutaneous techniques, radiofrequency ablation provides the longest pain relief with minimal side effects [1].

In 1983, Mullen and Lictor first described percutaneous balloon microcompression of the trigeminal ganglion. Despite multiple advances in the technique, the side effects involving postoperative numbness described as *anesthesia dolorosa* and weakness in the muscles of mastication, which can occur in about 66% of cases led to this technique to fall out of favor [9].

In the early 2000s, thermal ablation of the trigeminal nerve, by way of radiofrequency ablation modalities, began to be described [10]. Several authors report efficacious use of this modality with good benefit [11, 12]. The greatest benefit is thought to be obtained with combined use of continuous and pulsed radiofrequency ablation. Main adverse effects include formation of cheek hematomas, facial paresthesias or numbness, and motor impairments of the muscles of mastication.

Surgical Interventions

In 1891, Sir Victor Horsley described the first open surgical procedure for Trigeminal Neuralgia, which involved targeting the preganglionic rootlets of the nerve [1, 2].

In 1892, Hartley and Krause described the Hartley–Krause approach to section the nerve at the foramen ovale and rotundum. This approach was further modified by Frazier and Spiller, subsequently Spiller–Frazier procedure became the gold standard for TN for close to 50 years [13].

In 1925, Walter Dandy renowned neurosurgeon was not convinced by the Spiller–Frazier approach and advocated the partial sectioning of the nerve in the posterior cranial fossa. During that procedure, he observed that the nerve was being compressed by aberrant vascular malformations [13–15]. With the advent of the operative microscope, Peter Jannetta was finally able to further confirm this theory in 1967.

In 1967, Peter Jannetta was finally able to further confirm the theory of Walter Dandy with the advent of operative microscope [16]. He pioneered the technique of microvascular decompression (MVD), which is now considered the gold standard treatment for medically refractory TN. The success rates of MVD approach >90% with long-term durability [17–19].

In 1971, Lars Leksell described his experience and success with stereotactic radiosurgery for the treatment of TN [20]. This strategy since evolved into conventional gamma knife irradiation and was reported by several others [21–23]. Data suggest success rates of approximately 80% with minimal risk of facial paresthesias [24].

References

1. Patel SK, Liu JK. Overview and history of trigeminal neuralgia. Neurosurgery clinics of North America, vol. 27. Philadelphia: WB Saunders; 2016. p. 265–76.
2. Cole CD, Liu JK, Apfelbaum RI. Historical perspectives on the diagnosis and treatment of trigeminal neuralgia. Neurosurg Focus. 2005;18(5):E4.
3. Carnochan JM. On Tic Douloureux: "the painful affection of the face, Dolor Faciei Crucians," of Fothergill, with a new operation for its cure. Am J Dent Sci. 1860;10(2):254.

4. Adams H, Pendleton C, Latimer K, Cohen-Gadol AA, Carson BS, Quinones-Hinojosa A. Harvey Cushing's case series of trigeminal neuralgia at the Johns Hopkins Hospital: a surgeon's quest to advance the treatment of the "suicide disease". Acta Neurochir. 2011 May 17;153(5):1043–50.
5. Hutchinson BE. Cases of Tic Douloureux, cured by the carbonate of iron. Lond Med Phys J. 1825;54(320):281.
6. Bergouignan M. Cures heureuses de neurologies essentielles par le dephenyl hydantoinate de sounde. Rev Laryngol Otol Rhinol. 1942;63:34–41.
7. Qin Z, Xie S, Mao Z, Liu Y, Wu J, Furukawa TA, et al. Comparative efficacy and acceptability of antiepileptic drugs for classical trigeminal neuralgia: a Bayesian network meta-analysis protocol. BMJ Open. 2018 Jan 1;8:1.
8. Chir MK-AK. Undefined. Zur elektrochirurgie. 1931.
9. Mullan S, Lichtor T. Percutaneous microcompression of the trigeminal ganglion for trigeminal neuralgia. J Neurosurg. 1983 Dec 1;59(6):1007–12.
10. Yoon KB, Wiles JR, Miles JB, Nurmikko TJ. Long-term outcome of percutaneous thermocoagulation for trigeminal neuralgia. Anaesthesia. 1999 Aug;54(8):803–8.
11. Elawamy A, Abdalla EE, Shehata GA. Effects of pulsed versus conventional versus combined radiofrequency for the treatment of trigeminal neuralgia: a prospective study. Pain Phys. 2017;20(6):E873–81.
12. Ding Y, Li H, Hong T, Zhu Y, Yao P, Zhou G. Combination of pulsed radiofrequency with continuous radiofrequency thermocoagulation at low temperature improves efficacy and safety in V2/V3 primary trigeminal neuralgia. Pain Phys. 2018;21(5):E545–53.
13. Shelton M. Working in a very small place: the making of a neurosurgeon. Philadelphia: W. W. Norton & Company; 1989.
14. WE D. An operation for the cure of Tic Douloureux. Arch Surg. 1929 Feb 1;18(2):687.
15. Dandy WE. The treatment of trigeminal neuralgia by the cerebellar route. Ann Surg. 1932 Oct;96(4):787–95.
16. Jannetta PJ, McLaughlin MR, Casey KF. Technique of microvascular decompression. Technical note. Neurosurg Focus. 2005;18(5):E5.
17. Günther T, Gerganov VM, Stieglitz L, Ludemann W, Samii A, Samii M. Microvascular decompression for trigeminal neuralgia in the elderly: long-term treatment outcome and comparison with younger patients. Neurosurgery. 2009 Sep;65(3):477–82.
18. Fields HL. Treatment of trigeminal neuralgia. N Engl J Med. 1996;334:1125–6.
19. Barker FG, Jannetta PJ, Bissonette DJ, Larkins MV, Jho HD. The long-term outcome of microvascular decompression for trigeminal neuralgia. N Engl J Med. 1996 Apr 25;334(17):1077–83.
20. Leksell L. Stereotaxic radiosurgery in trigeminal neuralgia. Acta Chir Scand. 1971;37:311–4.
21. Leksell L. Stereotactic radiosurgery. J Neurol Neurosurg Psychiatry. 1983 Sep 1;46(9):797–803.
22. Kondziolka D, Lunsford LD, Flickinger JC, Young RF, Vermeulen S, Duma CM, Jacques DB, Rand RW, Regis J, Peragut JC, Manera L. Stereotactic radiosurgery for trigeminal neuralgia: a multiinstitutional study using the gamma unit. J Neurosurg. 1996 Jun 1;84(6):940–5.
23. Lindquist C, Kihlström L, Hellstrand E. Functional neurosurgery-a future for the gamma knife? Stereotact Funct Neurosurg. 1991;57(1–2):72–81.
24. Kondziolka D, Perez B, Flickinger JC, Habeck M, Lunsford LD. Gamma knife radiosurgery for trigeminal neuralgia: results and expectations. Arch Neurol. 1998 Dec 1;55(12):1524–9.

Anatomy of the Trigeminal Nerve

Michael Suer

Trigeminal Nerve Nuclei (Fig. 2.1)

The trigeminal nerve has both somatic and motor components with four distinct nuclei controlling neuronal signaling comprising the largest of the cranial nerve nuclei. The motor nucleus is a small, round structure within the pons; whereas the sensory nucleus is quite long extending into the medulla becoming continuous with the posterior horn of the spinal cord. Excluding the fibers to the mesencephalic nucleus, the sensory fibers from the trigeminal nerve travel along axons to their cell bodies in the trigeminal ganglion [1].

All motor and sensory fibers of the trigeminal ganglion enter the brainstem at the level of the mid-pons. The afferent fibers then travel to their respective nucleus in the medulla and even into the spinal cord via the spinal tract to synapse in the long sensory nucleus. Within this framework, the fibers within the brainstem are organized from rostral to caudal as proprioceptive followed by light touch and then pain. In total, the nucleus is divided into four parts from rostral to caudal: mesencephalic nucleus, chief/principal sensory nucleus, motor nucleus, and the spinal trigeminal nucleus. We will discuss each of these in turn [1, 2].

Mesencephalic Nucleus

The mesencephalic nucleus, the most rostral of the nuclei, contains cell bodies of neurons processing proprioceptive input regarding opposition of the teeth and dental pain; and it is the afferent limb for the jaw jerk reflex. The tract and nucleus are located within the caudal midbrain and rostral pons near the periaqueductal gray [1, 2].

M. Suer (✉)
Department of Orthopedics and Rehabilitation, University of Wisconsin, Madison, WI, USA
e-mail: suer@rehab.wisc.edu

© The Author(s), under exclusive license to Springer Nature Switzerland AG 2021
A. Abd-Elsayed (ed.), *Trigeminal Nerve Pain*,
https://doi.org/10.1007/978-3-030-60687-9_2

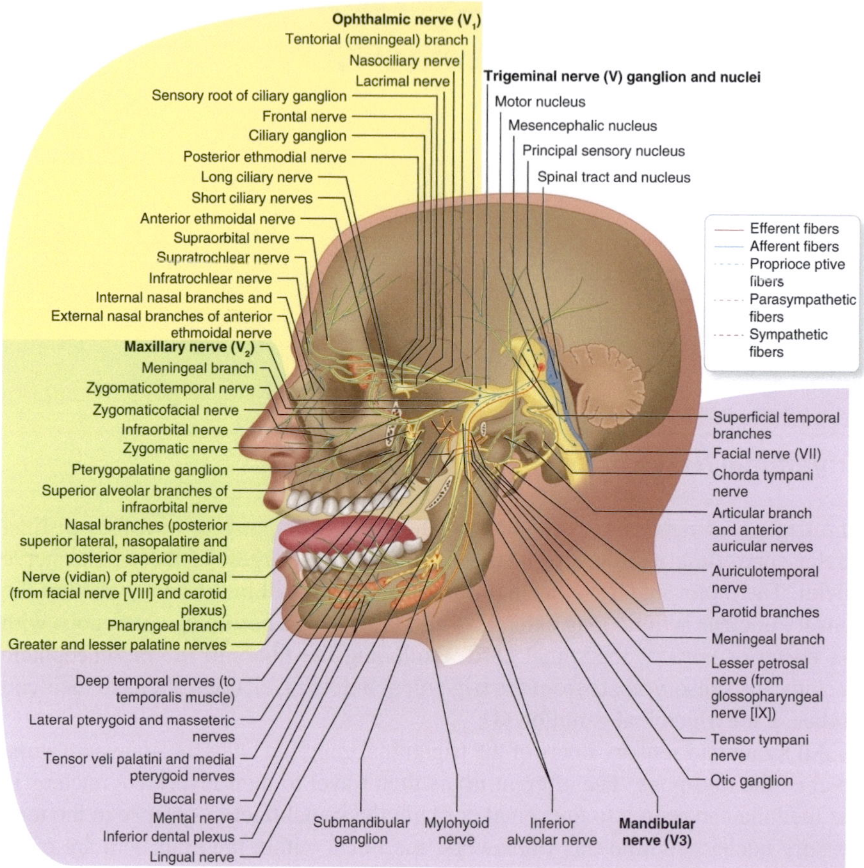

Fig. 2.1 Diagram of the trigeminal nerve nuclei and intracranial courses of the main branches of the trigeminal nerve

Unique to the mesencephalic nucleus, it contains no chemical synapses. Rather, the neurons are pseudounipolar receiving proprioceptive information from the mandible, sending projections to the trigeminal motor nucleus to mediate the monosynaptic jaw jerk reflex. Axons from the spinal and principal nucleus form the trigeminocerebellar tract ascending to the cerebellum [3]. This nucleus is the only central nervous system structure to contain the cell bodies of first-order neurons and can thus be considered as a sensory ganglion within the brainstem [4, 5].

Principal Sensory Nucleus

The principal sensory nucleus (chief sensory nucleus, main trigeminal sensory nucleus) receives discriminative sensation and light touch of the ipsilateral face and conscious proprioception from the jaw. It is located within the mid to caudal pons lateral to the trigeminal motor nucleus. The nucleus further divides into the dorso-medial and ventrolateral divisions. The former of these receives input only from the oral cavity. This information travels to the ipsilateral ventral posteromedial (VPM) nucleus of the thalamus via the dorsal trigeminothalamic tract. The ventrolateral division receives sensory input from all the divisions of the trigeminal nerve. Projections then decussate and second-order neuronal fibers convey information via the ventral trigeminothalamic tract to the contralateral VPM nucleus of the thalamus. Together, the second-order neurons of the ventral and dorsal trigeminal tracts are known as the trigeminal lemniscus conveying sensory information from the trigeminal system to the VPM of the thalamus [1, 2].

Spinal Trigeminal Nucleus

The spinal trigeminal nucleus (SpV or Sp5), a sensory tract located in the lateral medulla, is responsible for relaying sensation (deep or crude touch, pain, temperature) from the ipsilateral face. While the predominant afferent fibers are from the trigeminal nerve, it also receives input from the facial nerve (CN VII), glossopharyngeal nerve (CN IX), vagus nerve (CN X), and C1-C3 spinal segments [6]. Further dividing, SpV is separated into three subnuclei or pars. The subnucleus oralis is associated with fine touch from the orofacial region and is continuous with the principal sensory nucleus mentioned above. The subnucleus interpolaris is associated with transmission of touch and dental pain. And the subnucleus caudalis is associated with the transmission of painful and thermal stimuli from the ipsilateral face. The SpV projects to the ventral posteromedial (VPM) in the contralateral thalamus via the ventral trigeminal tract [1, 7].

The subnucleus caudalis is the most caudal segment of the trigeminal sensory nuclear complex. As it closely resembles the laminated structure of the dorsal horn of the spinal cord with which it is continuous, it is often termed the medullary dorsal horn. It is within this nucleus that the upper cervical afferent roots (C1–C3) interact with the descending trigeminal nociceptive afferents. These cervical afferent fibers receive input from the muscles, joints, and ligaments of the upper cervical segments; dura mater; posterior cranial fossa; and the vertebral artery. The bidirectional referral of painful sensations between the neck and trigeminal sensory receptive fields is due to this convergence of fibers [6].

Trigeminal Motor Nucleus

The final nucleus, the trigeminal motor nucleus, is in the dorsolateral pontine tegmentum at the mid-pons. It is located medial to the principal sensory nucleus and lateral to the mesencephalic nucleus. Coming from the primary motor cortex, branchial motor neurons innervate the muscles of mastication and palate to a lesser degree via the mandibular nerve (V3). Efferent motor fibers leaving the nucleus do not decussate; however, due to the bilateral cortical input, a unilateral transection of these nerves will not result in paralysis [2, 8].

Trigeminal Nerve and Distal Projections (Figs. 2.2 and 2.3a, b)

Ophthalmic Nerve

The ophthalmic nerve (V1) provides sensory innervation from the scalp, forehead, upper part of the sinuses, upper eyelid and associated mucous membranes, cornea, and bridge of the nose. Branches of the ophthalmic nerve include the nasociliary, lacrimal, and frontal nerves. Prior to branching into these three main divisions, the ophthalmic nerve gives off the tentorial (meningeal) branch.

Frontal Nerve

The largest of the main V1 branches, the frontal nerve, branches from the ophthalmic nerve immediately prior to entering the lateral portion of the superior orbital fissure traveling superolateral to the annulus of Zinn between the lacrimal nerve and the inferior ophthalmic vein. After entering the orbit, it divides further into the supratrochlear nerve and the supraorbital nerve. These branches briefly re-enter the frontal bone prior to exiting through their respectively named supratrochlear foramen and supraorbital foramen (or notch). They both ascend into the forehead between the corrugator supercilii and frontalis muscles dividing into a medial and lateral branch providing innervation to the forehead, upper eyelid, and conjunctiva.

Nasociliary Nerve

The nasociliary nerve, intermediate in size between the frontal and lacrimal nerves, enters the orbit between the two heads of the lateral rectus muscle between the superior and inferior rami of the oculomotor nerve (CN III). It branches into six terminal nerves including the communicating branch to the ciliary ganglion, long and short ciliary nerves, posterior ethmoidal nerve, anterior ethmoidal nerve, and becomes the infratrochlear nerve (the terminal branch).

Running through the short ciliary nerves, sensations from the eyeball including the cornea, iris, and ciliary body pass through the ciliary ganglion. Without forming synapses, they leave the ganglion in the sensory root joining the nasociliary nerve.

The long ciliary nerves, totaling 2 or 3 in number, accompany the short ciliary nerves from the ciliary ganglion providing sensation again from the eyeball. They also contain sympathetic fibers from the superior cervical ganglion to the dilator pupillae muscle, though the short ciliary nerves also contain sympathetic fibers.

The anterior ethmoidal nerve branches near the medial wall of the orbit traveling through the anterior ethmoidal foramen to the anterior cranial fossa. The anterior ethmoidal nerve provides sensation from the anterior and middle ethmoidal air cells and the meninges. It passes through the cribriform plate into the nasal cavity giving off branches to the roof of the nasal cavity. Here it bifurcates into the lateral internal nasal branch and the medial internal nasal branch. Within the nasal cavity, it provides sensation from the anterior part of the nasal septum. The external nasal branch of the anterior ethmoidal nerve also provides innervation from the skin on the lateral sides of the nose.

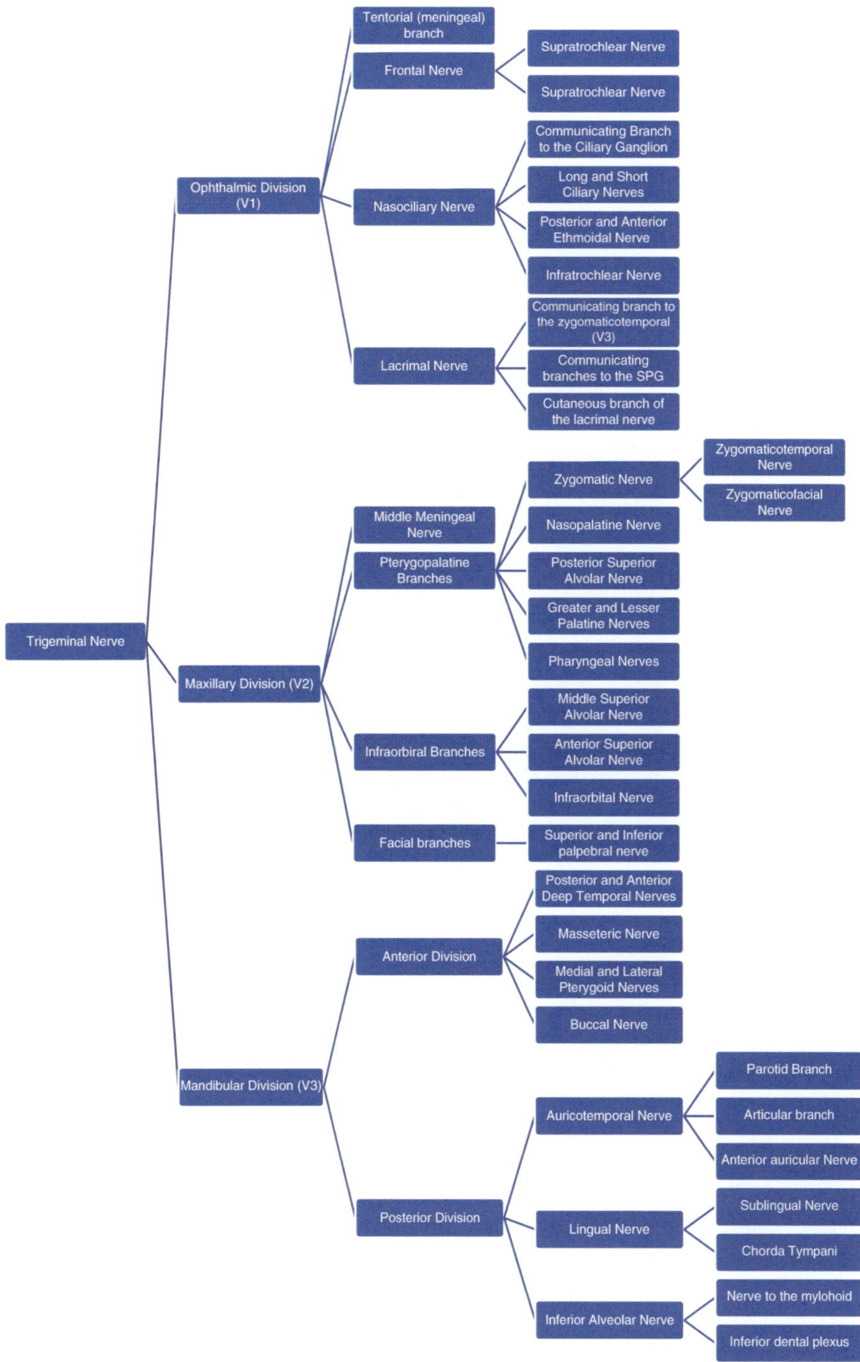

Fig. 2.2 Trigeminal nerve branches

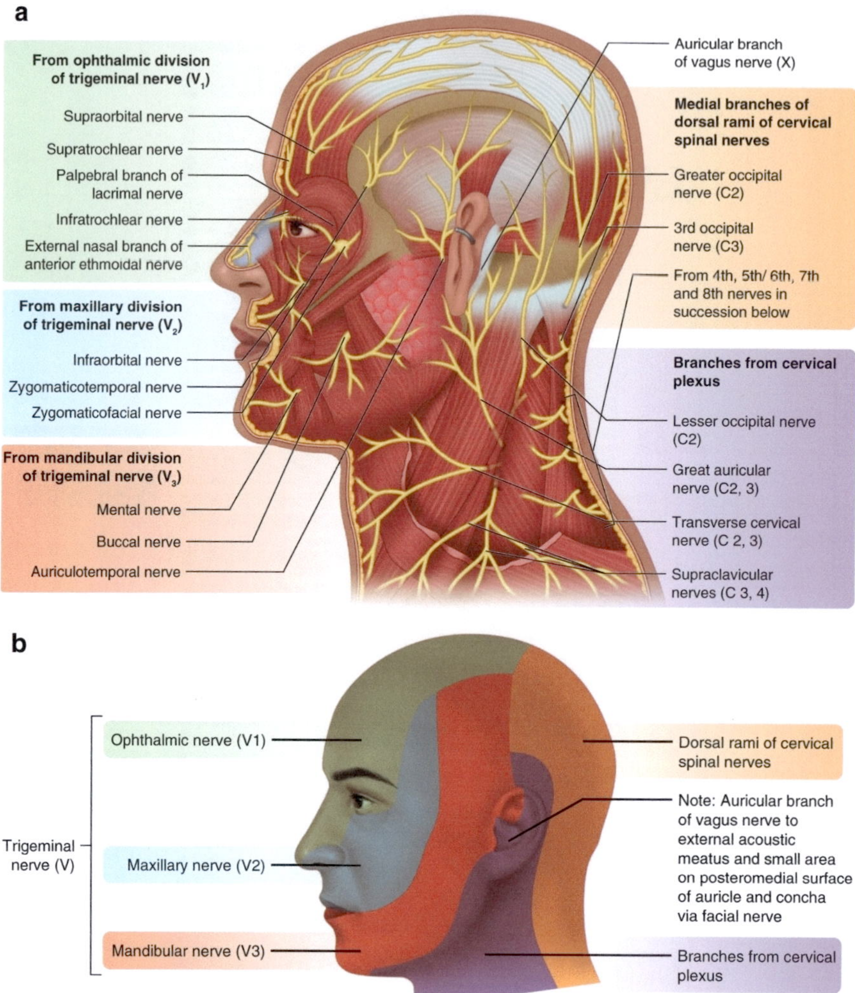

Fig. 2.3 (**a**) Cutaneous sensory branches of the head and neck. (**b**) Distribution of cutaneous sensation of the head and neck

The infratrochlear nerve travels anteriorly along the upper border of the medial rectus muscles beneath the trochlea exiting the orbit medially dividing into smaller sensory branches providing innervation from the skin of the eyelid, conjunctiva, lacrimal sac, lacrimal caruncle, and the side of the nose above the medial canthus.

Lacrimal Nerve

The smallest division of the ophthalmic nerve, the lacrimal nerve, branches immediately before traveling through the superior orbital fissure traveling along the lateral wall with the lacrimal artery and provides a communicating branch to the zygomaticotemporal (branch of V3). It then provides communicating branches carrying postganglionic parasympathetic axons from the pterygopalatine ganglion. The lacrimal nerve travels through the lacrimal gland providing sensory and parasympathetic branches to the gland and finally continues anteriorly as the cutaneous branch of the lacrimal nerve.

Maxillary Nerve

The maxillary nerve (V2) provides sensation from the lower eyelid and associated mucous membranes, middle portion of the sinuses, nasal cavity and middle part of the nose, cheeks, upper lip, some teeth of the upper jaw, and associated mucous membranes, and the roof of the mouth. It also carries parasympathetic preganglionic fibers (sphenopalatine) and postganglionic fibers (zygomatic, greater, and lesser palatine and nasopalatine) to and from the pterygopalatine ganglion.

The maxillary nerve begins as a flattened plexiform nerve passing through the lateral wall of the cavernous sinus and exiting the skull through the foramen rotundum where it becomes more cylindrical. After crossing the pterygopalatine fossa, it enters the orbit through the inferior orbital fissure and runs along the floor of the orbit in the infraorbital groove and the infraorbital canal. It terminates as the infraorbital nerve leaving the skull through the infraorbital foramen. Along this path, it gives off multiple branches providing sensation as noted above.

Intracranially, the first branch of the maxillary nerve is the middle meningeal nerve which branches immediately following its origin prior to entering the foramen rotundum. Accompanying the middle meningeal artery and vein, it enters the cranium through the foramen spinosum providing sensation from the dura mater.

Pterygopalatine Branches

After passing through the foramen rotundum, there are six branches from the maxillary nerve: the zygomatic, nasopalatine, posterior superior alveolar, greater and lesser palatine, and pharyngeal nerves. The zygomatic nerve branches at the pterygopalatine ganglion traveling through the fossa through the inferior orbital fissure into the orbit where it divides into the zygomaticotemporal and zygomaticofacial nerves which travel through the respectively named foramina into the zygomatic bone. This branch contains sensory axons providing innervation from the skin overlying the temporal and zygomatic bones. It also carries postganglionic parasympathetic axons that have their cell bodies in the pterygopalatine ganglion. As mentioned previously, these axons travel to the lacrimal nerve through a communicating branch.

The nasopalatine nerve (i.e., long sphenopalatine nerve) enters the nasal cavity through the sphenopalatine foramen. It passes across the roof of the nasal cavity to reach the septum. It descends along the roof of the mouth through the incisive canal and communicates with the nerve of the contralateral side and the greater palatine nerve. It provides sensation from the structures around the maxillary central incisors, lateral incisors, and canines. It also provides minor sensory signaling from the nasal septum via the medial superior posterior nasal branch.

The molars, by contrast, have sensory afferents through the posterior superior alveolar nerve. This nerve branches from the maxillary nerve just prior to the infraorbital groove descending on the tuberosity of the maxilla. It also provides sensation from the gingiva and mucous membrane of the cheek. After entering the alveolar canals on the maxilla, it communicates with the middle superior alveolar nerve and provides sensation from the maxillary sinus.

The greater (anterior) and lesser palatine nerves descend through the greater palatine canal. Within the pterygopalatine canal, the greater palatine nerve branches into the lateral posterior inferior nasal branch which enters the nasal cavity through the palatine bone ultimately distributing fibers to the soft palate. The greater palatine nerve exits through the greater palatine foramen onto the hard palate passing forward as far as the incisors. It provides sensation to the gingiva, mucous membrane of the hard palate, and communicates with the terminal filaments of the nasopalatine nerve. The lesser palatine nerve exits through the lesser palatine foramen providing sensation from the nasal cavity, soft palate, tonsils, and uvula.

The final branch in the area of the pterygopalatine fossa is the pharyngeal nerve. It passes through the palatovaginal canal and provides sensation from the nasal portion of the pharynx.

Infraorbital Branches

The first of the three main branches of the maxillary nerve within the infraorbital portion is the middle superior alveolar nerve which is present in a minority of individuals. In most, the anterior superior alveolar nerve provides sensation from this distribution. This middle branch provides sensation from the sinus mucosa and the roots of the maxillary premolars and first maxillary molar. The anterior superior alveolar nerve branches before the infraorbital nerve exits from the infraorbital foramen and descends within the anterior wall of the maxillary sinus. It then divides into branches which supply the incisors and canine teeth. In conjunction with the posterior superior alveolar nerve and the middle superior alveolar nerve, it forms the superior dental plexus providing sensation from the upper jaw.

The final infraorbital branch, the infraorbital nerve, is clinically relevant in headaches. This terminal branch arises onto the anterior surface of the maxilla through the infraorbital foramen where it divides into terminal branches—palpebral, nasal, and superior labial. The palpebral branch provides sensation from the lower eyelid; the nasal branch from the side of the nose and nasal septum; and the superior labial branch to the skin of the anterior cheek and upper lip. The infraorbital nerve also crosses and forms a plexus with the facial nerve [9].

Facial Branches

Facial branches of the maxillary nerve consist of the inferior palpebral nerve and the superior labial branches. The former of these supplies the skin and conjunctiva of the lower eyelid joining the facial and zygomaticofacial nerves at the lateral orbit. The latter provides sensation from the skin of the upper lip, the mucous membrane of the mouth, and labial salivary glands.

Mandibular Nerve

The mandibular nerve (V3) is the sole branch the provides both sensory and motor information. It provides sensation from the outer part of the ear, lower part of the mouth and associated mucous membranes, anterior 2/3 of the tongue, lower teeth and associated mucous membranes, lower lip, and chin. It should be noted that special sensation (taste) of the tongue is provided by the chorda tympani branch of the facial nerve. While the motor and sensory roots take a briefly separate course, they join prior to exiting the skull through the foramen ovale. It is near this junction that the meningeal (recurrent) branch of the mandibular nerve enters the skull via the foramen spinosum with the middle meningeal artery on its way to providing sensation from the dura mater and mastoid cells. The mandibular nerve then courses through the infratemporal fossa where it branches into anterior and posterior divisions.

Anterior Division

Immediately after the anterior-posterior split, the anterior division branches into several nerves. The posterior and anterior deep temporal nerves ascend above the lateral pterygoid muscle entering the temporal fossa. They provide motor innervation to the temporalis which elevates and retracts the mandible. The deep branch also provides an articular branch providing minor innervation to the temporomandibular joint (major supply is via the auriculotemporal nerve).

The masseteric nerve branches from the anterior division passing laterally just medial to the temporomandibular articulation and posterior to the tendon of the temporalis. Along with the masseteric artery, it crosses the mandibular notch to the deep surface of the masseter. The masseter elevates the mandible with bilateral contraction closing the jaws. The deep part of the masseter also retracts the jaw. Similarly, the masseteric nerve also provides minor innervation to the temporomandibular joint.

The medial and lateral pterygoid nerves, which innervate the respective pterygoid muscles, are the next branch of the anterior division. The medial also provides innervation to the tensor tympani (noise reduction during mastication) and tensor veli palatine (tensing of the soft palate) muscles. The latter of these is the only muscle of the soft palate—palatoglossus, palatopharyngeus, levator veli palatine, and musculus uvulae—which is not innervated by the pharyngeal plexus via the vagus nerve [10]. The lateral pterygoid nerve enters and provides motor stimulation to the lateral pterygoid muscle. The medial pterygoid muscles elevate and protrude the mandible with bilateral activation and provide side–side motion with unilateral activation. The lateral pterygoid muscles protrude the mandible depressing the chin with bilateral activation and similarly provide side–side motion with unilateral activation.

The sole sensory nerve of the smaller anterior division is the buccal nerve. After branching from the mandibular nerve after the foramen ovale, it descends under the tendon of the temporalis muscle and the masseter muscle. It provides sensory information from the cheek. The buccinator, a muscle of facial expression rather than mastication, is provided by the buccal branches of the facial nerve (CN VII).

Posterior Division

Soon after splitting from the anterior division, the posterior division gives rise to the lingual nerve and auriculotemporal nerves and becomes the inferior alveolar nerve.

Auricotemporal

Coming off the posterior division, two nerve roots encircle the middle meningeal artery prior to joining as a single auriculotemporal nerve. After giving off a secretomotor parotid branch, the nerve turns superior where it divides into the articular branch and anterior auricular nerves. It crosses superficial to the zygomatic process of the temporal bone and branches into multiple superficial temporal branches. In total, it supplies sensation from the auricle, external acoustic meatus, outer side of the tympanic membrane, and the skin in the temporal region. The posterior auricular nerve, which supplies the auricularis posterior muscle and supplies sensation from the occiput, is a branch of the facial nerve (CN VII).

Lingual Nerve

Responsible for providing sensation from the anterior 2/3 of the tongue, the lingual nerve branches from the posterior division descending between the medial pterygoid muscle and the angle of the ramus of the mandible. It is joined here by the chorda tympani nerve (branch of the facial nerve CN VII) at an acute angle which provides taste sensation from the anterior 2/3 of the tongue. After passing between the hyoglossus and the submandibular gland crossing the duct of the submandibular gland from lateral to medial, it runs along the tongue becoming the sublingual nerve. The posterior 1/3 of the tongue is supplied by the glossopharyngeal nerve.

Prior to branching from the lingual nerve toward the facial nerve, the fibers of the chorda tympani traverse with the lingual nerve carrying both sympathetic and parasympathetic nerve fibers. Near the posterior border of the mylohyoid muscle, the submandibular ganglion is suspended from the lingual nerve by two nerve filaments. It is through this ganglion that the sympathetic fibers cross and parasympathetic nerves synapse.

Inferior Alveolar Nerve

The final major branch of the posterior division of the mandibular nerve is the inferior alveolar nerve. Soon after forming this last branch prior to entering the mandibular foramen, the nerve to the mylohyoid takes off descending in a groove on the inner surface of the mandible innervating the mylohyoid muscle (tongue and hyoid elevation) and the anterior belly of the digastric muscle (elevates the hyoid).

The inferior alveolar nerve then passes through the mandibular foramen into the mandibular canal in the ramus of the mandible. Here it forms the inferior dental plexus giving off gingival and dental nerves to the lower molars and second premolar. At the level of the lower second pre-molars, it gives off the mental nerve which exits via the mental foramen providing sensation to the chin and lower lip. It continues as the mandibular incisive nerve providing sensation to the lower canines and incisors.

Associated Structures

Otic Ganglion

The otic ganglion is a 2–3-mm parasympathetic ganglion located within the infratemporal fossa just distal to the foramen ovale on the medial surface of the mandibular nerve at the junction of the motor and sensory roots. Preganglionic parasympathetic fibers of the inferior salivary nucleus of the glossopharyngeal nerve arrive at the otic ganglion synapsing with postganglionic fibers. These fibers, via communicating branches to the auriculotemporal nerve (branch of V3), proceed to the parotid gland where they produce vasodilatation and secretomotor effects.

Passing through the ganglion without synapsing, the postganglionic fibers from the superior cervical ganglion pass through to reach the parotid gland via the same auriculotemporal nerve. These produce vasomotor function within the parotid gland. As mentioned previously, motor nerves to the medial pterygoid, tensor palati, and tensor tympani also pass through the ganglion though do not synapse here.

Submandibular Ganglion

The submandibular ganglion, a small fusiform ganglion located near the posterior border of the mylohyoid muscle, is suspended from the lingual nerve (branch of V3) by two nerve filaments. Within this ganglion, preganglionic parasympathetic fibers from the superior salivary nucleus (chorda tympani via the lingual nerve) of the pons synapse. The postganglionic fibers transmit the parasympathetic secretomotor signals to the oral mucosa, submandibular salivary gland, and the sublingual salivary gland. Sympathetic fibers from the external carotid plexus pass through the submandibular ganglion.

Sphenopalatine Ganglion

The sphenopalatine ganglion (also known as pterygopalatine ganglion, Meckel's ganglion, or SPG) is a parasympathetic ganglion found within the sphenopalatine fossa. While it is mostly innervated by the facial nerve (via the greater petrosal nerve), it has projections through branches of the trigeminal nerve. Within the fossa, it is located just inferior to the maxillary nerve as it traverses the fossa. It supplies the lacrimal gland; paranasal sinuses; gingiva; and the mucosal glands of the nasal cavity, pharynx, and hard palate.

Two sphenopalatine branches of the maxillary nerve provide a few sensory fibers from the SPG. The majority of fibers from the SPG serve in the parasympathetic nerve system. Stemming from the facial nerve, preganglionic fibers from the greater petrosal nerve synapse with postganglionic parasympathetic fibers providing vasodilation and secretory efferent fibers. Sympathetic fibers pass through the ganglion without synapsing arriving from the superior cervical ganglion through the carotid plexus, then the deep petrosal nerve and greater petrosal nerve. Both the sympathetic and parasympathetic efferent fibers transmit via the infraorbital nerve, superior alveolar nerves, nasopalatine nerve, and the greater and lesser palatine nerves.

References

1. Yousry I, Moriggl B, Schmid UD, Naidich TP, Yousry TA. Trigeminal ganglion and its divisions: detailed anatomic MR imaging with contrast-enhanced 3D constructive interference in the steady state sequences. AJNR Am J Neuroradiol. 2005;26:1128–35.
2. Price S, Daly DT. Neuroanatomy, nucleus trigeminal [Updated 2019 Mar 24]. In: StatPearls [internet]. Treasure Island (FL), StatPearls Publishing; 2020 Jan. Available from https://www.ncbi.nlm.nih.gov/books/NBK539823/
3. Nolte J. The human brain - an introduction to its functional anatomy. 6th ed. New York: Elsevier; 2008. p. 499–509.
4. Shigenaga Y, Doe K, Suemune S, Mitsuhiro Y, Tsuru K, Otani K, Shirana Y, Hosoi M, Yoshida A, Kagawa K. Physiological and morphological characteristics of periodontal mesencephalic trigeminal neurons in the cat—intra-axonal staining with HRP. Brain Res. 1989 Dec 25;505(1):91–110.
5. Panneton WM, Pan B, Gan Q. Somatotopy in the medullary dorsal horn as a basis for orofacial reflex behavior. Front Neurol. 2017;8:522.
6. Bogduk N. The anatomical basis for cervicogenic headache. J Manip Physiol Ther. 1992;15:67–70.
7. Patel NM, Das MJ. Neuroanatomy, spinal trigeminal nucleus. [Updated 2019 Mar 19]. In: StatPearls [Internet]. Treasure Island (FL), StatPearls Publishing; 2020 Jan. Available from https://www.ncbi.nlm.nih.gov/books/NBK539729/
8. Kim JS, Lee JH, Lee MC. Patterns of sensory dysfunction in lateral medullary infarction. Clinical-MRI correlation. Neurology. 1997 Dec;49(6):1557–63.
9. Hwang K, Yang SC, Song JS. Communications between the trigeminal nerve and the facial nerve in the face: a systematic review. J Craniofac Surg. 2015;26(5):1643–6. https://doi.org/10.1097/SCS.0000000000001810.
10. Drake RL, Vogl AW, Mitchell AWM, illustrations by Richard M. Tibbitts and Paul Richardson. Gray's anatomy for students. Philadelphia: Elsevier/Churchill Livingstone; 2005.

Epidemiology

3

Hemant Kalia, Omar Viswanath, and Alaa Abd-Elsayed

Introduction

Trigeminal Neuralgia (TN) has been described in the literature as one of the most debilitating presentations of orofacial pain.

International classification of headache disorder third edition defines TN as recurrent paroxysms of unilateral facial pain in the distribution(s) of one or more divisions of the trigeminal nerve, with no radiation beyond [1], and fulfilling criteria B and C

A. Pain has all of the following characteristics:
   1. Lasting from a fraction of a second to 2 min [2].
   2. Severe intensity [3].
   3. Electric shock-like, shooting, stabbing, or sharp in quality.

H. Kalia
Rochester Regional Health System, Rochester, NY, USA

O. Viswanath
Department of Anesthesiology, Louisiana State University Health Shreveport, Shreveport, LA, USA

Department of Anesthesiology, Creighton University School of Medicine, Omaha, NE, USA

Valley Pain Consultants – Envision Physician Services, Phoenix, AZ, USA

Department of Anesthesiology, University of Arizona College of Medicine-Phoenix, Phoenix, AZ, USA

A. Abd-Elsayed (✉)
Department of Anesthesiology, University of Wisconsin School of Medicine and Public Health, Madison, WI, USA
e-mail: abdelsayed@wisc.edu

© The Author(s), under exclusive license to Springer Nature Switzerland AG 2021
A. Abd-Elsayed (ed.), *Trigeminal Nerve Pain*,
https://doi.org/10.1007/978-3-030-60687-9_3

B. Precipitated by innocuous stimuli within the affected trigeminal distribution [4].
C. Not better accounted for by another ICHD-3 diagnosis.

Classic TN is defined as following all above-described features without apparent cause other than neurovascular compression [5].

Secondary TN is defined as caused by any underlying disease affecting trigeminal ganglion. Clinical examination shows sensory changes in a significant proportion of these patients [5].

Idiopathic TN is defined as a type of TN with neither electrophysiological tests nor MRI showing significant abnormalities [5].

Prevalence and Incidence Rates

TN is considered a rare orofacial pain condition. There is still considerable debate in the literature surrounding its true prevalence and incidence rates. Most of the studies overestimate the prevalence due to convenience sampling. De Toledo et al. [6] designed their study with a specific focused question, "What are the prevalence and epidemiological characteristics of TN in the general population?" After careful analysis of three studies which met the criteria of the Agency for Healthcare Research and Quality for observation studies, they came to the following conclusions [6]:

- The prevalence rate of TN ranges between 0.03% and 0.3%.
- Females are more likely to be affected by TN than men.
- People who are 37–67 years old are more likely to be afflicted by TN.
- V2 and V3 are the most commonly affected branches of TN.

There also appears to be a predilection of the right side in TN as compared to other orofacial pain conditions, but there are no anatomical reasons for the blood vessel loop to be present more frequently on the right side of the cranial fossa [7]. Moreover, TN without an aberrant blood vessel and vascular loops in asymptomatic patients have been reported, thereby arguing against the theory that vascular compression is the main etiology for TN. The maxillary nerve exits out of foramen rotundum, which has shown to be smaller on the right side in numerous radiological and anatomical studies [8]. Neto et al. [8] concluded that due to these anatomical findings corroborated by demographic and epidemiological data the entrapment of maxillary nerve is much more common on the right side as it crosses the foramen rotundum. Burchiel et al. [9] reported 36 out of 42 patients with TN were found to have anatomical distortions of the nerve by an artery, vein, bony prominence, or a combination of factors.

In another review on malignant peripheral sheath tumors by Schmidt et al.; the average age on onset was found to be 44.6 years. The tumors were more prevalent in males (77.1%) and 36.1% of all tumors involved trigeminal ganglion. Mandibular branch was most commonly involved (72%), followed by maxillary (60%) and the ophthalmic (32%), close to 50% of the patients had two or more branches involved [10].

Mandibular nerve can get entrapped at multiple sites along its course; foramen ovale being the most common one especially if the diameter of the foramen is too small or the size of the nerve segment across the foramen is too large. Again, anatomically right-sided foramen ovale tends to be narrower than the left side thereby explaining potential preponderance of the right side as compared to the left [8].

Another common site of entrapment for mandibular nerve along its course is at the infratemporal fossa, partial or complete calcification of pterygoalar or pterygospinous ligaments can lead to compression of the posterior trunk of the nerve. The nerve can be compressed between medial and lateral pterygoid muscles or displaced by the lateral pterygoid plate [11].

Relationship between mandibular nerve involvement and temporomandibular joint (TMJ) was explored by Costen et al. in 1934. Costen's Syndrome is characterized by symptoms of impaired hearing, ear "stuffiness," ear pain, dizziness, sinus like pain, headaches, and trismus [12].

Hypertension is one of the key risk factors for vascular compression. Most often, trigeminal neuralgia occurs where the nerve root is compressed near the pons [13].

The reported estimates of incidence rates of TN range between 11 and 42 cases per 100,000 people per year with female preponderance [6]. Classic TN is generally diagnosed in elderly population with peak incidence between 50 and 60 years.

Another reason for significant variation in both prevalence and incidence rates in the literature is due to lack of consensus on diagnostic criteria of TN. International Headache Society (IHS) published their recommendations in the third edition of ICHD in 2013. This consensus report provides a standardized nomenclature to appropriately diagnose TN, and will enhance the quality of research by minimizing heterogenous subject groups.

Although TN is more commonly seen in adults, pediatric TN represents <1.5% of all cases. Pediatric TN differs from Adult TN primarily being bilateral in nature (42%) and associated with compression of multiple cranial nerves (46%) [14].

Some of the other conditions that can mimic symptoms of TN and are useful for a differential diagnosis include cluster headaches, migraines, dental pain, giant cell arteritis, glossopharyngeal neuralgia, postherpetic neuralgia, occipital neuralgia, sinus infections (sinusitis), middle ear infections (otitis media), and temporomandibular joint syndrome.

Disparities in Management of Trigeminal Neuralgia

Disparity is often misconstrued in the context limited to differences between race and ethnicity, there are many dimensions of disparity in the United States, particularly in relation to health. Social determinants of health play a vital role on health outcomes of specific populations. Reiner et al. analyzed 652 patients from one of the nation's largest comprehensive health care systems in Detroit, MI, and concluded that racial disparity affected a patient's ability to undergo a procedure for TN. Although, this was primarily related to different patterns of referral to neurosurgery and neurology in the health system. There were also underlying cultural beliefs and perceptions about surgical and nonsurgical treatments modulating these referral patterns [15].

It is imperative to use the common definition for both clinical and research purposes to accurately diagnose TN and its subtypes. This will allow well-designed epidemiological studies, even if they are retrospective analysis/systematic to accurately define true prevalence and incidence rates of TN.

References

1. Benoliel R, Eliav E, Sharav Y. Self-reports of pain-related awakenings in persistent orofacial pain patients. search.ebscohost.com [Internet]. 2009. [cited 2020 May 9]. Available from http://search.ebscohost.com/login.aspx?direct=true&profile=ehost&scope=site&authtype=crawler&jrnl=10646655&asa=Y&AN=45078353&h=qgcFqQuXnzpwgQ0SxocXz2mAhc455p7f%2BwlFJcI2yNLMYkntUIya6uVMTAka1zUKfZ6dLtC96g5C81Mi0Rt7aQ%3D%3D&crl=c

2. Finnerup N, Svensson P. Trigeminal neuralgia. New classification and diagnostic grading for practice and research. 2016 [cited 2020 May 9]. Available from http://dl.umsu.ac.ir/handle/Hannan/122412

3. Di Stefano G, Maarbjerg S, Nurmikko T, Truini A, Cruccu G. Triggering trigeminal neuralgia. journals.sagepub.com [Internet]. 2018 May 14 [cited 2020 May 9];38(6):1049–56. Available from https://journals.sagepub.com/doi/abs/10.1177/0333102417721677

4. Drangsholt M. Practice ET-J of EBD, 2001 undefined. Trigeminal neuralgia mistaken as temporomandibular disorder. Elsevier [Internet]. [cited 2020 May 9]. Available from https://www.sciencedirect.com/science/article/pii/S1532338201700826

5. Olesen J, Bes A, Kunkel R, Lance JW, Nappi G, Pfaffenrath V, et al. The international classification of headache disorders, 3rd edition (beta version). Cephalalgia. 2013 Jul 1;33(9):629–808.

6. Porto De Toledo I, Conti Réus J, Fernandes M, Luís Porporatti A, Peres MA, Takaschima A, et al. Prevalence of trigeminal neuralgia: a systematic review. 2016 [cited 2020 Apr 26]. Available from https://doi.org/10.1016/j.adaj.2016.02.014

7. Katusic S, Williams DB, Beard M, Bergstralh EJ, Kurland LT. Epidemiology and clinical features of idiopathic trigeminal neuralgia and glossopharyngeal neuralgia: similarities and differences, Rochester, Minnesota, 1945-1984. Neuroepidemiology [Internet]. 1991 [cited 2020 Apr 26];10(5–6):276–281. Available from https://www.karger.com/Article/FullText/110284

8. Neto HS, Camilli JA, Marques MJ. Trigeminal neuralgia is caused by maxillary and mandibular nerve entrapment: greater incidence of right-sided facial symptoms is due to the foramen rotundum and foramen ovale being narrower on the right side of the cranium. Med Hypotheses. 2005 Jan 1;65(6):1179–82.

9. Burchiel KJ, Steege TD, Howe JF, Loeser JD. Comparison of percutaneous radiofrequency gangliolysis and microvascular decompression for the surgical management of Tic Douloureux. Neurosurgery [Internet]. 1981 Aug 1 [cited 2020 May 24];9(2):111–9. Available from https://academic.oup.com/neurosurgery/article/9/2/111/2746908

10. Malignant peripheral nerve sheath tumors of the trigeminal nerve: a systematic review of 36 cases in: Neurosurgical Focus Volume 34 Issue 3 (2013) [Internet]. [cited 2020 May 24]. Available from https://thejns.org/focus/view/journals/neurosurg-focus/34/3/article-pE5.xml

11. Piagkou M, Demesticha T, Skandalakis P, Johnson EO. Functional anatomy of the mandibular nerve: Consequences of nerve injury and entrapment. Clin Anat [Internet]. 2011 Mar 1 [cited 2020 May 24];24(2):143–50. Available from https://doi.org/10.1002/ca.21089

12. Costen JB. I. A syndrome of ear and sinus symptoms dependent upon disturbed function of the Temporomandibular joint. Ann Otol Rhinol Laryngol [Internet]. 1934 Mar 28 [cited 2020 May 24];43(1):1–15. Available from https://doi.org/10.1177/000348943404300101
13. Trigeminal neuralgia - UpToDate [Internet]. [cited 2020 May 24]. Available from https://www.uptodate.com/contents/trigeminal-neuralgia
14. Linskey ME, Grannan BL, Zhang W, Songjun R, Li W, Williams Z. CNS oral presentations 143 pediatric trigeminal neuralgia (TN): Results with Early Microvascular Decompression (MVD) stereotactic and functional neurosurgery resident award 144 prefrontal neurons modulate motor behavior by targeting distinct mediolateral cortical sites [Internet]. [cited 2020 May 31]. Available from www.neurosurgery-online.com
15. Reinard K, Nerenz DR, Basheer A, Tahir R, Jelsema T, Schultz L, et al. Racial disparities in the diagnosis and management of trigeminal neuralgia. J Neurosurg. 2017 Feb 1;126(2):368–74.

Trigeminal Neuralgia and Other Trigeminal Nerve Conditions

4

Susanne Seeger

Introduction

The presentation of pain in the distribution of the trigeminal nerve is highly variable. Trigeminal neuralgia is a common cause of facial pain, characterized by electrical shock-like pain attacks in the distribution of one or more trigeminal nerve branches. Trigeminal neuropathy is pain in the distribution of one or more trigeminal nerve branches caused by several underlying conditions. Other pain disorders can result in facial or oral pain. The etiology and clinical features of these conditions are discussed in this chapter. Trigeminal nerve anatomy as well as epidemiology, diagnostic tests, and treatment of these pain conditions will be discussed elsewhere in this publication.

Trigeminal Neuralgia

Diagnostic Criteria

Diagnostic criteria for trigeminal neuralgia (TN) have been established by the International Classification of Headache Disorders, Third Edition [1]:

(A) Recurrent paroxysms of unilateral facial pain in the distribution of one or more divisions of the trigeminal nerve, with no radiation beyond, and fulfilling criteria B and C.

S. Seeger (✉)
Department of Neurology, UW School of Medicine and Public Health, Madison, WI, USA
e-mail: seeger@neurology.wisc.edu

A. Abd-Elsayed (ed.), *Trigeminal Nerve Pain*,
https://doi.org/10.1007/978-3-030-60687-9_4

(B) Pain has all of the following characteristics:
   1. Lasting from a fraction of a second to 2 min.
   2. Severe intensity.
   3. Electrical shock-like, shooting, stabbing, or sharp in quality.
(C) Precipitated by innocuous stimuli within the affected trigeminal distribution.
(D) Not better accounted for by another ICHD-3 diagnosis.

Classification

Trigeminal neuralgia (TN) is further categorized as classic TN, secondary TN, and idiopathic TN. See Table 4.1.

Classic TN develops without apparent cause other than neurovascular compression, fulfilling criteria for trigeminal neuralgia and requiring demonstration on MRI or during surgery of neurovascular compression (not simply contact), with morphological changes in the trigeminal nerve root [1].

Secondary TN is defined as TN caused by underlying disease. Common causes include multiple sclerosis, cerebellopontine angle tumor, and arteriovenous malformation [1].

Idiopathic TN is defined as TN with neither neurophysiological tests nor MRI showing significant abnormalities [1].

Etiology and Pathophysiology

Classic TN is caused by neurovascular compression of the trigeminal nerve root at the root entry zone at the level of the pons [2, 3]. Secondary TN is caused by compression of the nerve by lesions close to the nerve entry zone, such as cerebellopontine angle tumors, or arteriovenous malformations (AVMs). Compression of the nerve ultimately results in circumscribed demyelination, which interferes with impulse transmission [4, 5]. This may cause ectopic impulses [4]. Additionally, there is evidence for central sensitization of pain processing in the trigeminal pathways, suggesting a coexisting central pain mechanism [6, 7].

Table 4.1 Trigeminal neuralgia classification

	Classic TN	Secondary TN	Idiopathic TN
Clinical presentation	Pain fulfilling ICHD 3 criteria for TN	Pain fulfilling ICHD 3 criteria for TN	Pain fulfilling ICHD 3 criteria for TN
Underlying cause	Neurovascular compression at the trigeminal nerve root entry zone demonstrated on MRI or during surgery	• Multiple sclerosis • Cerebellopontine angle tumor • Arteriovenous malformation	No underlying cause identified on MRI or electrophysiological testing

Secondary TN due to multiple sclerosis (MS) is caused by a demyelinating plaque at the trigeminal nerve root entry zone at the pons, resulting in demyelination of trigeminal nerve nuclei [8].

Clinical Features

TN has an incidence of 4–13/100,000 people [9, 10]. This neuralgia is frequently seen in the elderly, most commonly after the age of 50 years. It is more common in women with a male: female ratio between 1:1.5 and 1:1.7 [10].

Pain due to trigeminal neuralgia is characterized by paroxysms of pain, described as sharp, superficial, stabbing, or electrical shock-like. It is usually intense and can affect one or more branches of the trigeminal nerve. The intensity of the pain may increase over time. The pain is maximal at onset and lasts several seconds. Pain lasting longer than 2 min is rare. Paroxysms of pain may occur repeatedly followed by a several minute refractory period. During the refractory period pain attacks cannot be precipitated by the usual triggers [11, 12]. An important feature that distinguishes TN from other facial pain disorders is that it does not occur at night.

The pain of TN is typically unilateral. Rarely does it occur bilaterally but not usually simultaneously. The maxillary (V2) and mandibular (V3) branches are affected in most cases. In less than 5% of cases is the ophthalmic (V1) branch affected in isolation [11, 13].

Most patients are pain-free between pain attacks. Some patients with a long-standing history of TN may describe persistent mild pain. Patients may experience additional symptoms such as spams of the facial muscles during the pain attacks. These spasms resemble facial tics and therefore TN used to be called tic douloureux.

Other possible associated symptoms include autonomic symptoms, such as lacrimation or conjunctival injection with TN of the V1 branch [11, 14, 15]. If autonomic symptoms are prominent the differential diagnosis includes short-lasting unilateral neuralgiform headache attacks with conjunctival injection and tearing (SUNCT) or short-lasting unilateral neuralgiform headache attacks with cranial autonomic symptoms (SUNA).

Another typical feature of TN is the presence of triggers and trigger zones. Typical triggers include cold air, brushing teeth, chewing, or talking. Trigger zones are areas in the distribution of the affected nerve branch, close to the midline. Even light touch of these trigger zones can provoke paroxysms of pain [11, 12]. Avoidance of triggers can lead to weight loss or dehydration.

The severity and frequency of TN pain may fluctuate over time. Most patients have recurrent episodes lasting several weeks to months followed by pain-free intervals, although in some cases less severe background pain may persist [11, 13].

The diagnosis of TN can often be made solely on clinical grounds, however, diagnostic tests should be performed to evaluate for underlying causes. Diagnostic studies are covered in Chap. 5.

The Differential Diagnosis of TN is broad and includes other trigeminal nerve disorders or headache disorders that mimic TN. A thorough history is usually helpful in distinguishing these disorders described below.

Dental Pain

Pain related to dental causes can sometimes be confused with TN in the V2 or V3 distribution. The pain related to TN is sharp, electrical shock-like with a refractory period. Pain related to TN does not awaken patients from sleep. Dental pain is often dull and throbbing. It is continuous without a refractory period. It does not resolve at night [16].

First Bite Syndrome

This condition is characterized by brief facial pain attacks triggered by the first bite of a meal. The pain lessens with subsequent bites. Another trigger can be the smell of food. There are no cutaneous triggers, which distinguishes this disorder from TN. This condition can be seen with neck and throat cancer or after neck dissection for cancer [17].

Painful Trigeminal Neuropathy

Pain due to trigeminal neuropathy occurs in the distribution of one or more branches of the trigeminal nerve. This pain is often continuous, but there may be superimposed paroxysms of pain. It is often described as burning, aching, or squeezing. Clinically, one can find sensory deficits in the distribution of the trigeminal nerve branch. Allodynia and cold hyperalgesia are common [1]. This condition is rarely idiopathic. It is caused by injury of the trigeminal nerve due to an underlying condition, such as trauma, acute herpes zoster, or postherpetic neuralgia.

1. Painful Trigeminal Neuropathy attributed to herpes zoster: Acute herpes zoster is caused by reactivation of the varicella zoster virus (VZV). The virus remains dormant in the dorsal root ganglia after the acute infection. Any condition that weakens the immune system (age, malignancy, immunosuppressive agents, etc.) can allow the virus to travel along the peripheral nerve and cause hemorrhagic inflammation of the nerve and corresponding nerve root and dorsal root ganglion [18]. This pain is accompanied by the clinical signs of acute herpes zoster. It is characterized by unilateral facial pain in the distribution of one or more branches of the trigeminal nerve, lasting less than 3 months. Herpes zoster in the distribution of the trigeminal nerve occurs in the ophthalmic branch (V1) branch in 80% of cases [18]. The pain is severe and burning. Pain may occur before the rash develops or even without a rash [18]. Therefore, it is important to consider acute

herpes zoster in patients with new-onset pain in the V1 distribution. Other cranial nerve palsies affecting the oculomotor (III), trochlear (IV), or abducens (VI) nerves may occur.

2. Trigeminal Postherpetic Neuralgia: This diagnosis is made if pain persists more than 3 months after the resolution of the herpes zoster rash. In some patients, the pain may persist for years. The pain is described as burning and severe. Itching can be quite prominent [19, 20]. Following the acute inflammation of the peripheral nerve, dorsal root, and dorsal root ganglion axonal and myelin loss can be observed. Peripheral sensitization of dorsal root neurons can lead to spontaneous neuronal activity and may explain the persistent pain [20].

3. Painful Post-Traumatic Trigeminal Neuropathy (previously known as anesthesia dolorosa): This pain develops after an injury to the trigeminal nerve or its branches. In addition to pain, there are signs of trigeminal nerve dysfunction such as sensory loss, hyperalgesia, or allodynia. This diagnosis is suggested by a history of direct trauma to the nerve, which could be mechanical or radiation induced. Surgical procedures in the face or the sinuses can also result in painful trigeminal neuropathy. Additionally, it can develop as a complication of neuro-ablative treatment for TN [1, 21].

4. Painful trigeminal neuropathy attributed to other disorders: Painful trigeminal neuropathy may develop in the context of other medical conditions, such as multiple sclerosis, a connective tissue disorder, or a space-occupying lesion [1].

Paratrigeminal Oculosympathetic Syndrome (Raeder's Syndrome)

This condition is characterized by constant unilateral pain in the ophthalmic (V1) branch of the trigeminal nerve. The pain is often described as burning and is accompanied by hypoesthesia or dysesthesia. The pain worsens with eye movement. It is accompanied by ipsilateral Horner syndrome: ptosis and miosis [1]. Underlying causes include mass lesions in the middle cranial fossa, syphilis, or sinusitis. Another important underlying cause is carotid artery dissection [1, 22, 23].

Burning Mouth Syndrome

This condition is characterized by a constant burning sensation of the tongue or the oral mucosa. It is usually bilateral, most commonly affecting the tip of the tongue. Accompanying symptoms include dryness of the mouth and altered taste. An underlying cause cannot be found in idiopathy burning mouth syndrome, although trigeminal small fiber sensory neuropathy has been suggested [1, 24, 25]. Postmenopausal women are affected predominantly [26]. Underlying causes, such as candidiasis, diabetes mellitus, vitamin deficiencies, or connective tissue disorders need to be ruled out. The pain can improve spontaneously in up to half of all patients [25].

Persistent Idiopathic Facial Pain (Previously Known as Atypical Facial Pain)

This facial or oral pain is persistent, occurs daily for at least 2 hours per day for more than 3 months. It is described as dull, aching, or nagging [1]. It is often poorly localized and does not strictly follow the distribution of a peripheral nerve [1]. Pain may start in the nasolabial fold or one side of the chin. It may spread throughout the face and neck. The neurological examination should be normal and no underlying causes should have been identified. This is therefore a diagnosis of exclusion. While mood disorders, such as depression can be present in many patients, depression is not considered the etiology of this pain disorder. Persistent idiopathic facial pain is considered a central pain syndrome [27, 28].

Central Neuropathic Facial Pain

In contrast to persistent idiopathic facial pain central neuropathic facial pain has an underlying cause. It can be attributed to multiple sclerosis or poststroke pain [1].

Neuralgia in the Distribution of Other Cranial Nerves

Neuralgia of the nervus intermedius, glossopharyngeal nerve, occipital, or greater auricular nerve can cause pain in the head or neck, however, a careful history with emphasis on the location of the pain should help distinguish these neuralgias from TN. Painful optic neuritis or recurrent painful ophthalmoplegic neuropathy (formerly known as ophthalmoplegic migraine) may also result in pain in the head or face, but the accompanying clinical features will point to a diagnosis other than a trigeminal nerve disorder.

Headache Disorders that Can Mimic TN

Migraine

The pain associated with migraine is described as throbbing or pulsating, lasts between 4 and 72 hours and is of moderate to severe intensity. It can be aggravated by routine physical activity and is accompanied by either nausea or photo- and phonophobia [1]. The pain is often unilateral, but can be bilateral. Migraine pain may radiate to the face and is often most intense in the forehead or periorbital region. A careful history with emphasis on the pattern, duration, and accompanying symptoms should help distinguish a migraine disorder from TN.

Trigeminal Autonomic Cephalalgias

Cluster Headache

This is the most common Trigeminal Autonomic Cephalalgia (TAC). Pain attacks are short but excruciating. Pain is unilateral, and accompanied by autonomic signs and symptoms. The pain is periorbital or orbital. Another important feature is the presence of restlessness or agitation during the pain attacks [1].

Other TACs

The pain attacks of the other TACs are of higher frequency and shorter duration than cluster headaches and some show a dramatic response to indomethacin treatment.

In particular, short-lasting unilateral neuralgiform headache attacks with conjunctival injection and tearing (SUNCT) or short-lasting unilateral neuralgiform headache attacks with cranial autonomic symptoms (SUNA) can mimic the pain associated with TN given their short duration and high frequency. The associated autonomic signs and symptoms and response to treatment may help with the differential diagnosis. See Table 4.2.

Cluster-Tic Syndrome

This condition is characterized by the presence of pain attacks that resemble TN or cluster headaches or both [29–31].

Table 4.2 Trigeminal neuralgia and trigeminal autonomic cephalalgias

	Cluster headache	Paroxysmal hemicrania	SUNCT[a] SUNA[b]	Hemicrania continua	Trigeminal neuralgia
Female: Male	1:4.3	1.1–2.7:1	1:1.5	2:1	1.5–1.7:1
Attack frequency	Once every other day to 8/day	1–40/day	1–200/day	Chronic pain with acute exacerbations	Several hundred/day
Attack duration	15–180 min	2–30 min.	5 s –6 min	Chronic pain	Fraction of second to 2 minutes
Abortive treatment	Sumatriptan Oxygen	N/A	N/A	N/A	N/A
Preventive treatment	Prednisone Verapamil Lithium Others	Indomethacin	Lamotrigine Topiramate Gabapentin	Indomethacin	Carbamazepine Oxcarbazepine Others

[a]SUNCT: short-lasting unilateral neuralgiform headache attacks with conjunctival injection and tearing
[b]SUNA: short-lasting unilateral neuralgiform headache attacks with cranial autonomic symptoms

References

1. Headache Classification Committee of the International Headache Society (IHS). The international classification of headache disorders, 3rd edition. Cephalalgia 2018; 38:1.
2. Love S, Coakham HB. Trigeminal neuralgia: pathology and pathogenesis. Brain. 2001;124:2347.
3. Hamlyn PJ. Neurovascular relationships in the posterior cranial fossa, with special reference to trigeminal neuralgia. 2. Neurovascular compression of the trigeminal nerve in cadaveric controls and patients with trigeminal neuralgia: quantification and influence of method. Clin Anat. 1997;10:380.
4. Love S, Hilton DA, Coakham HB. Central demyelination of the Vth nerve root in trigeminal neuralgia associated with vascular compression. Brain Pathol. 1998;8:1.
5. Hilton DA, Love S, Gradidge T, Coakham HB. Pathological findings associated with trigeminal neuralgia caused by vascular compression. Neurosurgery. 1994;35:299.
6. Fromm GH, Terrence CF, Maroon JC. Trigeminal neuralgia. Current concepts regarding etiology and pathogenesis. Arch Neurol. 1984;41:1204.
7. Obermann M, Yoon MS, Ese D, et al. Impaired trigeminal nociceptive processing in patients with trigeminal neuralgia. Neurology. 2007;69:835.
8. Truini A, Prosperini L, Calistri V, et al. A dual concurrent mechanism explains trigeminal neuralgia in patients with multiple sclerosis. Neurology. 2016;86:2094.
9. MacDonald BK, Cockerell OC, Sander JW, Shorvon SD. The incidence and lifetime prevalence of neurological disorders in a prospective community-based study in the UK. Brain. 2000;123(Pt4):665.
10. Katusic S, Beard CM, Bergstralh E, Kurland LT. Incidence and clinical features of trigeminal neuralgia, Rochester, Minnesota, 1945-1984. Ann Neurol. 1990;27:89.
11. Maarbjerg S, Gozalov A, Olesen J, Bendtsen L. Trigeminal neuralgia - a prospective systematic study of clinical characteristics in 158 patients. Headache. 2014;54:1574.
12. Di Stefano G, Maarbjerg S, Nurmikko T, et al. Triggering trigeminal neuralgia. Cephalalgia. 2018;38:1049.
13. Zakrzewska JM, Linskey ME. Trigeminal neuralgia. BMJ. 2014;348:g474.
14. Sjaastad O, Pareja JA, Zukerman E, et al. Trigeminal neuralgia. Clinical manifestations of first division involvement. Headache. 1997;37:346.
15. Pareja JA, Barón M, Gili P, et al. Objective assessment of autonomic signs during triggered first division trigeminal neuralgia. Cephalalgia. 2002;22:251.
16. Graff-Radford SB. Facial pain. Neurologist. 2009;15:171.
17. Linkov G, Morris LG, Shah JP, Kraus DH. First bite syndrome: incidence, risk factors, treatment, and outcomes. Laryngoscope. 2012;122:1773.
18. Liesegang TJ. Herpes zoster ophthalmicus. Natural history, risk factors, clinical presentation, and morbidity. Ophthalmology. 2008;115(2 Suppl):S3–S12.
19. Watson CP, Evans RJ, Watt VR, Birkett N. Postherpetic neuralgia: 208 cases. Pain. 1988;35:289.
20. Truini A, Galeotti F, Haanpää M, et al. Pathophysiology of pain in postherpetic neuralgia: a clinical and neurophysiological study. Pain. 2008;140:405–10.
21. Benoliel R, Zadik Y, Eliav E, et al. Peripheral painful traumatic neuropathy: clinical features in 91 cases and proposal of novel diagnostic criteria. J Orofac Pain. 2012;26:49–58.
22. Shoja MM, Tubbs RS, Ghabili K, et al. Johan Georg Raeder and paratrigeminal sympathetic paresis. Childs Nerv Syst. 2010;26:373–6.
23. Solomon S. Raeder syndrome. Arch Neurol. 2001;58:661–2.
24. Lauria G, Majorana A, Borgna M, et al. Trigeminal small-fiber sensory neuropathy causes burning mouth syndrome. Pain. 2005;115:332.
25. Scala A, Checchi L, Montevecchi M, et al. Update on burning mouth syndrome: overview and patient management. Crit Rev Oral Biol Med. 2003;14:275–91.
26. Kohorst JJ, Bruce AJ, Torgerson RR, et al. A population-based study of the incidence of burning mouth syndrome. Mayo Clin Proc. 2014;89:1545.

27. Cranial neuralgias and central causes of facial pain. In: Lance JW, Goadsby PJ, editors. Mechanism and management of headache. Philadelphia: Elsevier Butterworth Heinemann; 2005. p. 333.
28. Boes CJ, Copobianco DJ, Cutrer FM, et al. Headache and other craniofacial pain. In: Bradley WG, Daroff RB, Fenichel GM, et al., editors. Neurology in clinical practice. Philadelphia: Butterworth Heinemann; 2004. p. 2055.
29. Watson P, Evans R. Cluster-tic syndrome. Headache. 1985;25:123.
30. Alberca R, Ochoa JJ. Cluster tic syndrome. Neurology. 1994;44:996.
31. Mulleners WM, Verhagen WI. Cluster-tic syndrome. Neurology. 1996;47:302.

Michael Suer

Introduction

Trigeminal nerve disorders are a common cause of facial pain with highly variable clinical presentations. Establishing trigeminal nerve diagnoses can prove challenging given the overlap amongst these disorders. The focus of this chapter is on the diagnosis of these conditions based on history, physical examination, and neuroimaging studies. Where able, we will discuss the differential diagnoses of these conditions and differentiate the key clinical features of each entity. Trigeminal nerve anatomy, etiology, and clinical features of these conditions are discussed in the previous chapter. Treatment of these pain conditions will be discussed elsewhere in this publication.

Trigeminal Neuralgia

History

As Established by the International Classification of Headache Disorders, Third Edition (ICHD-3), the Diagnosis of Trigeminal Neuralgia (TN) is Established on Clinical Findings [1]

1. Recurrent paroxysms of unilateral facial pain in the distribution(s) of one or more divisions of the trigeminal nerve, with no radiation beyond, and fulfilling criteria B and C
2. Pain has all of the following characteristics:
   (a) Lasting from a fraction of a second to 2 min

M. Suer (✉)
Department of Orthopedics and Rehabilitation, University of Wisconsin, Madison, WI, USA
e-mail: suer@rehab.wisc.edu

© The Author(s), under exclusive license to Springer Nature Switzerland AG 2021
A. Abd-Elsayed (ed.), *Trigeminal Nerve Pain*,
https://doi.org/10.1007/978-3-030-60687-9_5

    (b) Severe intensity
    (c) Electric shock-like, shooting, stabbing or sharp in quality
3. Precipitated by innocuous stimuli within the affected trigeminal distribution
4. Not better accounted for by another ICHD-3 diagnosis

Pain with TN is typically unilateral in a V2 and/or V3 distribution; although occasionally, patients will exhibit bilateral alternating pain and rarely bilateral pain simultaneously [2]. Interestingly, TN affects the right side of the face 5 times more often than the left. Autonomic symptoms—lacrimation, conjunctival injection, rhinorrhea—can occur with attacks in a V1 trigeminal distribution [2]. The presence of autonomic features is more suggestive of the syndromes of short-lasting unilateral neuralgiform headache attacks with conjunctival injection and tearing (SUNCT) and short-lasting unilateral neuralgiform headache attacks with autonomic symptoms (SUNA) [1].

Some patients exhibit pre-trigeminal neuralgia syndrome for weeks to years prior to fulfilling diagnostic criteria for TN [3]. Common complaints including unrelenting sinus pain or toothache lasting for hours triggered by jaw movements or drinking [3]. TN pain and severity may fluctuate over time with most patients having recurrent episodes lasting weeks to months. While most patients have pain-free intervals, some exhibit less severe background pain between episodes. The number of attacks may vary from less than 1 per day up to hundreds per day. TN is a notable exception to the general rule that nerve injuries cause constant pain and/or allodynia. [2, 4]

The presence of triggers or trigger zones is also typical of TN and is a valuable clue to the diagnosis of TN. Trigger zones are in the distribution of the affected nerve branch often close to the nose or mouth and patients will carefully avoid the area. Even light touch of these zones can evoke pain. Other common triggers include cold air, brushing teeth, chewing, talking, or smiling. In other facial pain syndromes, by contrast, patients will often exhibit relief with massage or thermal modalities [2, 4].

Once the diagnosis of TN is suspected per the above criteria, secondary causes should be vetted. In most instances, painful trigeminal neuropathy can be differentiated from TN by a comprehensive history and physical exam. Painful trigeminal neuropathy is defined as facial pain in the distribution(s) of one or more branches of the trigeminal nerve that is caused by another disorder and is indicative of neural damage and will be outlined further below [1].

See Fig. 5.1 for the diagnostic evaluation of suspected trigeminal neuralgia.

Red Flag Symptoms

As with any pain complaint, one must be constantly vigilant for symptoms that could forewarn a more sinister ailment. See Table 5.1 for red flag symptoms and possible diagnoses to consider.

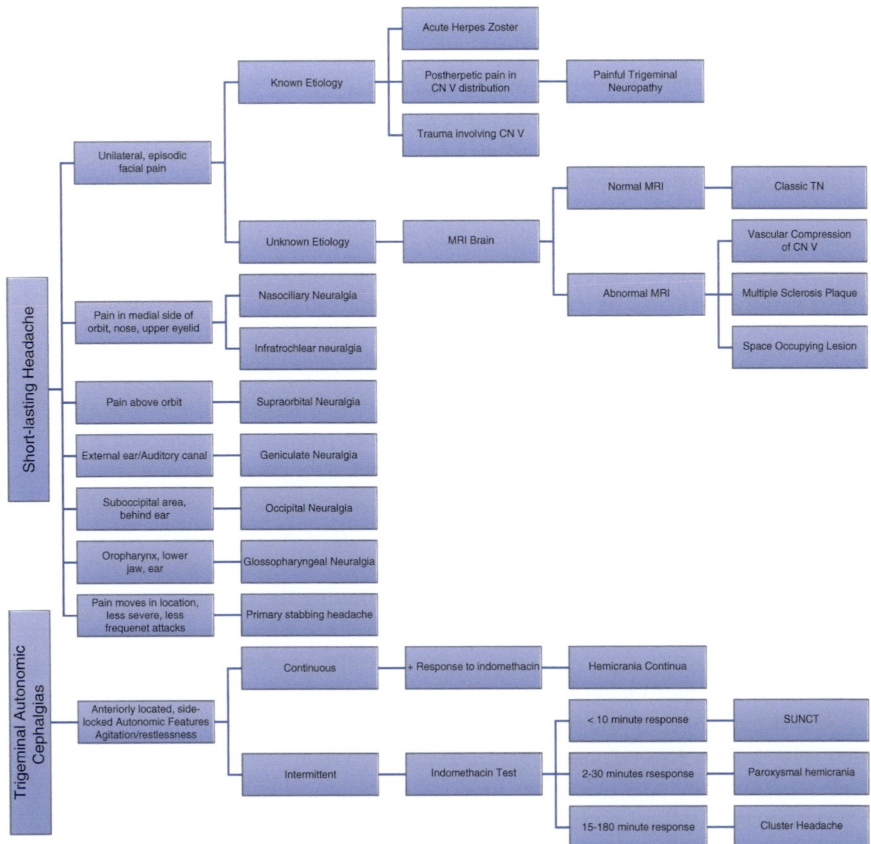

Fig. 5.1 Diagnostic Algorithm

Table 5.1 Red flag symptoms in workup for headache

Symptom	Considerations
Rapid onset	Arterial dissection, TIA, SAH, sinus venous thrombosis, seizure
Thunderclap	Reaching maximum intensity in less than 1 min SAH, hemorrhagic stroke, RCVS, pituitary apoplexy
Neurologic symptoms	Arterial dissection, stroke, giant cell arteritis, glaucoma
Prominent neck pain ± fever	Meningitis
Age > 50 at onset	Giant cell arteritis, intracranial tumor/metastasis, hypertension
Worsening with position or Valsalva	IIH, sinus thrombosis, intracranial tumor/metastasis, CSF leak
New/worsening headache with history of migraine	Medication overuse, hypertension, intracranial tumor/metastasis

TIA transient ischemic attack; *SAH* subarachnoid hemorrhage; *RCVS* reversible cerebral vasoconstriction syndrome; *IIH* idiopathic intracranial hypertension; *CSF* cerebrospinal fluid

Differential Diagnosis

The differential diagnosis of TN includes conditions such as acute herpes zoster, postherpetic neuralgia, trauma to the trigeminal nerve, dental pain, and others. While the ophthalmic branch (V1) is the most common trigeminal branch affected by postherpetic neuralgia, it is rare in TN with less than 5% of cases showing isolated V1 symptoms [5]. See Table 5.2 for differentiating features of diagnoses to consider in workup for TN.

Physical Examination

The physical examination for TN can prove challenging, especially if patients are in the midst of a pain episode. Patients may limit the examination for fear of stimulating trigger zones. An astute clinician must observe patient behavior prior to initiating the physical exam and should seek permission for the exam prior to commencing. If at all possible, one should avoid touching trigger zones in patients with TN.

The goal of the physical examination is to eliminate alternative diagnoses as there should be no abnormalities unless there is a prior or concomitant neurologic process. A thorough neurologic examination including the cranial nerves with particular note on facial sensation, masseter bulk, masseter strength, and corneal reflex should be performed. One should also examine the head and neck including the mouth, teeth, temporomandibular joint, and ears to rule out other conditions.

Sensation of each of the three branches of the trigeminal nerve should be evaluated with a light touch (cotton wool), pinprick, vibration, heat, cold, and finally deep pressure. Lewy and Grant in 1938 [6] and later confirmed in other papers [7, 8] reported that 25% of patients with TN will have sensory abnormalities although they may be unaware of the deficits. One can also find temporal summation (abnormal increase in the intensity of pain with constant-strength stimulus after cessation of stimulus) which is a hallmark of neuropathic pain [9]. While typical trigger zones verify the diagnosis of trigeminal neuralgia, one should not be encouraged to provoke these areas unnecessarily as doing such may cause a significant increase in the patient's pain.

Patients with sensory abnormalities in the trigeminal area, loss of corneal reflex, or weakness in the facial muscles should trigger the physician to further evaluate for secondary causes of trigeminal neuralgia or facial pain. See below for further insight into the physical exam for trigeminal neuropathy. Features on physical examination that should elicit concern for other causes of pain include:

1. Abnormal neurological examination
2. Abnormal oral, dental, or ear examination
3. Age younger than 40 years
4. Bilateral symptoms
5. Dizziness or vertigo
6. Hearing loss or abnormality
7. Numbness

Table 5.2 Differential diagnosis of trigeminal neuralgia

Diagnosis	Differentiating features from TN
Cluster headache	Longer-lasting pain Orbital or supraorbital pain May wake from sleep Autonomic symptoms
Dental pain	Localized Related to biting, hot/cold foods Visual abnormalities on dental exam
Giant cell arteritis (temporal arteritis)	Persistent pain Temporal Often bilateral Jaw claudication
Glossopharyngeal neuralgia	Pain in tongue, mouth, throat Triggered by coughing, yawning, swallowing May be unable to speak during attacks, avoids moving lips/tongue Involuntary startle during attempt to touch affected side is diagnostic
Intracranial tumor (acoustic neuromas, cerebral aneurysms, trigeminal neuromas, and meningiomas)	May have neurological signs or symptoms
Migraine	Longer-lasting pain Photophobia and/or phonophobia Family history
Multiple sclerosis	Eye symptoms Other neurological symptoms
Otitis media	Pain localized to the ear Abnormalities on exam and tympanogram
Paroxysmal hemicrania	Pain in forehead or eye Autonomic symptoms (conjunctival injection, lacrimation) Indomethacin responsive Does not respond to carbamazepine
Postherpetic neuralgia	Continuous pain Tingling History of zoster Often V1 distribution
Sinusitis	Persistent pain Nasal symptoms
SUNCT[a] SUNA[b]	Ocular or periocular Autonomic symptoms
Temporomandibular joint syndrome	Persistent pain Localized tenderness Jaw abnormalities
Trigeminal neuropathy	Persistent pain Associated sensory loss
Occipital neuralgia	Pain in posterior head

(continued)

Table 5.2 (continued)

Diagnosis	Differentiating features from TN
Tic convulsif	Prominent hemifacial spasm Dilated and ectatic basilar artery or other vascular malformation compressing the trigeminal nerve

[a]SUNCT: short-lasting unilateral neuralgiform headache attacks with conjunctival injection and tearing

[b]SUNA: short-lasting unilateral neuralgiform headache attacks with cranial autonomic symptoms

8. Pain episodes persisting longer than 2 min
9. Pain outside of trigeminal nerve distribution
10. Visual changes

Neuroimaging

There are no routinely indicated neuroimaging or laboratory tests as patients with characteristic history and normal neurologic examination may be treated without further workup. However, distinguishing between classic and symptomatic forms of TN is not always clear and thus imaging studies are often undertaken. As computer tomography (CT) is limited in evaluating the brainstem and cisterns, magnetic resonance imaging (MRI) is the modality of choice. The most common abnormalities on neuro-imaging are vascular contact, cerebellopontine angle tumors, and multiple sclerosis (MS) [10, 11].

MRI is the imaging modality of choice and is indicated in patients younger than 60 years of age, its utility is mainly in excluding a tumor or MS. Some physicians recommend elective MRI for all patients to exclude mass lesion or aberrant vessel compressing the nerve roots. According to a report of the Quality Standards Subcommittee of the American Academy of Neurology and the European Federation of Neurological Societies [12], routine head imaging identifies structural causes in up to 15% of patients (Level C). There was insufficient evidence to support or refute the usefulness of identifying neurovascular compression of the trigeminal nerve (Level U).

In such cases that vascular compression is seen, it is important to note if the contacting vessel is an artery or vein and if it is contacting the proximal or distal portion of the cisternal portion of the trigeminal nerve. A dedicated protocol including T2 or T1 volumetric acquisition techniques with thin slices in all three planes should be helpful. Magnetic resonance angiography (MRA) can assist in locating the vascular compression though it has low sensitivity. Newer techniques, such as high-resolution, 3-dimensional MRA, and 3-D fast asymmetric spin-echo sequences with multiplanar reconstruction have been evaluated but no recommendations have been made [12, 13]. Overall, the sensitivity of MR on neurovascular insults has shown significant variability in outcomes and techniques and is thus not considered reliable [12, 14].

Isolated cranial nerve palsies bare special mentioned due to their relationship with MS. While brainstem involvement is common at MS onset, truly isolated cranial nerve palsies are somewhat rare. Of these, a study by Zadro et al. [15] demonstrated the trigeminal nerve was most commonly involved as a presenting symptom of MS (trigeminal neuralgia in 1.9% and sensory neuropathy in 2.9%). Interestingly, only 26 of 50 patients had positive brain MRI in their study. However, with newer MRI techniques (their study utilized 1.5 T MRI) the sensitivity may improve [16].

Pediatric Considerations

Pediatric TN, which accounts for 1.5% of TN cases [17], differs from adult in that bilateral and multiple cranial nerve compressions are more common at 42% and 46%, respectively. Pediatric TN is commonly caused by neurovascular compression in the prepontine cistern as a result of abnormal vessels, vascular malformation, tumors, cysts, aneurysm, or arachnoiditis [18].

Painful Trigeminal Neuropathy

As described in Chap. 4, pain due to trigeminal neuropathy occurs in the distribution of one or more branches of the trigeminal nerve. While the pain is often continuous, there are often superimposed attacks of pain described as burning, aching, or squeezing as well as allodynia or hyperalgesia [1]. This entity is oft caused by injury to the trigeminal nerve due to an underlying condition as we will discuss below [1]. Classically, patients will exhibit pain in an area of the face which exhibits impaired or absent sensation; however, other signs of neuropathy and/or centralized pain may be present. In differentiating trigeminal neuropathy from trigeminal neuralgia, as the underlying disorder progresses in trigeminal neuropathy, more neurons are destroyed resulting in the appearance of numbness and/or weakness.

For further details on the underlying pathology, please refer to Chap. 4. See Table 5.3 for differential diagnosis of trigeminal neuropathy.

Physical Exam

Presented here as a general outline for the workup of trigeminal neuropathy are guidelines for the exam in patients with facial pain and/or numbness. The concepts presented here are true for any of the etiologies of trigeminal neuropathy and for trigeminal nerve exams in general. The exam should include comprehensive neurological evaluation and inspection of the ears, nose, throat, and cerebrovascular structures.

Table 5.3 Differential diagnosis of trigeminal neuropathy [19]

History	Diagnoses to consider
Trauma	Accidental Surgical Dental (especially third molar) Chemical Radiation
Inflammatory/autoimmune	Undifferentiated and mixed connective tissue disease Progressive systemic scleroderma Sjogren's syndrome Sarcoidosis Multiple sclerosis
Vascular	Pontomedullary ischemia or hemorrhage Vascular malformation
Neoplastic	Intra- or extra-cranial compression Perineural spread Metastases Carcinomatous meningitis
Infectious	Leprosy Varicella zoster virus Herpes simplex virus Lyme disease Syphilis Fungi
Degenerative	Kennedy's disease
Metabolic	Stilbamidine Trichloroethylene Oxaliplatin Diabetes mellitus
Congenital	Skull base anomalies Congenital trigeminal anesthesia with or without Goldenhar–Gorlin syndrome or Mobius syndrome
Other	Amyloidosis Pseudotumor cerebri

General Inspection

Visual inspection and manual palpation may reveal atrophy in the temporalis and/or masseter muscles. Other muscles to consider include the mylohyoid and tensor veli palatine. Observe jaw movements looking for symmetry as the jaw will deviate toward the side of a weakened pterygoid. Oral breathing may also be present if the patient has jaw-drop leading to dry mouth and thickened secretions. Jaw movements may also be limited if the patient has a malignancy in the masticator space (opening) or rostral brainstem or bilateral cerebral disease (jaw protrusion and deviation) [20].

Neurologic Examination

A complete neurologic examination should begin with cranial nerve testing. Sensation of each of the three branches of the trigeminal nerve should be evaluated with a light touch (cotton wool), pinprick, vibration, heat, cold, and finally deep pressure. In trigeminal neuropathy, one may find partial or complete sensory loss, allodynia, or hyperalgesia. The finding of tactile triggers would favor TN over trigeminal neuropathy although sensory abnormalities may be seen in either of these entities. Within the clinical setting of nerve dysfunction, neuroimaging can prove critical as the predictive value of clinical neurosensory testing has some limitations. One must also be mindful of a central neurologic process such as sensory trigeminal nucleus versus spinal trigeminal nuclear lesions [19, 20].

Reflexes

Jaw Jerk

Also knows as the masseteric T reflex, the jaw jerk is performed with the mouth held in a slightly open position. The mandible is tapped at a downward angle just below the lips. Sensory afferent neurons project to the trigeminal mesencephalic nucleus in series with the ipsilateral efferent arc through the pontine trigeminal motor nucleus which innervates the masseter [19, 20].

The reflex is considered a monosynaptic dynamic stretch reflex used to judge the integrity of the upper motor neurons projecting to the trigeminal motor nucleus. In individuals with an upper motor neuron lesion, the jaw will jerk; while the reflex is normally absent [19, 20].

Corneal (Blink) Reflex

The corneal reflex is an involuntary direct and consensual (contralateral) blinking of the eyelids elicited by stimulation of the cornea. It is mediated by sensory afferents of the nasociliary branch of the ophthalmic nerve to synapses within the spinal trigeminal nucleus in the brainstem which project to the facial nucleus. The temporal and zygomatic branches of the facial nerve (CN VII) initiate the motor response (efferent fiber) [21].

This reflex is performed by having the patient look away while the cornea is touched by a cotton tip or drop of saline. One should observe both eyes blink immediately following stimulation. If no blink response is observed, a sensory lesion is most likely present. When the untested eye does not blink, a contralateral facial nerve palsy may be present. If the tested eye does not blink, but the untested eye does, an ipsilateral facial nerve palsy may be present. One must use caution in individuals who regularly wear contact lenses as this reflex may be diminished [21].

Painful Trigeminal Neuropathy Attributed to Herpes Zoster

History

Acute herpes zoster (shingles) is an acute viral disease affecting the trigeminal nerve (CN V) as a result of reactivation of the varicella zoster virus that has remained dormant in the trigeminal nerve root ganglion. The diagnosis of acute herpes zoster can be established based on the patient's medical history and clinical findings. One should obtain a detailed history including a history of chickenpox or acute herpes zoster. Within the latter of these, note:

- Location of the lesion (does it cross midline, which dermatome)
- Symptoms associated with the lesions
- Trigger points or zones that aggravate pain
- Swelling on the affected side

One should also note the type of pain experienced paying particular attention to symptoms of neuropathic pain (paresthesia, dysesthesia, allodynia, and/or hyperalgesia) [1, 22].

Herpes zoster occurs in the ophthalmic branch (V1) of the trigeminal nerve in approximately 80% of cases. Pain may occur before the rash develops even without a rash; however, it must be present for less than 3 months (it is otherwise categorized as post-herpetic neuralgia). Other cranial nerve palsies that can be seen include oculomotor (III), trochlear (IV), or abducens (VI) nerves [22].

Physical Exam

Vesicles typically appear along the path of a single dermatome with the ophthalmic division (V1) most commonly affected. The rash presents initially as macules and papules progressing into vesicles and pustules that eventually dry, leaving a crusting appearance after 5–7 days. Vesicles in the cornea may lead to ulceration and warrant specialist consultation [22].

A rare entity, Ramsay Hunt syndrome (or herpes zoster oticus), presents as facial palsy, loss of taste (ageusia), buccal ulcerations, and appearance of rash within the auditory canal. This is a result of an outbreak affecting the facial nerve rather than the trigeminal [22].

Neuroimaging

While neuroimaging is not necessary for diagnosis, one could consider laboratory tests such as direct immunofluorescence assay for VZV antigen or polymerase chain reaction (PCR) for VDV DNA for atypical rash [22].

Trigeminal Postherpetic Neuralgia

History

Post-herpetic neuralgia (PHN) is pain which persists more than 3 months after resolution of the vesiculopapular rash [1]. While it resolves in most cases spontaneously over a course of weeks to months after resolution of the rash, the pain can persist longer. There have been reports of onset of pain months or years after the initial episode of herpes zoster has resolved. This neuropathic pain may include reports of itching, stabbing, sharp, burning sensation, allodynia, and/or hyperalgesia [22, 23].

The patient may reveal conditions that help in the differential diagnosis including a recent history or the presence of herpes simplex virus, impetigo, candidiasis, contact dermatitis, insect bites, autoimmune blistering disease, dermatitis herpetiformis, and drug-related eruptions. Pain following a documented episode of acute herpes zoster normally provides a clear diagnosis although the rash is not required for diagnosis. Other risk factors that should raise awareness for PHN include advanced age, prodromal pain, and symptoms of allodynia. Fatigue, anorexia, weight loss, insomnia, reduced physical activity, depression, anxiety, and a decrease in social contacts are commonly associated with PHN [24, 25].

Physical Exam

The physical exam may or may not reveal evidence of previous infection as some areas of previous AHZ infection may manifest as cutaneous scarring. Areas may also display hypersensitivity or hyposensitivity to pain or allodynia. As such, practitioners should be cautious and seek permission prior to testing sensation. Similar to TN, one should begin with light touch and progress through other modalities to deep pressure, stopping if the patient experiences significant discomfort. Autonomic changes may also occur in the area, notably increased sweating [23–25].

Neuroimaging

PHN diagnosis does not require lab or imaging workup.

Painful Post-traumatic Trigeminal Neuropathy

History

Painful trigeminal neuropathy is defined by head and/or facial pain in the distribution of one or more branches of the trigeminal nerve caused by another disorder and indicative of neural damage [1]. Diagnostic criteria per the ICHD-3 [1] are as follows:

1. Facial and/or oral pain in the distribution of one or both trigeminal nerves
2. History of an identifiable traumatic event to the trigeminal nerve, with clinically evident positive (hyperalgesia, allodynia) and/or negative (hypoesthesia, hypoalgesia) signs of trigeminal nerve dysfunction
3. Evidence of causation demonstrated by both of the following:
    (a) Pain is located in the distribution(s) of the trigeminal nerve(s) affected by the traumatic event
    (b) Pain has developed within 6 months of the traumatic event
4. Not better accounted for by another ICHD-3 diagnosis

The causative trauma may be of mechanical, chemical, thermal, or radiation origin and one should seek to further establish this. Painful post-traumatic trigeminal neuropathy most occurs in an iatrogenic nature as a complication of rhizotomy or thermocoagulation done to treat trigeminal neuralgia. It can, at times, be more intolerable than the pain from TN itself [1, 26].

Physical Exam

As with the above entities, a complete cranial nerve exam should be performed including testing sensation beginning with light touch (cotton swab) progressing to sharp, deep pressure last. As indicated in the ICHD-3 [1] criteria, the physical exam should coincide with the history of neuropathy. Similar to the previously discussed trigeminal neuropathies, traumatic trigeminal neuropathy may exhibit hyperalgesia, allodynia, hypoesthesia, and/or hypoalgesia.

Neuroimaging

Similar to the above entities of painful trigeminal neuropathy, neuroimaging is not required for diagnosis due to trauma.

Painful Trigeminal Neuropathy Attributed to Other Disorder

History

In the absence of the above entities as underlying causes of trigeminal neuropathy, one must further delve into the patient's history and review of systems for other rarer causes of trigeminal neuropathy. Factors to consider in the history include: hypo- or complete anesthesia, dry eyes, diminished taste, and weakness or difficulty with chewing [27].

Also consider soft palate dysfunction and hearing deficits or Eustachian tube dysfunction as the medial pterygoid nerve innervates the tensor veli palatine muscle. Cool temperatures may also trigger visual disturbances (blurring) due to corneal edema in the ipsilateral eye [19].

Physical Exam

As with the above entities and outlined at the head of the section, the physical exam should be complete looking for signs of nerve dysfunction as well as assessing for other etiologies that could cause trigeminal neuropathy.

Neuroimaging

Lesions producing symptoms of trigeminal neuropathy can occur anywhere along the path of the trigeminal nerve from the brainstem to the distal projections. Radiological evaluation should therefore include each of these areas—brainstem including upper cervical ganglion, skull base, trigeminal ganglion, cavernous sinus, and along the extra-cranial pathways—to be considered optimal. While CT has a role in the assessment of peripheral nerve segments and bony skull base, MRI with and without contrast is the imaging modality of choice as mentioned previously [28].

Paratrigeminal Oculosympathetic Syndrome (Raeder's Syndrome)

This condition is characterized by constant unilateral pain in the ophthalmic (V1) branch of the trigeminal nerve accompanied by an ipsilateral Horner syndrome [1]. Horner's syndrome is characterized by miosis (i.e., constricted pupil), partial ptosis, and loss of hemifacial sweating (i.e., anhidrosis), as well as enophthalmos (sinking of the eyeball into the bony cavity that protects the eye).

History

The patients will typically describe pain, sensory or motor deficits, and/or ipsilateral Horner's syndrome (oculosympathetic paresis) with ptosis and miosis. Unlike Horner syndrome, there is no anhidrosis and pain is present due to the preservation of trigeminal sensory irritation. Enopthalmos may be present [29].

Autonomic features may also be reported as conjunctival tearing or erythema. Pain is often described as boring with intermittent lancinating pain and is localized in or around the eye. It is often less well-defined than pain associated with TN [29].

Physical Exam

As with other entities discussed in this chapter, a complete exam including cranial nerves must be performed as other parasellar cranial nerves (oculomotor (III), trochlear(IV), facial (V), and abducens (VI) nerves) may be involved. Rare instances of internal carotid pathology have also resulted in Raeder's syndrome without parasellar cranial nerve involvement [30, 31].

Further complicating the examination of Raeder syndrome, Horner's syndrome can occur in other pathologies including cluster headache, carotid dissection, or carotid aneurysm. Unilateral Horner's syndrome and trigeminal nerve involvement are the hallmark features on the exam [29–31].

Neuroimaging

Workup should include MRI and MR angiography (MRA) of the brain to help exclude secondary causes such as dissection, vascular anomaly, and aneurysm. Originally believed to be due to space-occupying lesions in the paratrigeminal area of the middle cranial fossa, benign forms without paratrigeminal cranial nerve involvement have also been reported [32].

Raeder syndrome localizes lesions of the middle cranial fossa involving the oculopupillary sympathetic fibers traveling with the trigeminal and oculomotor nerves. Painful oculosympathetic palsy involves the location where these fibers join the ophthalmic division of the trigeminal nerve. At this location, multiple cranial nerve deficiencies (CN II-VI) have been described. Careful imaging of this area is highly recommended [32].

Supraorbital and Infraorbital Neuralgia

Supraorbital and infraorbital neuralgia are somewhat rare entities characterized by persistent pain in the orbital region. Pain is described as either persistent or persistent with shock-like paresthesias in the area of the respective nerve distribution. These can follow trauma (blow to the head, previous black eye, etc.) although they can also be idiopathic.

Physical examination will reveal no cranial nerve pathology. Glaucoma may also cause intermittent ocular pain and may cause permanent loss of vision if untreated so ophthalmic examination is strongly recommended. Similarly, for infraorbital neuralgia, one should consider sinus and dental pathology [33].

In the absence of other headaches, pain with Tinel's over the nerve with pain radiating into the forehead (supraorbital neuralgia) or infraorbital area (infraorbital neuralgia) is suggestive of the respective neuralgia. The supraorbital notch can be identified with the patient lying in a supine position and looking straight forward. The notch will be located at the inferior margin of the orbit directly superior to the pupil. The infraorbital foramen may be identified with the patient in the same position. However, the foramen is palpated along the inferior rim of the infraorbital ridge along a line drawn sagittal from the pupil downward. Diagnosis can be confirmed with pain relief following a small volume supraorbital nerve block [33, 34].

References

1. Headache Classification Committee of the International Headache Society (IHS). The international classification of headache disorders, 3rd edition. Cephalalgia. 2018;38(1):1–211. https://doi.org/10.1177/0333102417738202.
2. Zakrzewska JM, Linskey ME. Trigeminal neuralgia. BMJ. 2014;348:g474.
3. Fromm GH, Terrence CF, Chattha AS, Glass JD. Baclofen in trigeminal neuralgia: its effect on the spinal trigeminal nucleus: a pilot study. Arch Neurol. 1980 Dec;37(12):768–71.
4. Di Stefano G, Maarbjerg S, Nurmikko T, et al. Triggering trigeminal neuralgia. Cephalalgia. 2018;38:1049.
5. Maarbjerg S, Gozalov A, Olesen J, Bendtsen L. Trigeminal neuralgia—a prospective systematic study of clinical characteristics in 158 patients. Headache. 2014;54:1574.
6. Lewy FH, Grant FC. Physiopathologic and pathoanatomic aspects of major trigeminal neuralgia. Arch Neurol Psychiatr. 1928;40:1126–34.
7. Eide PK, Rabben T. Trigeminal neuropathic pain: pathophysiological mechanisms examined by quantitative assessment of abnormal pain and sensory perception. Neurosurgery. 1998;43:1103–10.
8. Nurmikko TJ. Altered cutaneous sensation in trigeminal neuralgia. Arch Neurol. 1991;48:523–7.
9. Casey KF. Role of patient history and physical examination in the diagnosis of trigeminal neuralgia. Neurosurg Focus. 2005;18(5):E1. https://doi.org/10.3171/foc.2005.18.5.2.
10. Majoie CB, Hulsmans FJ, Castelijns JA, Verbeeten B Jr, Tiren D, van Beek EJ, et al. Symptoms and signs related to the trigeminal nerve: diagnostic yield of MR imaging. Radiology. 1998 Nov;209(2):557–62.
11. Tash RR, Sze G, Leslie DR. Trigeminal neuralgia: MR imaging features. Radiology. 1989;172(3):767–70. https://doi.org/10.1148/radiology.172.3.2772186.
12. Gronseth G, Cruccu G, Alksne J, Argoff C, Brainin M, Burchiel K, et al. Practice parameter: the diagnostic evaluation and treatment of trigeminal neuralgia (an evidence-based review): report of the quality standards Subcommittee of the American Academy of Neurology and the European Federation of Neurological Societies. Neurology. 2008 Oct 7;71(15):1183–90.
13. Tanaka T, Morimoto Y, Shiiba S, Sakamoto E, Kito S, Matsufuji Y, et al. Utility of magnetic resonance cisternography using three-dimensional fast asymmetric spin-echo sequences with multiplanar reconstruction: the evaluation of sites of neurovascular compression of the trigeminal nerve. Oral Surg Oral Med Oral Pathol Oral Radiol Endod. 2005 Aug;100(2):215–25.

14. Montano N, Conforti G, Di Bonaventura R, Meglio M, Fernandez E, Papacci F. Advances in diagnosis and treatment of trigeminal neuralgia. Ther Clin Risk Manag. 2015;11:289–99. https://doi.org/10.2147/TCRM.S37592.
15. Zadro I, Barun B, Habek M, Brinar VV. Isolated cranial nerve palsies in multiple sclerosis. Clin Neurol Neurosurg. 2008;110(9):886–8. https://doi.org/10.1016/j.clineuro.2008.02.009.
16. Comi G, Filippi M, Rovaris L, Leocani L, Medaglini S, Locatelli T. Clinical, neurophysiological, and magnetic resonance imaging correlations in multiple sclerosis. J Neurol Neurosurg Psychiatry. 1998;64(Suppl 1):S21–5.
17. Resnick DK, Levy EI, Jannetta PJ. Microvascular decompression for pediatric onset trigeminal neuralgia. Neurosurgery. 1998;43(4):804–7.
18. Linskey ME. 143 pediatric trigeminal neuralgia (TN): results with early microvascular decompression (MVD). Neurosurgery. September 2017;64:234. https://doi.org/10.1093/neuros/nyx417.143.
19. Kim JS, Lee JH, Lee MC. Patterns of sensory dysfunction in lateral medullary infarction. Clinical-MRI correlation. Neurology. 1997;49:1557–63.
20. Wiebers DO. Mayo Clinic examinations in neurology. 7th ed. St. Louis: Mosby; 1998.
21. Peterson DC, Hamel RN. Corneal reflex. [Updated 2019 Jun 22]. In: StatPearls [Internet]. StatPearls Publishing, Treasure Island (FL); 2020 Jan. Available from https://www.ncbi.nlm.nih.gov/books/NBK534247/
22. Liesegang TJ. Herpes zoster ophthalmicus. Natural history, risk factors, clinical presentation, and morbidity. Ophthalmology. 2008;115(2 Suppl):S3–S12.
23. Feller L, Jadwat Y, Bouckaert M. Herpes zoster post-herpetic neuralgia. SADJ J South Afr Dental Assoc. 2005;60(10):432–7.
24. Nalamachu S, Morley-Forster P. Diagnosing and managing postherpetic neuralgia. Drugs Aging. 2012;29:863–9. https://doi.org/10.1007/s40266-012-0014-3.
25. Sampathkumar P, Drage LA, Martin DP. Herpes zoster (shingles) and postherpetic neuralgia. Mayo Clin Proc. 2009;84(3):274–80. https://doi.org/10.4065/84.3.274.
26. Heros RC, Heros DA, Schumacher JM, Marsden CD. Principles of neurosurgery. In: Bradley WG, Daroff RB, Fenichel GM, editors. Neurology in clinical practice. Philadelphia: Butterworth Heinemann; 2004. p. 963.
27. Smith JH, Cutrer FM. Numbness matters: a clinical review of trigeminal neuropathy. Cephalalgia. 2011;31(10):1131–44. https://doi.org/10.1177/0333102411411203.
28. Hutchins LG, Harnsberger HR, Hardin CW, Dillon WP, Smoker WR, Osborn AG. The radiologic assessment of trigeminal neuropathy. AJR Am J Roentgenol. 1989;153(6):1275–82. https://doi.org/10.2214/ajr.153.6.1275.
29. Nolph MB, Dion MW. Raeder's syndrome associated with internal carotid artery dilation and sinusitis. Laryngoscope. 1982 Oct;92(10):1144–8.
30. Shoja MM, Tubbs RS, Ghabili K, et al. Johan Georg Raeder (1889-1959) and paratrigeminal sympathetic paresis. Childs Nerv Syst. 2010;26:373–6.
31. Raeder JG. "Paratrigeminal" paralysis of oculo-pupillary sympathetic. Brain. 1924;47:149–58.
32. Solomon S, Lustig JP. Benign Raeder's syndrome is probably a manifestation of carotid disease. Cephalgia. 2001;21:1–11.
33. Vasudha J, Divakar P, Manohar M. Supraorbital neuralgia. Case Rep. 2014;7(2):208–10.
34. Knight GC. Infra-orbital neuralgia. Proc R Soc Med. 1948;41(9):587–92.

Non-Pharmacological Management

6

Behnum Habibi, Travis Cleland, and Chong Kim

Introduction

Trigeminal Neuralgia (TN) is an uncommon facial pain syndrome. It can be associated with increasing age, hypertension, and other chronic conditions (e.g., Multiple Sclerosis). Reports of its incidence vary from 4 to 28.9 cases per 100,000 people [1]. It occurs more commonly on the right side of the face and it is more frequently diagnosed in women than in men. The condition was originally described as a form of "sensory epilepsy," suggestive of its symptomatology. Clinically, TN is characterized by recurrent episodes of facial pain of a short duration that are typically one-sided and in the distribution of one or more branches of the trigeminal nerve [2]. The mandibular and maxillary branches are more commonly affected than the ophthalmic branch. Painful episodes can be triggered by small movements of the jaw and facial muscles or stimulation of the face [3]. Radiological investigations may reveal causative structural lesions. Common structural etiologies include vascular compression or abnormalities, cysts, and tumors. Other etiologies may not be detectable with currently available diagnostic testing. As a first-line treatment, the anti-seizure medication Carbamazepine is often recommended [4], due to its use and success in multiple controlled trials since the 1960s. Interventional therapies including surgery and percutaneous nerve blocks/ablations are often used in refractory cases. The most common surgical treatment is microvascular decompression of the trigeminal nerve via the posterior fossa. Percutaneous trigeminal branch nerve blocks and radiofrequency ablations are alternatives to surgical treatment. In this chapter, non-pharmacologic and non-interventional treatments will be discussed using an evidence-based approach. These treatments date back to 1677 when the

B. Habibi · T. Cleland · C. Kim (✉)
Case Western Reserve University School of Medicine/MetroHealth, Cleveland, OH, USA
e-mail: tcleland@metrohealth.org; ckim3@metrohealth.org

© The Author(s), under exclusive license to Springer Nature Switzerland AG 2021

A. Abd-Elsayed (ed.), *Trigeminal Nerve Pain*,
https://doi.org/10.1007/978-3-030-60687-9_6

prominent political philosopher Dr. John Locke documented his treatment of the Countess of Northumberland, wife of the British Ambassador to France, who suffered from severe acute pain on the right side of her face. This chapter will focus on more modern home remedies, the B vitamins, acupuncture, and laser therapy. Demographics, pathophysiology, clinical features, and common treatments (oral medications, local injections, surgeries, psychological interventions, and physical therapy) are discussed in more detail elsewhere.

Home Remedies

The American Academy of Neurology (AAN) provides clinical guidelines for the management of trigeminal neuralgia. These guidelines do not comment specifically on home remedies, though they do recommend against the use of topical ophthalmic anesthesia as a treatment (Grade B recommendation, per the AAN strength of recommendation guide available at www.neurology.com) [5]. The International Headache Society does not have published guidelines for the management of trigeminal neuralgia. In 2019, the European Academy of Neurology (EAN) published guidelines for the treatment of TN based on a systematic review of existing evidence [6]. With regard to home treatments, they report that transcutaneous electrical stimulation was successful in relieving symptoms of TN, but this modality has not been compared to standard treatments. Other common home remedies are not discussed at length in these clinical guidelines or systematic reviews. These clinically common remedies include trigger avoidance, which is an important tool for patients (though its specifics are not well researched). Another home remedy, aromatherapy (e.g., lavender) is also anecdotally useful for patients given its ease of use. However, it has not been specifically studied for TN. Finally, topical pressure/cold/heat therapies (e.g., warm bean bags placed over the painful area for 10 min) have been reported useful by patients with TN, but safety and therapeutic profiles have not been thoroughly studied.

Data on alternative medicinal home remedies include some basic science studies and small non-controlled trials. For example, Wu-tou decoction (WTD) is a traditional Chinese medicine that has been used for trigeminal neuralgia as well as other neuropathic pain syndromes. Animal data suggest that WTD acts by increasing the expression of neurotrophic factors and decreasing the expression of C-C chemokine receptor type 5 (CCR5) [7]. Go-rei-san, a Japanese traditional medicine was described in a case series of four patients with intractable trigeminal pain who could not tolerate Carbamazepine [8]. It was reportedly effective.

In an animal model of trigeminal neuralgia, established by inducing a chronic contusion injury in the infraorbital branch of the trigeminal nerve, another traditional Chinese medicine was shown to be effective. The drug, Corydalis yanhusuo, is proposed to work via the upregulation of cannabinoid CB1 receptors as described in the same animal study in the Chinese publication The Journal of Southern Medical University [9]. Another Japanese medicine Yokukansan has been described in the Japanese Journal of Anesthesiology as a treatment for neuropathic pain, including TN [10]. Its proposed mechanism is the downregulation of 5-hydroxy-tryptamine (5-HT) 2A receptors in the prefrontal cortex and improved stability of myelin sheaths.

Collagen and Coenzyme Q10 have been suggested as treatments for neuropathic pain and TN. An online patient support group, the Facial Pain Association, has a single blog entry describing a decrease in pain intensity and frequency with simultaneous over-the-counter Collagen and Co-enzyme Q10 consumption. There is a paucity of data to support this practice.

Elderberry syrup has been anecdotally suggested as a treatment for TN. The proposed mechanism of action is via "antioxidants" concentrated in the berry and/or unnamed anti-inflammatory compounds. The syrup, in the only description found by this author, is a concentrate of the berry mixed with alcohol, confounding its therapeutic benefit. Peppermint candies have also been discussed anecdotally as TN treatments but in multiple unpublished reports, these candies worsened symptoms of TN. Data supporting these and other alternative home remedies are limited in quality and quantity. However, these and other treatments may warrant further study and serve as alternatives for those with otherwise limited treatment options.

Vitamin B

There is evidence that the B vitamins can relieve neuropathic pain. Treatment of TN with Vitamin B12, for example, was reviewed in The Lancet in 1954 [11]. In 1952 the journal *Neurology* reported that a large dose of Vitamin B12 relieved trigeminal pain [12]. More recently, a 2012 study in the journal *Life Sciences* investigated vitamin B use in an animal model of TN [13]. Treatment with Vitamins B1 (thiamine), B6 (pyridoxine), and B12 (cyanocobalamin) ameliorated distinct nociceptive behaviors in male Wistar rats. In particular, B12 worked synergistically with Carbamazepine to reduce nociception in this animal model. In a Chinese controlled clinical trial, an injection of Vitamin B12 was compared to oral carbamazepine [14]. One hundred and four patients with trigeminal neuralgia were included in the study. The efficacy of Vitamin B12 (98.2%) was significantly better than the efficacy of the control Carbamazepine (80.9%; $p < 0.01$). Several other studies have been published on vitamin B use in trigeminal neuralgia, but they were primarily published in German and Italian languages and clustered in the 1950s and 1960s.

Acupuncture

Acupuncture is generally viewed as a safe and effective treatment for headaches of multiple etiologies [15]. However, mechanisms for acupuncture's effectiveness in TN are not clear. No clinical guidelines or Cochrane reviews describe the use of acupuncture for TN. As of March 2020, few systematic reviews were available on the use of acupuncture for TN. Hu et al. published one such systematic review of seven databases in 2019 [16]. The group found 33 randomized controlled trials and concluded that acupuncture may improve symptoms of TN. In particular, the studies suggest that acupuncture combined with Carbamazepine was more effective than Carbamazepine alone. Another review published in the British Medical Journal— Clinical Evidence in 2009 commented on acupuncture for TN but could not make conclusions on its efficacy [17]. Finally, a review published in 2010 in the journal *Alternative Therapies in Health and Medicine* searched English and Chinese databases for trials of acupuncture in TN [18]. Twelve studies met inclusion criteria in which acupuncture treatment arms (506 patients total) were compared to control groups receiving Carbamazepinc (414 patients total). Four of the studies concluded that acupuncture was superior to Carbamazepine. Eight studies showed no difference between the two groups. The review also concluded the evidence to be of low methodological quality precluding meta-analysis. Overall, compared to home remedies and laser therapy, there is a greater quantity and quality of literature in support of acupuncture for the treatment of TN. However, this body of literature is of overall limited quality and further study would be useful. In addition to traditional acupuncture, the practice of stimulating "pressure points" has been anecdotally suggested as a treatment for TN. Reflexology, wherein pressure is applied with varying force to different areas of the body, is a practice similar to pressure point stimulation. While no peer-reviewed studies have been published on these practices in cases of TN, there are many practitioners, typically with "Chinese" or "Traditional" medicine backgrounds, who provide such treatments. Traditional medicine practices may also use herbal steams which may be beneficial in TN and date back to at least the nineteenth century. Again, while no peer-reviewed evidence supports their use, these treatments are likely safe and may confer benefits to patients.

Laser Therapy

Laser therapy has been discussed in the literature as a promising treatment for TN. For example, the previously mentioned systematic review [17] in BMJ Clinical Evidence commented on laser therapy for TN but could not make conclusions on its efficacy. Laser therapy typically utilizes single-wavelength light sources to generate laser radiation and monochromatic light which may alter physiology on cellular and tissue levels [19, 20]. Like acupuncture, no clinical guidelines or Cochrane reviews describe the use of laser therapy for TN. As of March 2020, one systematic review was available on the use of laser therapy for TN in the United States National Library of Medicine. This review by Falaki et al. searched multiple databases for English language articles describing the effect of low-level laser therapy on TN. Articles published prior to 2011 were reviewed. One study by Walker in 1983 showed successful treatment of symptoms after 30 sessions of laser therapy. Another article by the same Walker published in 1988 in the Clinical Journal of Pain showed improved symptoms with one-year of follow-up [21]. A distinct form of laser therapy, GaAlAs laser was tested by Vernon and Hasbun in two patients with TN and was effective for up to 12 months. These results were published in Practical Pain

Management in 2008. Side effects in these studies were minimal and overall, laser therapy may be considered as an option for refractory cases of TN or in patients who do not tolerate the side effects of more common treatments.

Other Therapies

Multiple other non-pharmacologic therapies for TN exist that do not fit into the above categories. These will briefly be reviewed here. Yoga, Tai chi, and similar practices have benefits similar to light exercise. Patients with cervical disc disease and glaucoma should be advised that inverted positions employed with yoga should be avoided. Yoga may be particularly beneficial for patients unable to tolerate more intensive exercise, as an alternative to a sedentary lifestyle. No published studies exist regarding yoga and TN in the US National Library of Medicine (PubMed).

Extracorporeal shock wave therapy is a noninvasive ultrasound modality that typically targets soft tissues. One case report [22] has been published in the American Journal of Physical Medicine and Rehabilitation on the use of shock wave therapy for TN, with 10 Hz ultrasound waves targeted at the surface projection of the trigeminal ganglion. Pain scores decreased in this patient at 1, 2, and 5 months after baseline from 8, to 3, 1, and 1, respectively. No adverse event was reported.

Meditation is a common anecdotal, potentially therapeutic, modality for TN. There are no published reports of its use for TN. To date, there is one English language randomized controlled study comparing mindfulness mediation to a control group among patients with postherpetic neuralgia [23]. While not similar in etiology to TN, postherpetic neuralgia also causes neuropathic pain and the results from this study may be generalizable to other neuropathic pain syndromes. The total number of patients in the study was 27. Questionnaires were used to assess pain levels at enrollment, 2 weeks post-enrollment, and 6 weeks post-enrollment. Meditation was performed 1–2 times per day at increasing durations, starting from 3-min sessions up to 16 min. Pain and physical function levels improved significantly in the treatment group. This suggests meditation may be a useful adjunctive therapy in cases of neuropathic pain, including TN.

Biofeedback therapy is another alternative treatment modality that has been suggested for TN [24]. It is related to relaxation training and uses physiological measures (often EEG, EMG, and/or galvanic skin response) to aide in relaxation. Again, the evidence for this practice is limited. Reviews for its use in TN have not been published. In a 2018 Cochrane review of non-pharmacological therapy for pain related to Multiple Sclerosis, biofeedback was noted to have "very low-level evidence" supporting its use [25]. In contrast, in 2004 the US Headache Consortium gave the highest level of evidence to biofeedback in a review of its use in migraine treatment [26]. Hypnotherapy, like biofeedback therapy, is a type of relaxation-inducing behavioral treatment. A case series of its use for TN was published in the journal *Anesthesia Progress* in 1985 [27]. Two patients were treated with hypnotherapy for refractory TN. Treatments consisted of daily therapy for 1 week followed by weekly therapy as well as independent home therapy sessions. One patient was able to taper her Carbamazepine and Baclofen doses due to the therapy and the other was able to increase her physical and social functioning. The patients were followed for 3 years and reported persisting benefits. It is plausible to this author that biofeedback and other forms of relaxation therapy can improve the perception of pain in patients with TN.

Anecdotally, patients have reported trigeminal nerve pain relief with the use of orthotics. Mouthguards, for instance, may provide some relief for TN, perhaps by altering trigeminal nerve signaling via activation of its motor fibers. No published studies on the use of mouthguards for TN exist. Another orthotic, the earplug, has been suggested to patients with TN via a blog entry on the Facial Pain Association website. The potential mechanism of action is unclear. The same blog post also suggests a cervical collar placed over the scalp as a potential treatment, as well as an elastic "cranial cap." Again, potential mechanisms of action for these orthotics are unclear.

In conclusion TN is a relatively uncommon pain disorder. This has limited the study of alternative therapies. However, TN is a very painful condition that can significantly affect the activities of daily living and overall function of patients. Therefore, it is important to consider alternative therapies for patients who cannot or do not wish to pursue pharmacologic or interventional treatments. Among these alternative therapies, treatment with vitamin B has the highest quality evidence, with studies published in the journals Lancet and Neurology. However, most of the published work on vitamin B and TN is from the mid-twentieth century and more modern trials are limited in number. Acupuncture is another safe and effective alternative therapy for TN. Several systematic reviews have concluded that there is supporting evidence for acupuncture in TN though the quality of the reviewed studies is generally of low methodological quality and the mechanism by which acupuncture is supposed to work for TN is unclear. Home remedies such as Wu-tou decoction, Go-rei-san, Corydalis yanhusuo, and Yokukansan have also been studied and are promising alternative treatments for TN. As with other alternative therapies, the evidence for their use is mostly limited to case series' and animal studies. Laser therapy is another alternative treatment for TN. Again, the evidence is limited to case series and case reports, and the mechanism of action is unclear. Like the other topics discussed in this chapter, laser therapy may be a reasonable alternative when patients cannot tolerate better-studied treatments. Finally, easy to use treatments such as trigger avoidance, aromatherapy, and topical pressure/heat/cold may be advisable given the apparent lack of risk and anecdotally reported benefits. These non-pharmacologic therapies may also serve as useful adjuncts to more common treatments.

References

1. White T, Rastogi R, Singh TSS. Trigeminal neuralgia. In: Abd-Elsayed A, editor. Pain. Cham: Springer; 2019.
2. Zakrewska JM, Chen HI, Lee JYK. Trigeminal and glossopharyngeal neuralgia. In: McMahon SB, editor. Wall and Melzack's textbook of pain. Amsterdam: Elsevier; 2013.

3. Rasmussen P. Facial pain. IV. A prospective study of 1052 patients with a view of: precipitating factors, associated symptoms, objective psychiatric and neurological symptoms. Acta Neurochir. 1991;108:100–9.
4. Cruccu G, Gronseth G, Alksne J, et al. AAN-EFNS guidelines on trigeminal neuralgia management. Eur J Neurol. 2008;15:1013–28.
5. Gronseth G, Cruccu G, Alksne J, Argoff C, Brainin M, Burchiel K, Nurmikko T, Zakrzewska JM. Practice parameter: the diagnostic evaluation and treatment of trigeminal neuralgia (an evidence-based review). Neurology. 2008. https://n.neurology.org/content/71/15/1183. Accessed 25 Mar 2020.
6. Bendtsen L, Zakrzewska JM, Abbott J, et al. European Academy of Neurology guideline on trigeminal neuralgia. In: Wiley Online Library. 2019. https://onlinelibrary.wiley.com/doi/full/10.1111/ene.13950. Accessed 25 Mar 2020.
7. Guo Q, Mizuno K, Okuyama K, Lin N, Zhang Y, Hayashi H, Takagi N, Sato T. Antineuropathic pain actions of Wu-tou decoction resulted from the increase of neurotrophic factor and decrease of CCR5 expression in primary rat glial cells. Biomed Pharmacother. 2020. https://www.ncbi.nlm.nih.gov/pubmed/31945696. Accessed 25 Mar 2020.
8. Kido H, Komasawa N, Fujiwara S, Minami T. Efficacy of Go-rei-san for pain management in four patients with intractable trigeminal neuralgia. Masui Jpn J Anesthesiol. 2017. https://www.ncbi.nlm.nih.gov/pubmed/30380286. Accessed 25 Mar 2020.
9. Huang J-Y, Fang M, Li Y-J, Ma Y-Q, Cai X-H. Analgesic effect of Corydalis yanhusuo in a rat model of trigeminal neuropathic pain. J South Med Univ. 2010. https://www.ncbi.nlm.nih.gov/pubmed/20855279. Accessed 25 Mar 2020.
10. Nakamura Y, Tajima K, Kawagoe I, Kanai M, Mitsuhata H. Efficacy of traditional herbal medicine, Yokukansan on patients with neuropathic pain. Masui Jpn J Anesthesiol. 2009. https://www.ncbi.nlm.nih.gov/pubmed/19860227. Accessed 25 Mar 2020.
11. Surtees S, Hughes R. Treatment of trigeminal neuralgia with vitamin B12. Lancet. 1954;263:439–41.
12. Fields WS, Hoff HE. Relief of pain in trigeminal neuralgia by crystalline vitamin B12. Neurology. 1952;2:131.
13. Kopruszinski CM, Reis RC, Chichorro JG. B vitamins relieve neuropathic pain behaviors induced by infraorbital nerve constriction in rats. Life Sci. 2012;91:1187–95.
14. Zhou C-S, Kong D-Q, Han Z-Y. Clinical observation on acupoint injection of VitB12 for treatment of trigeminal neuralgia. Zhongguo Zhen Jiu. 2007. https://www.ncbi.nlm.nih.gov/pubmed/17926620. Accessed 26 Mar 2020.
15. Zhao CH, Stillman MJ, Rozen TD. Traditional and evidence-based acupuncture in headache management: theory, mechanism, and practice. Headache J Head Face Pain. 2005;45:716–30.
16. Hu H, Chen L, Ma R, Gao H, Fang J. Acupuncture for primary trigeminal neuralgia: a systematic review and PRISMA-compliant meta-analysis. Complement Ther Clin Pract. 2019;34:254–67.
17. Zakrzewska JM, Linskey ME. Trigeminal neuralgia. BMJ Clin Evid. 2009. https://www.ncbi.nlm.nih.gov/pmc/articles/PMC2907816/. Accessed 26 Mar 2020.
18. Liu H, Li H, Xu M, Chung K-F, Zhang SP. A systematic review on acupuncture for trigeminal neuralgia. Alternative therapies in health and medicine. 2010. https://www.ncbi.nlm.nih.gov/pubmed/21280460. Accessed 26 Mar 2020.
19. Ilbuldu E, Cakmak A, Disci R, Aydin R. Comparison of laser, dry needling, and placebo laser treatments in Myofascial pain syndrome. Photomed Laser Surg. 2004;22:306–11.
20. Constantini D, Delogu G, Tomasello C, Sarra M. The treatment of cranio-facial pain by electroacupuncture and laser irradiation. Ann Ital Chir. 1997;68:505–9.
21. Walker J, Akhanjee L, Cooney M, Goldstein J, Tamayoshi S, Segal-Gidan F. Laser therapy for pain of trigeminal neuralgia. Clin J Pain. 1988;3:183–7.
22. Zhang D, et al. Radial extracorporeal shock wave therapy in an individual with primary trigeminal neuralgia: a case report and literature review. Am J Phys Med Rehabil. 2018;97(5):e42–5. https://doi.org/10.1097/PHM.0000000000000831.

23. Meize-Grochowski R, Shuster G, Boursaw B, DuVal M, Murray-Krezan C, Schrader R, Smith BW, Herman CJ, Prasad A. Mindfulness meditation in older adults with postherpetic neuralgia: a randomized controlled pilot study. Geriatr Nurs. 2015;36(2):154–60. https://doi.org/10.1016/j.gerinurse.2015.02.012. Epub 2015 Mar 14. PMID: 25784079; PMCID: PMC4488325.
24. Feller L, et al. "Postherpetic Neuralgia and Trigeminal Neuralgia." Pain Research and Treatment, vol. 2017; 2017. https://doi.org/10.1155/2017/1681765.
25. Bhasker A, et al. "Non-pharmacological Interventions for Chronic Pain in Multiple Sclerosis." The Cochrane Database of Systematic Reviews, vol. 2018, no. 12, Dec. 2018, https://doi.org/10.1002/14651858.CD012622.pub2.
26. Cristina T, et al. "Assessing and Treating Primary Headaches and Cranio-Facial Pain in Patients Undergoing Rehabilitation for Neurological Diseases." The Journal of Headache and Pain, vol. 18, no. 1, Sept. 2017. https://doi.org/10.1186/s10194-017-0809-z.
27. Bernard G. "Trigeminal Neuralgia: Management of Two Cases with Hypnotherapy." Anesthesia Progress. 1985;32(5):206–08. https://www.ncbi.nlm.nih.gov/pmc/articles/PMC2175410/.

Tiffany M. Houdek

Introduction

Trigeminal neuralgia is in a group of diagnoses that result in facial pain. Physical therapy cannot effectively treat trigeminal neuralgia alone. The severe pain associated with trigeminal neuralgia leads to changes in the mechanical and myofascial system of the head, face, neck, and shoulders. Over time postural changes, disuse atrophy, avoidance of activity result in muscular weakness leading to new secondary dysfunction. Eventually, this will lead to a potential trigger or ability to aggravate the trigeminal nerve again as compression and abnormal forces can develop in the face, head, neck, and shoulders. When these changes occur, it is extremely challenging to reverse these changes without physical therapy intervention. These secondary impairments can lead to continued activity limitations and participation restrictions due to persistent facial pain. In clinical practice, many patients have a secondary facial pain syndrome, in addition to trigeminal neuralgia (Fig. 7.1).

Physical therapists are experts in the diagnosis and treatment of the movement system of the human body. For optimal functional outcomes, all aspects of the condition including the secondary changes and dysfunction need to be addressed. This results in optimal treatment effects and outcomes for the whole person. The interplay between the many parts of the human body affected by trigeminal neuralgia will be reviewed. This chapter serves to demonstrate the role of physical therapy on the healthcare team and its ability to treat primary and secondary dysfunctions related to trigeminal neuralgia.

T. M. Houdek (✉)
UW Health, University of Wisconsin Hospital and Clinics, Madison, WI, USA
e-mail: THoudek@uwhealth.org

A. Abd-Elsayed (ed.), *Trigeminal Nerve Pain*,
https://doi.org/10.1007/978-3-030-60687-9_7

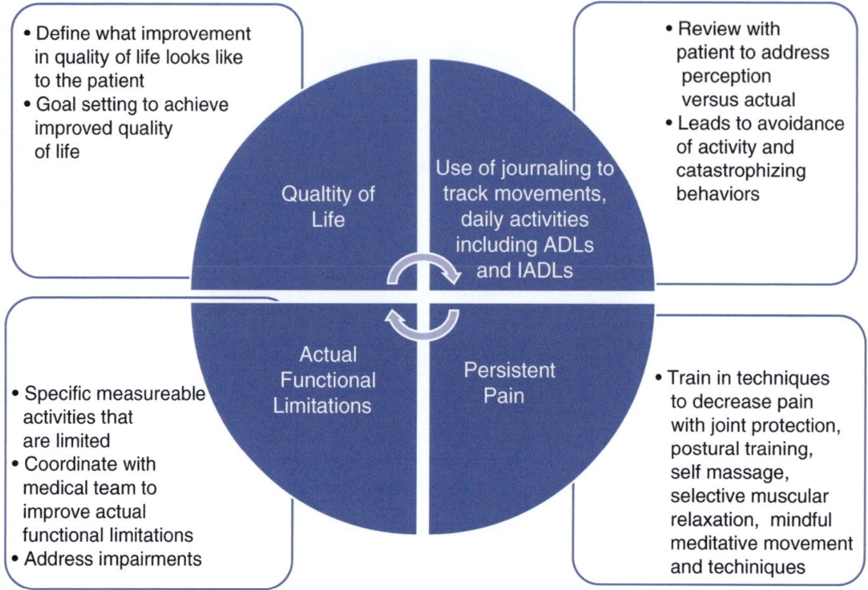

Fig. 7.1 Cycle of persistent pain, functional limitations, and quality of life

Physical Therapy and Role on Health Care Team

American Physical Therapy Association describes physical therapy practice using an established theoretical and scientific base of knowledge. Innovative approaches to address movement system dysfunction are an integral part of the profession. Physical therapists use clinical applications in the restoration, maintenance, and promotion of optimal physical function. Physical therapists are health care professionals who establish a movement diagnosis to treat individuals throughout the lifespan.

Physical therapists:

- Diagnose and manage movement dysfunction and enhance physical and functional abilities
- Restore, maintain, and promote not only optimal physical function but optimal wellness and fitness and optimal quality of life as it relates to movement and health
- Prevent the onset, symptoms, and progression of impairments, functional limitations and disabilities that may result from diseases, disorders, conditions, or injuries

The terms "physical therapy" and "physiotherapy," and the terms "physical therapist" and "physiotherapist," are synonymous [1].

Physical therapists assess "the movement system, which is the integration of body systems that generate and maintain movement at all levels of bodily function. Human movement is a complex behavior within a specific context, and is influenced by social, environmental, and personal factors. Recognition and validation of the movement system is essential to understand the structure, function and potential of the human body. The physical therapist is responsible for evaluating and managing an individual's movement system across the lifespan to promote optimal development; diagnose impairments, activity limitations, participation restrictions; and provider interventions targeted at preventing or ameliorating activity limitations and participation restrictions" [2].

As in medicine, physical therapists can specialize in various aspects of the human movement system. Orthopedic physical therapists often work with patients in pain. Typical orthopedic physical therapists will help a patient recover from surgery, a trauma (such as a motor vehicle accident), sprains, strains, and other conditions that cause acute pain. Orthopedic physical therapists can specialize to work with patients who suffer from conditions that result in persistent pain. The role of the pain physical therapist is to contribute to the health care team's treatment plan to decrease pain and address any other identified impairments. Often impairments of muscular spasm, trigger points, myofascial restriction, muscular weakness, flexibility deficits, postural imbalance, physical deconditioning are found in patients with trigeminal neuralgia. These are secondary impairments and dysfunction that result due to the recurrent severe pain experienced by the patient with trigeminal neuralgia.

It has been shown that multi-modal treatment of persistent painful conditions is necessary for the best outcomes. There is no current research to guide the physical therapist in the specific treatment of trigeminal neuralgia. However, regional interdependence has been well studied in physical therapy. The health care team is needed to provide a multi-modal treatment approach for optimal outcomes. Integrating medical interventions to address the pain of trigeminal neuralgia, psychological interventions, physical therapy treatment of movement system applying the right intervention at the right time. This leads to increased tolerance to perform physical therapy interventions that the patient would not have otherwise tolerated. The team works together to consistently work toward functional and quality of life improvement.

Regional Interdependence: Health Care Team

The term regional interdependence has been used to describe one event or intervention that can influence a seemingly unrelated intervention. Therefore, the communication and collaboration across the health care team is extremely important when working with patients with persistent pain. Trigeminal neuralgia is characterized by sudden severe pain attacks. Triggers for these attacks can be absent or very difficult to ascertain. Patients may attribute these pain attacks to a recent event such as a physical therapy exercise or medication change (Fig. 7.2). Collaboration across the team helps to find the best treatment and understanding any and all downstream effects. This addresses the potential negative effects of our treatment plans that the patient experiences remote from the desired effect (Fig. 7.3).

Fig. 7.2 Negative impact on patients

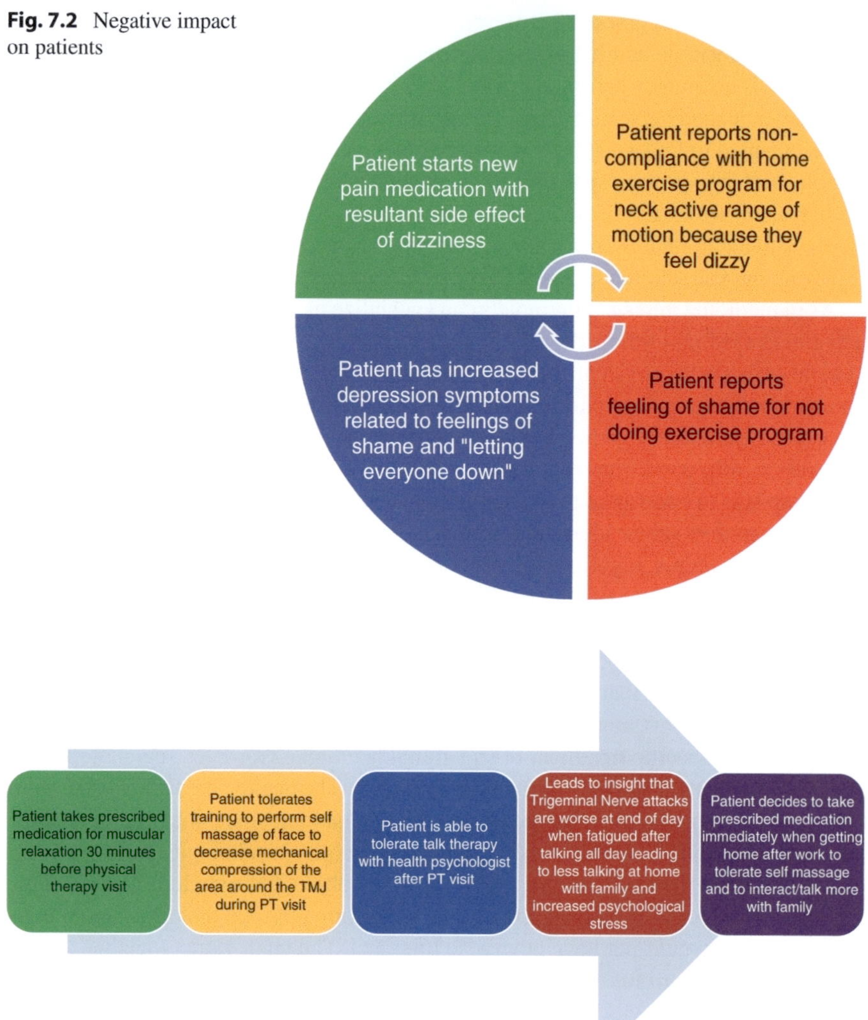

Fig. 7.3 Positive effects on pain, activity limitation and participation restrictions leading to less disability

Regional Interdependence

Movement System

With respect to musculoskeletal problems, regional interdependence refers to the concept that seemingly unrelated impairments in a remote anatomical region may contribute to, or be associated with, the patient's primary complaint [3]. In this

Fig. 7.4 Areas of
movement system

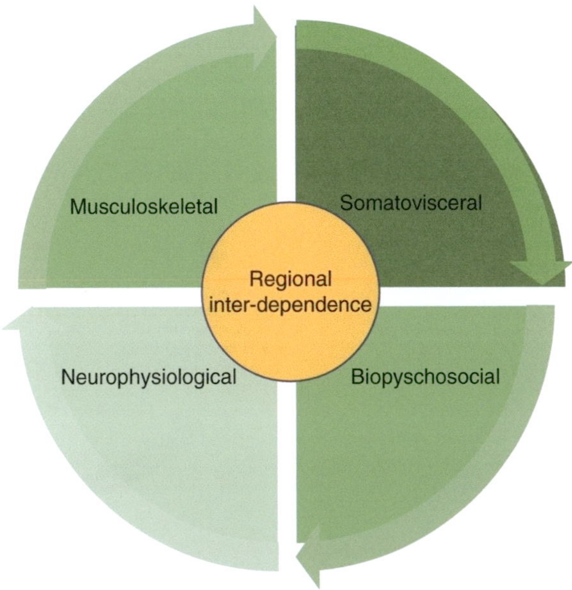

case, trigeminal neuralgia may be directly or indirectly affected by impairments from other body regions. The distance of these body regions to each other does not reflect the level of significance on the symptoms the patient is experiencing. The physical therapist will first assess the area of pain complaint but then, based on the best available research, should evaluate and identify impairments that may be amenable to treatment especially when first-line treatments are ineffective. This is especially important for persistent pain conditions, such as trigeminal neuralgia. Figure 7.4 shows how areas of the movement system can be affected over time leading to additional impairments that will not respond to treatments aimed at the trigeminal nerve.

For trigeminal neuralgia, the concept of regional interdependence is used as the mainstay of the best evidence-informed treatment philosophy for physical therapy intervention. Current physical therapy evidence supports clinically relevant relationships between regions [4]. Specific to trigeminal neuralgia, it is clinically relevant to perform a thorough evaluation of mechanical, myofascial, central, and peripheral neurological systems of the cervical spine, thoracic spine and ribs, and shoulders (Fig. 7.5). Clinically important changes and subsequent outcomes can be best achieved when the concept of regional interdependence is utilized. Physical therapists use this model to treat areas away from the painful area yet make an impact in the body as a whole. This can be especially valuable when the patient does not tolerate treatment at the site of pain.

In addition, altered muscular function leads to new symptoms and a variety of other effects that lead to decreased quality of life. Figure 7.6 demonstrates how altered muscle function can lead to significant activity limitations and participation restrictions significantly decreasing a patient's quality of life.

Fig. 7.5 Impact on musculoskeletal system

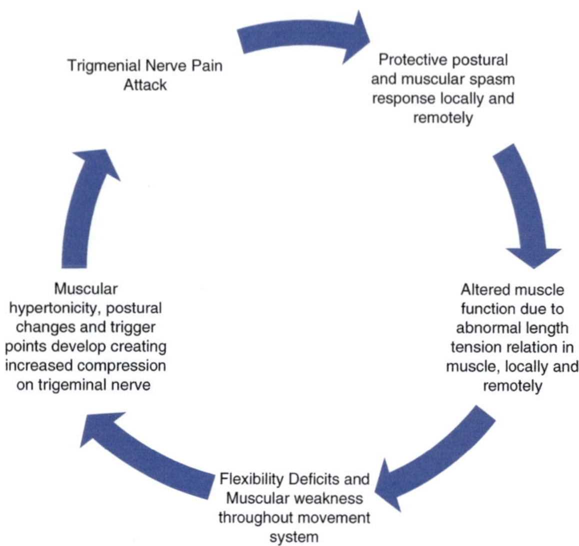

Physical therapists address each of the solid blue arrows causing change in the noted impairment through multiple physical therapy interventions. This shows how addressing breathing mechanics can have a significant change on quality of life without treating the trigeminal neuralgia pain directly.

Use of skilled physical therapy interventions for back pain while addressing postural imbalance that resulted from protective pain muscular response. Trigeminal nerve pain attacks decrease the ability to participate in daily activities. The use of pacing of daily activities decreases fatigue and muscular overuse.

Training in selective muscular relaxation, self-soft tissue mobilization, clinical myofascial release, use of dry needling, mindfulness activities addressing facial, neck, upper back and shoulder tension, meditative movement improve the length–tension relationship of the muscles of the upper quarter of the body all serve to change the tension–pain cycle which leads to improvement in function.

Physical Therapy Evaluation

Physical therapy evaluation is multi-faceted to understand the whole person and their environment. The evaluation centers around the movement system as it relates to activity limitations and participation restrictions. Functional limitations and impairments are identified with a thorough subjective interview and objective examination. Integrating these the physical therapist determines a movement system diagnosis and treatment plan. On the health care team, the physical therapist contributes to the team plan of care and goals to improve the function and quality of life of the patient.

Fig. 7.6 Impact on muscle function and quality of life

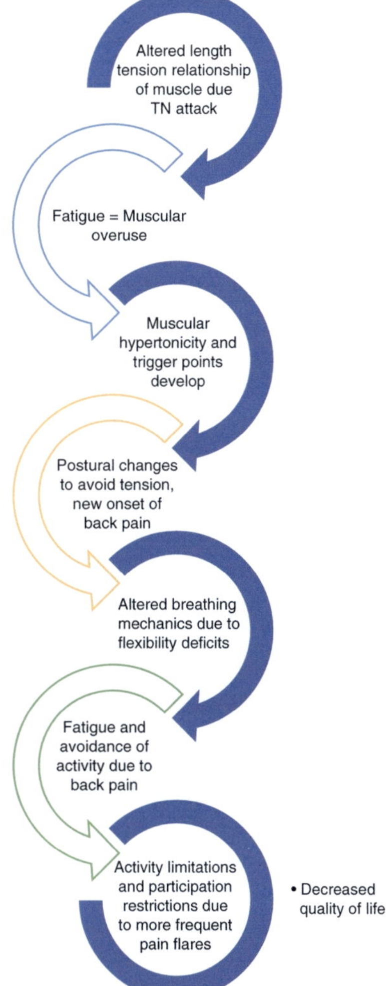

A thorough subjective interview is important to obtain at the initial visit. The history of the symptoms of the pain symptoms, in addition to prior injuries or surgeries, are relevant as noted by regional interdependence. Functional limitations consisting of activity limitations and participation restrictions are obtained through the subjective interview and use of patient-reported outcome tools such as the Neck Disability Index and/or the Quick DASH. Assessment of quality of life through the use of patient-reported outcome tools such as the VR-12 or SF-36 helps to identify and quantifies the patient's experience in the clinic, including sleep. Clear understanding of the patient's pain and effect on life important to obtain at the initial clinic visit. The physical therapist refers to this initial visit frequently throughout the plan of care to assess for change.

Subjective reports of pain are more complex than a rating on the 0–10 numerical pain scale. Physical therapists address this by inquiring about different descriptions of the pain. Pain is assessed at rest, with different activities, lowest level, highest level, and an average level. Frequency and intensity of the pain symptoms are reported as this can also be measured as change. For instance, constant facial pain and headache can accompany trigeminal neuralgia. The patient may report 10/10 severe pain attacks that fade over time and occur 7–10 times per day. They also report dull aching pain in the head, neck, and shoulders constantly rated at 6/10, made worse by prolonged sitting and standing. Pain with eating especially chewing items like steak or gum increases unilateral facial pain to 9/10 but talking increases bilateral facial pain to 7/10. Rest relieves the talking pain but has no effect on the severe pain attacks. The patient may also complain of constant squeezing pain on the top of head pain at 3/10 unrelated to the dull aching pain. All these pain descriptions, frequency, and intensity are opportunities for change, which is why a thorough subjective interview is extremely important.

When considering regional interdependence, a thorough history of other musculoskeletal and neurological conditions and review of systems for medical screening need to be performed. Physical therapists are extensively trained in medical screening to determine appropriateness for physical therapy and communicate any concerning red flags to the medical team.

Review of medications is important as many medications affect the movement system. A physical therapist needs to be knowledgeable regarding these medications. Understanding of the pharmacodynamics of a drug's action, and how it influences the patients physiological and biochemical systems, allows the physical therapist to tailor their treatment to maximize these effects. Timing of medications and physical therapy interventions have been used utilized in orthopedic surgery for decades as acute pain after surgery can be severe. Patients need pain relief to tolerate activities required by the rehabilitation team. This leads to greater improvement in function over time. Poor timing can lead to refusal to participate with physical therapy and deleterious effects of disuse atrophy, physical deconditioning, and development of contractures. Pain physical therapy relies on the medical team's treatment plan, working with the team to use prescribed medications and procedures performed by the medical doctors to improve patient participation in the physical therapy plan of care. Balancing the physiological and biochemical effects of a medication or procedure on nerve function, muscular tone, balance, dizziness, sensation among others needs to be monitored by the physical therapy as well to watch for outcomes unintended or that limit physical therapy interventions as well.

Objective examination of the movement system focuses on these main elements: observational analysis, palpatory assessment, measurement of range of motion, objective measure of strength, joint play assessment, flexibility assessment, balance assessment, and other orthopedic or neurological special tests as needed. A neurological screen is performed to ensure symptoms are consistent with clinical findings of referring medical doctor.

Observational analysis focuses on postural alignment, gait, transfers, and movement analysis based on functional limitations noted in subjective interviews.

Functional tasks may be performed with motion analysis with special attention on compensatory strategies. Signs of muscular weakness, flexibility deficits, and balance impairment can be noted during the observational analysis leading to further examination.

Palpation assessment during an examination for trigeminal neuralgia focuses on assessment of the head, face, neck, shoulder girdle. Sensitivity to touch, numbness, and pressure pain threshold may be assessed. Assessment of myofascial restrictions, resting muscular tone, presence of active or latent trigger points all may be present. Special focus should address all primary and accessory breathing muscles as altered muscular function is common. Patients also will demonstrate poor muscular activation and timing due to the inhibitory effect of persistent pain. Palpating the timing of the muscular contraction in the movement system informs the physical therapist as to the underlying biomechanical forces acting on the surrounding structures. When altered biomechanics are present, abnormal forces especially in the face result in overuse and compression of surrounding structures.

Range of motion (ROM) of the spine, TMJ, shoulders should be assessed for potential limitations. American Academy of Orthopedic Surgeons has defined normative values for AROM that most physical therapists use. For reference, see Norkin and White's publications [5]. Limitations in active range of motion (AROM) may be due to muscular weakness, flexibility deficits, joint mobility restrictions. Assessment of pain resistance sequence allows the physical therapist to determine the structure involved in AROM limitation. Passive range of motion (PROM) is also assessed to know what is available for motion at a certain joint. Limitations in PROM may be improved with certain treatments. Limitations in PROM may also determine the effectiveness of a physical therapy treatment. For instance, advanced osteoarthritis of the TMJ will limit PROM. This is not likely to improve with physical therapy intervention therefore the physical therapist will adjust their treatment intervention to compensatory strategies and joint protection, instead of restoration of normal joint motion.

Muscular strength assessment as defined by Kendall [6] is typically used by the physical therapist. As a point of reference: Kendall's manual muscle test is a procedure that uses a 5-point grading scale, measurement requires a 5 s hold at mid-range of the muscle's action in an anti-gravity position. Frequently a 5-point grading scale is used in health care for strength assessment from different authors. Often the muscle being tested is not in a mid-range, anti-gravity position or held for the full 5 s. It is important to note this as strength assessment using different authors by different providers of the health care team may result in differences noted in the medical record. Physical therapists use the Kendall assessment of muscular strength to obtain a fully functional strength assessment.

Strength assessment for a person with trigeminal neuralgia should focus on the entire upper quarter and facial muscles including assessment of cross-body patterns. It is common to see contralateral lower extremity strength deficits from the side of pain. Disuse atrophy, muscular weakness, and physical deconditioning also can present due to persistent pain leading to avoidance of activity.

Joint play assessment should focus on the cervical spine, tempo mandibular joints (TMJ), thoracic spine, rib cage, glenohumeral joints, acromioclavicular joints, and sternoclavicular joints. Regional interdependence in physical therapy states that at least one joint above and below the affected region should be assessed. Innovative approaches in pain management have also noted that ground reaction forces of the lower extremity can affect upper quarter symptoms due to poor absorption of these forces during functional activities of gait when joint mobility deficits, muscular weakness, and flexibility deficits are present. The typical presentation would be the patient's report of "my face hurts when I walk." Addressing the lower extremity impairments can lead to dissipation of the ground reaction with less force transmitted through the body.

Flexibility deficits of the bilateral upper quarter muscles including all breathing muscles. Flexibility is the muscle's ability to change length compared to muscular tone which is the resting length of the muscle. Hypertonicity and trigger points can lead to a flexibility deficit; however, a flexibility deficit does not produce hypertonicity and trigger points. Flexibility deficits appear over time as an adaptation compared to muscular hypertonicity, spasm, and trigger points can be transient or persistent. Addressing the true impairment will lead to improved functional outcomes in the physical therapy plan of care.

After a thorough examination, a movement system diagnosis is established, a treatment plan is determined considering and working with the medical team's plan of care as noted previously to maximize effects. An example of a physical therapy movement system diagnosis could be: Medical diagnosis of trigeminal neuralgia leading to a movement system diagnosis of central sensitization of the face, postural dysfunction, myofascial restriction with active trigger points in the ipsilateral altered motor function of the facial muscles leading to upper cross syndrome affecting the bilateral upper quarters.

Physical Therapy Treatment Interventions

A variety of treatment interventions are used to treat the nerve pain associated with trigeminal neuralgia and secondary diagnoses. Outlined here are the suggested treatment options:

Desensitization: a process by which physical touch is applied in a systematic approach to the painful areas to decrease the pain response. A variety of textures, temperatures, and pressures are used systematically with the patient application during home program frequently very important to the efficacy of this treatment to retrain the pain response to the physical stimuli. Objective statements and use of visual biofeedback during desensitization are used to retrain the system.

Desensitization of the Face To set a baseline: you will need to determine what you can handle for desensitization. Every person is different and pain response is different. It is important to objectively quantify the sensations in your face for type of sensation (hot, cold, pressure, numb, tingle, sharp, dull, stabbing, electrical, aching, burning, etc.). Track how you feel on a chart to look for patterns that can assist the physical therapist with modifications of the desensitization program.

There are different types of sensations that will need to be desensitized. Typically working on the easiest to tolerate, working up to the most difficult to tolerate.

- *Pressure:* this is highly variable and can be addressed in multiple ways. Included below is an example of how to prescribe this intervention.
- *Temperature*: Typically, a temperature will be more or less tolerated. There can be a baseline temperature change or a perceived response to a stimulus that can all be affected. For instance, warm stimuli with a perception of a painful cold. Start with a lukewarm temperature and start to gradually increase in a stepwise progression to warmer and colder to tolerate change in temperature.
- *Texture*: It is very common to have difficulty tolerating different textures. Most people respond best to progress from very smooth to very inconsistent. A typical progression is as follows: silk, polyester, polyester/cotton blend, cotton, smooth washcloth, old used washcloth, corduroy, back of the corduroy, carpet piece, burlap. You can also use a fluid such as a lotion, cream lotion, 50/50 cream sugar scrub, 100% sugar scrub, apricot scrub.

An example of pressure desensitization program is outlined below. The same concept is applied to temperature and texture. Start with a tolerated sensation and make it "boring" to the nervous system by being consistent and frequent. After 7–10 days, change to a sensitive pressure, temperature, or texture and repeat. Continue to progress every 7–10 days until all pressures, temperature, and textures are tolerated.

Pressure Sensation Set the timer for 5 min, start with 3 times per day with the goal being 5 min of every hour awake.

During the desensitization, it is important to acknowledge the sensation of pain; however, train the patient to look for other sensations related to the amount of pressure. The patient should apply the pressure, being in control of how much pressure and for what duration. As they are practicing, it is important to refocus thoughts on the actual experience rather than the perceived experience.

Tell the patient to try to focus on the sensation/feeling of your hand touching your face. Objective statements: "My hand is touching my face," "My hand is touching my face with firm consistent pressure," "My hand is lightly tapping my face."

Perform in cycles (1→3, then repeat 1→3) until the time is up.

Monitor symptoms afterward: no change = good, improvement in symptoms = good. Increase in symptoms for more than 15 minutes = consult a physical therapist to adjust parameters. Every 7–10 days increase the duration, frequency, or pressure.

Cycle

1. Firm static pressure: Left hand on left side of face, add right-hand right side of face, remove left hand, return left hand. Repeat up to 10 cycles
2. Light consistent moving touch: Both hands at the same time, start at eyebrows to the cheekbone, cheekbone to the top lip, top of lip to angle of jaw to the bottom lip Repeat up to 10 repetitions
3. Light tapping consistent moving touch: Both hands at the same time, start at eyebrows to the cheekbone, cheekbone to the top lip, top of lip to angle of jaw to the bottom lip Repeat up to 10 repetitions
4. In Fig. 7.7, arrows will show the introduction of a new desensitization technique every 3 days with a change in temperature every 9 days as an example of how to prescribe this intervention. It will take the patient consistent compliance to achieve results. Total time per type of desensitization: 5 minutes, frequency: once per hour with the goal that each type of sensation is worked on at least 3×/day.

Graded Motor Imagery [7, 8] This is a three-stage process of treatment where the proposed mechanism is the retraining of the somatosensory cortex and central pain response to physical stimuli and movement. The first stage focused on laterality training. Laterality training focuses on the retraining of the patient's ability to determine right versus left. This is accomplished by measuring accuracy and reaction time when looking at pictures of the human body. As treatment progresses, the complexity of the picture increases to require more cognitive processing. Technology has allowed for the development of applications that the patient can use on their smartphone or tablet to work on this training. The second stage is explicit motor imagery that focuses on imagined movements or tasks that typically result in pain. The patient will imagine the movements, working on decreasing the expectation of pain with a movement or stimuli. This is especially important as the range of motion or light touch can trigger a pain response in a person with central sensitization making other physical therapy interventions difficult to tolerate. A systematic approach to imagined movements works with desensitization to decrease pain response. The third stage is mirror therapy. In this stage, a mirror is used to visually

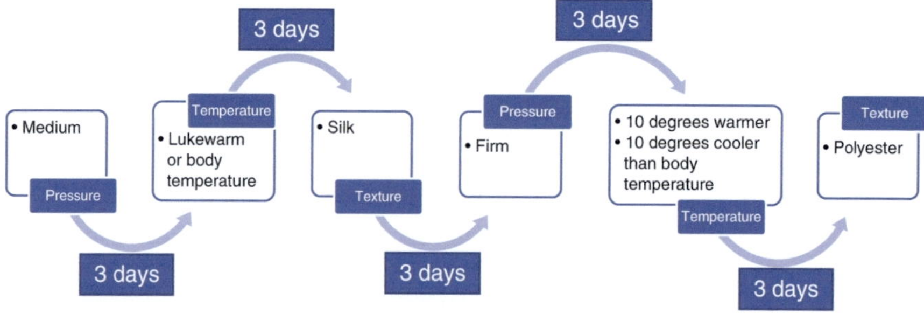

Fig. 7.7 Introduction of a new desensitization technique every 3 days

see a task, motion, or facial expression of the unaffected side in the mirror which will appear as the affected side, i.e., Mirror image. Visually this allows the patient to "see" a normal side in the mirror. Over time the mirror is moved in position to allow for the patient to see their affected side performing tasks, motion, or facial expression as the retraining progresses.

Myofascial treatment including manual clinical soft tissue mobilization, trigger point release with dry needling with or without electrical stimulation, myofascial release of the face, head, neck, and shoulders. Manual therapy may also include other joint mobilization to affected joints that have lost mobility due to lack of movement. Figure 7.8a–c shows a home exercise program to train patients for home myofascial treatment. Physical therapist in the clinic will use a similar technique, however will add in more trigger point release.

Postural retraining is very important to improve the line of gravity through the human body during a variety of positions (Fig. 7.9). The human body is adapted to be upright against the gravitational pull of the earth with many pulleys to increase the ability to generate a large amount of force for movement and sustained postures. This complex orientation of muscles, fascia, joints, and ligaments also has a great capacity for compensation leading to abnormal forces through the body. These abnormal forces over time can lead to persistent pain. Restoration of optimal posture decreases these forces and in turn pain response.

Postural Correction: Sternal Lift in Sitting

- Place your hand on your sternum or breastbone.
- Lift sternum up toward the ceiling.
  - You should feel your weight transfer onto your ischial tuberosities (sit bones) of your pelvis.
  - Shoulder blades will naturally pull down and back, a slight curve will occur at the low back and abdominals should become engaged.
  - Head and neck position will improve with a slight chin tuck.

Perform this correction every 5–6 min throughout your day or 10× per hour.

Many people find it helpful to link postural correction to an environmental cue, such as adjusting his/her eyeglasses, checking time/email, or answering the phone. For example, every time he/she adjusts the eyeglasses, postural correction is performed.

Postural correction is essential when driving or performing prolonged seated activities. Deflate lumbar support in seat if available. Perform sternal lift, inflate lumbar support, adjust rearview mirror. If during your travel, you can no longer see through the rearview mirror—perform postural correction. Perform postural correction at stoplights and/or stop signs.

The frequency of postural correction is important as you develop postural musculature strength. Your body will learn the best alignment and make good posture a

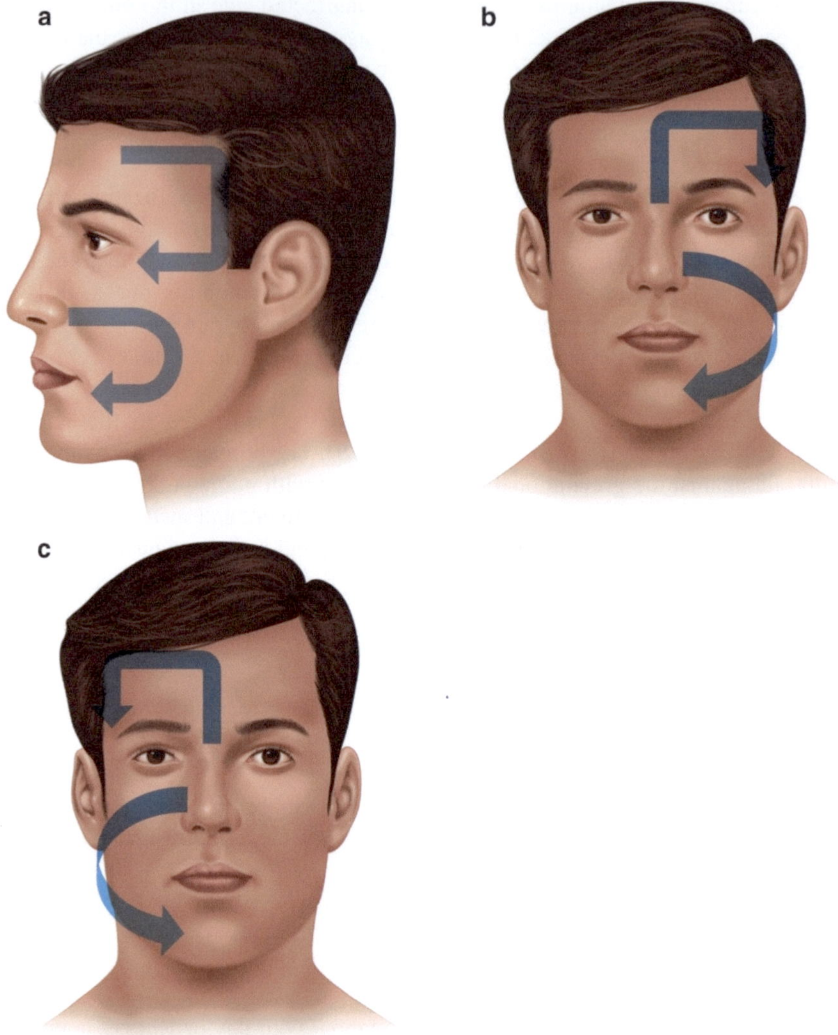

Fig. 7.8 (**a–c**) Application of pressure for myofascial release of the face

habit. Fidgeting is encouraged. Try to avoid performing a seated task without postural change for more than 30 min to decrease stress on joints.

Neuromuscular re-education of the face is used to decrease compensation which develops from persistent pain. Selective muscular relaxation of the head, neck, shoulder, face is used. Visual, physical, and verbal biofeedback is used to retrain how the face is used in daily life.

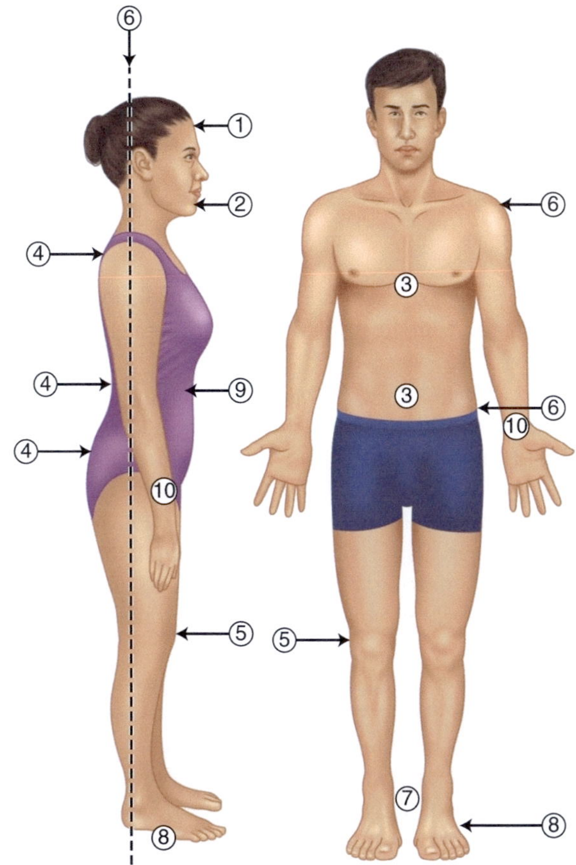

Fig. 7.9 Standing postural alignment: ideal. 1. Eyes level, 2. Chin slightly tucked in, 3. Abdominals engaged, 4. Tall spine with spinal curves maintained, 5. Knees straight, without hyperextension, 6. Level pelvis and shoulders, aligned through body, 7. Arches of feet maintained, 8. Feet on ground with pressure along the whole footprint, 9. Ribs pulled in, 10. Wrists relaxed

Transcutaneous electrical nerve stimulation and neuromuscular electrical stimulation can be used to accomplish the above-noted treatments with decreased pain or facilitation of the affected muscles. These modalities alone will not change the patient's movement system diagnosis but may serve as tools to assist in the application of the treatment plan.

Transcutaneous Electrical Stimulation (TENS) unit Instruction (Sample Instruction Sheet for Patients)

Placement: Place the electrodes on clean dry skin, no lotion. Place electrodes around the painful area in one of the following patterns. Make sure the electrodes are far enough apart from each other (the distance of the electrode itself). Usually about 2 inches apart in every direction.

***

Safety consideration: Avoid any areas of broken (open) skin such as healing incisions, cuts, abrasions, or skin that has a rash, eczema, psoriasis. Do not place on the front side of the chest or neck. Do not place on the face or genitals. Be sure you check that the electrodes and device are clean and in good working condition before use.

Parallel: electrical stimulation (in yellow) travels between electrodes (1, 2, 3, 4), wires are arrows ($\leftrightarrow$).

1 $\leftrightarrow$ 2
3 $\leftrightarrow$ 4

Interferential: Connect electrodes 1 to 4 and 2 to 3. This creates an X of electrical stimulation with the result of a larger treatment area.

Spine Placement for Extremity Pain You may also place the electrodes at your spine to treat an arm or leg area of pain. Please discuss with your therapist the best placement for you.

Programs or Pulse frequency/Pulse width/Waveform: Many TENS units have pre-set programs for you to choose from. Other TENS units need manual settings that require moving a dial. Please refer to the TENS unit owner's manual to use. Possible programs you may have on your unit may include:

- *Continuous*: constant/consistent electrical stimulation often described as a "buzzing." This type of stimulation is hypothesized to block the danger message from your body to your brain, therefore decreasing the pain response.
- *Burst*: cycles of bursts of electrical stimulation often described as "quick beats." This type of stimulation is hypothesized to stimulate the release of the brain's natural chemical pain relievers (such as endorphins).
- *Modulation*: changing intensity of electrical stimulation to avoid getting used to the TENS. Often feels as if the electrical stimulation is moving around. Modulation programs will typically use a continuous application.
Some devices combine different types of stimulation into one program.

Discuss the options your TENS unit has with your therapist to find the best application for you.

Intensity: The intensity needed for benefit from TENS varies from person to person and program to program. This may also change TENS session to TENS session. As we are trying to manipulate the nervous system for pain relief and improved function, the baseline level of pain, and other factors can affect how much TENS intensity you need at a given time.

The point at which you feel the electrical stimulation is called your threshold. The point at which you can no longer stand the electrical stimulation is your tolerance. When the electrical stimulation becomes painful, we describe this as noxious stimulation. For the purposes of TENS for pain relief and improved function, we want to be somewhere in the middle of threshold and tolerance, without noxious stimulation. It is recommended to find your threshold and then increase 1–2 points above this and adjust during your first TENS session to understand how you feel. If it gets too intense, you will know. Just lower the intensity as you need. Current research supports a *"strong sensation without pain"* for best results.

Safety Consideration If you feel funny during TENS application, please discontinue and talk to your therapist. You should discontinue use immediately if you feel any increased pain, stinging, or burning under the electrodes. Your therapist will perform a medical screen and discuss with your health care team prior to recommending TENS for pain relief. Persons who are *pregnant, have indwelling nerve stimulators, pacemakers, epilepsy, known active cancer, or infection*—need physician approval prior to the application of TENS. If you are placing electrodes over an area of decreased skin sensation, use caution as our prescription is to how much stimulation you feel. The electrodes are adhesive in most cases; therefore, allergies to adhesive or other components of the electrodes need to be considered.

Duration: The amount of time that you apply TENS is patient specific. You can use TENS as little or as much as you need for pain relief. Some people find that a 30-minute session of TENS can be helpful; while others may only use TENS for when pain increases. Talk to your therapist about what is the right duration for you. Typically, start with 15 minutes, 3×/day.

Safety Consideration You should discontinue use of TENS when you are sleeping, when the risk of getting your device wet is present, or when you are taking medication that makes it hard to concentrate.

Electrode care: Most electrodes are multi-use. Once you remove the electrodes place back into the plastic bag and seal. Typically, electrodes will last about 10–15 sessions. If your electrodes are nearing the end of their stickiness, *make sure they are not plugged into the device*, then put a couple drops of water on the sticky side and rub into the electrode. This will reactivate the adhesive to allow for 1–3 additional sessions of use (Fig. 7.10a–c).

Mindful meditative movement: Tai chi-based exercise, yoga-based exercise, qiong-based exercise also can be used as tools in the whole-body approach to the treatment of persistent pain. These ancient exercise forms inherently utilize breathing, mindfulness, and joint position sense. Physical therapists also apply neuromuscular re-education during these types of exercise to address fear avoidance behaviors and pain catastrophizing behaviors. Stimulation of the vagus nerve and sympathetic nervous system down training are the treatment effects that physical therapists target with these interventions.

Physical Therapy Goals

Patients suffering from trigeminal neuralgia present with significant impairments, activity limitations, and participation restrictions in addition to the pain from the

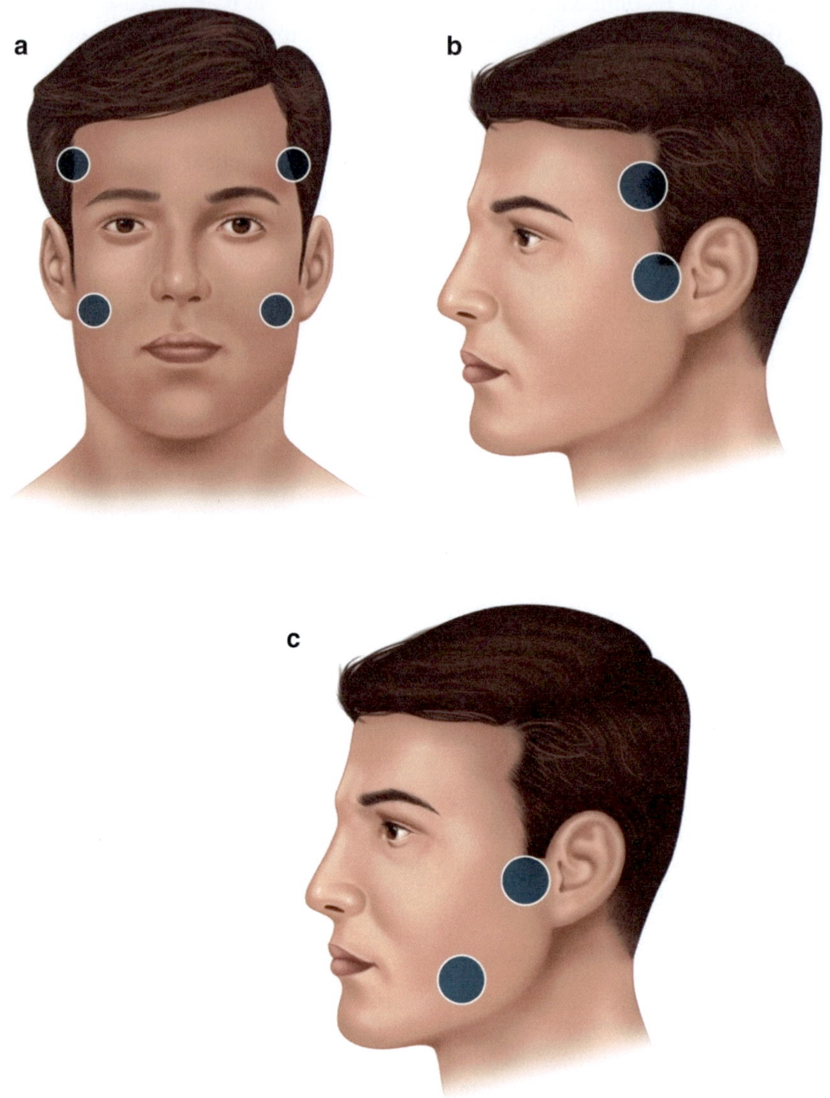

Fig. 7.10 (**a–c**) Sample placements of electrodes for TENS application

diagnosis. The physical therapist works with the health care team and the patient to provide patient-centered care in an interprofessional model focusing on regional interdependence to achieve the goals of improved function and quality of life. This chapter serves as an outline for the evaluation and treatment.

References

1. Guide to physical therapist practice, 2nd ed (2003).
2. www.apta.org/Vision/. Accessed 24 Apr 2020, vision statement last updated on 25 September 2019.
3. Wainner RS, Flynn TW, Whitman JM. Spinal and extremity manipulation: the basic skill set for physical therapists. San Antonio, TX: Manipulations, Inc; 2001.
4. Sueki DG, Cleland JA, Wainner RS. A regional interdependence model of musculoskeletal dysfunction: research, mechanisms, and clinical implications. J Man Manip Ther. 2013;21(2):90–102. https://doi.org/10.1179/2042618612Y.0000000027.
5. Norkin CC, White DJ. Measurement of joint motion: a guide to goniometry. Philadelphia: F.A. Davis Company; 2016.
6. Kendall FP, Kendall FP, editors. Muscles: testing and function with posture and pain. Baltimore, MD: Lippincott Williams & Wilkins; 2005.
7. Moseley GL. Graded motor imagery for pathologic pain. Neurology. 2006;67:1–6.
8. Moseley GL, Butler DS, Beames TB, Giles TJ. The Graded Motor Imagery Handbook. Adelaide Noigroup; 2012.

Elizabeth Lake

First-Line Treatments (Table 8.1)

Carbamazepine

Carbamazepine was initially shown to be more effective than a placebo for treating trigeminal neuralgia in a randomized placebo-controlled trial published in 1966 [1]. At that time, doses from 100 mg three times per day to 200 mg four times per day were used. Patients using carbamazepine for 2 weeks had a 58% improvement in pain when compared to a 26% improvement in the placebo group, which was statistically significant. Carbamazepine also decreased the number of pain paroxysms by 68% and decreased triggers including eating (71%) and contact (82%). About 50% of patients on carbamazepine experience side effects, with the majority of those reporting giddiness (feeling unbalanced/lightheaded). This tended to improve the longer the patient was on the medication.

In an analysis of four placebo-controlled trials of carbamazepine performed in the late 1960s, the number needed to treat was 1.7–1.8 and the medication decreased both frequency and intensity of pain attacks [2]. This analysis also found a number needed to harm of 3 for mild adverse events and 24 for serious events.

Carbamazepine is an anticonvulsant medication that works as a sodium channel blocker. It stabilizes the neural membrane to decrease neural firing and propagation of synaptic signaling. It is metabolized primarily by CYP3A4, found in the liver and small intestine. Carbamazepine also induces CYP3A4; therefore, as patients

E. Lake (⊠)
University of Wisconsin School of Medicine and Public Health, Madison, WI, USA
e-mail: lake@neurology.wisc.edu

© The Author(s), under exclusive license to Springer Nature Switzerland AG 2021
A. Abd-Elsayed (ed.), *Trigeminal Nerve Pain*,
https://doi.org/10.1007/978-3-030-60687-9_8

Table 8.1 Medications for the treatment of trigeminal neuralgia

Medication	Level of evidence	Common dosing	Side effects	Monitoring
Carbamazepine	I/II	600–800 mg/day	Hyponatremia, aplastic anemia, liver failure, Stevens–Johnson syndrome (SJS)	CBC, Sodium, LFTs, HLA-B*1502
Oxcarbazepine	II	300–600 mg bid	Hyponatremia, aplastic anemia, liver failure, SJS	CBC, Sodium, LFTs, HLA-B*1502
Baclofen	II	15–80 mg/day	Sedation, GI upset	N/A
Lamotrigine	II	100 mg bid	SJS, sedation, nausea	N/A
Pimozide	II	4–12 mg/day	Extrapyramidal symptoms (EPS), QT prolongation, neuroleptic malignant syndrome	ECG, fasting glucose and lipids, CBC, CMP, monitoring for EPS, ocular exams
Levetiracetam	III	1500–3000 mg –divided bid	Suicidal ideation, agitation	N/A
Gabapentin	III	300–1200 mg tid	Sedation, dizziness, lower extremity edema, weight gain	N/A
Pregabalin	III	300–600 mg divided bid	Sedation, dizziness, lower extremity edema, weight gain	Platelets if patient predisposed to thrombocytopenia
Clonazepam	III	6–8 mg divided two to three times per day	Sedation, ataxia, memory impairment	N/A
Valproate	III	500–1500 mg/day	Hepatotoxicity, pancreatitis, fetal malformations, weight gain	Total and free valproate level, LFTs, CBC, ammonia
Fosphenytoin	III	15–20 mg/kg	Ataxia, sedation	None (loading dose only)

increase the dose, initially metabolism of the drug will increase. Consider lower doses in patients with liver disease. No adjusts needed in patients with renal failure.

Serious side effects of the medication include hyponatremia, aplastic anemia, and liver failure, with recommendations to monitor sodium, CBC, and liver function tests at baseline and periodically afterward (consider checking at 3 months, then once every 6–12 months). More common side effects can include drowsiness, ataxia, and nausea. Minor side effects can usually be addressed by starting at a low dose and titrating slowly.

Special considerations before starting this medication include the risk of developing Stevens–Johnson syndrome or toxic epidermal necrolysis. Patients are at high risk for this if they carry the HLA-B variant HLA-B*1502. This variant is found predominantly in patients of Asian ancestry; therefore, it is reasonable to screen patients with appropriate background and avoid carbamazepine if this variant is identified.

Typically, carbamazepine can be started at 50 mg twice a day in the elderly population, or 100 mg twice a day in the younger population. The goal is to increase to 600–800 mg per day although up to 1200 mg per day have been used. Dose changes can be made every few days. The extended-release form, dosed twice per day, is easier for patients to adhere to; however, if immediate release is all that is available to the patient, it can also be dosed from two to four times per day. If using in patients of reproductive age, realize that this medication can reduce serum estrogen derivative concentrations, making oral birth control ineffective.

Oxcarbazepine

In general, patients do as well on oxcarbazepine as carbamazepine, with fewer side effects. However, patients who have not seen improvement on carbamazepine may still see improvement on oxcarbazepine. In a study of typical trigeminal neuralgia unresponsive to carbamazepine, oxcarbazepine monotherapy provided pain relief in 37.1% of patients and reduced the number of pain days by at least 50% in 67.5% of them [3].

Oxcarbazepine is an anticonvulsant that is a structural derivative of carbamazepine and works by blocking sodium channels. It also inhibits high-threshold N-type calcium channels and high-frequency firing of cutaneous afferent fibers following repetitive stimulation. Because of this, it is thought to work on both peripheral and central sensitization pathways [4].

Oxcarbazepine is quickly metabolized to its active form, a 10-monohydroxy metabolite (MHD), by the liver. This form does not autoinduce metabolism of oxcarbazepine like carbamazepine does, thus drug levels will continue to increase as the dose is increased. Consider decreased dosing in patients with liver disease. No adjustments are needed in patients with kidney disease. In the immediate release form, oxcarbazepine reaches a serum peak at 2 h, while the MHD peaks at 4.5 h. Hyponatremia is a serious side effect of this medication and occurs to a greater extent than with carbamazepine. Use cautiously in patients over the age of 65. Otherwise, side effects are similar to those of carbamazepine, but patients are less likely to develop liver and blood abnormalities.

Like with carbamazepine, patients are at higher risk of developing Stevens–Johnson syndrome or toxic epidermal necrolysis if they carry the HLA-B variant HLA-B*1502. Consider screening for this variant in patients of Asian ancestry before starting oxcarbazepine. Also note that if using in patients of reproductive age, this medication can reduce serum estrogen derivative concentrations, making oral estrogen-containing birth control ineffective.

Oxcarbazepine is started at 150 mg twice a day. Doses can be increased every few days by 300 mg to a goal of 300–600 mg twice a day. The maximum recommended dose of oxcarbazepine is 1800 mg per day. If converting between carbamazepine to oxcarbazepine, use a 2:3 conversion (e.g., If the patient is on carbamazepine 200 mg bid, convert to oxcarbazepine 300 mg bid).

Second-Line Treatments

Baclofen

Similar to carbamazepine, baclofen has been shown to depress the response to stimulation of the mechanoreceptor neurons in the spinal trigeminal nucleus oralis. When a conditioning stimulus is given to the maxillary nerve of a cat 100 ms before a test stimulus, segmental inhibition is elicited. When the animal is given baclofen (this also occurs with carbamazepine or phenytoin), the segmental inhibition is facilitated and the response to an unconditioned maxillary nerve stimulus is depressed as well [5].

Baclofen has been shown to reduce the number of daily spasms in a double-blinded crossover trial of ten patients. Seven patients had a reduction in the number of spasms per day, with a statistically significant decrease from an average of 11 spasms per day to 2.22 per day. In an expansion to an open-label trial that enrolled an additional 50 patients that were refractory to or unable to tolerate carbamazepine, 74% of patients had a decrease in intensity and frequency of attacks at 2 weeks. Patients also did better with a combination of baclofen and carbamazepine or phenytoin than on baclofen or the other medications alone [6].

Baclofen is a derivative of the neurotransmitter γ-aminobutyric acid (GABA) and thus is an agonist for the $GABA_B$ receptor. It is predominantly secreted in the urine unchanged; 15% of the dose is metabolized by the liver by deamination. Consider medication adjustment in patients with renal failure. Serum concentrations peak at 1 h, with elimination half-life at about 4 h. Because of this, three times a day dosing schedule is necessary for good pain control. Serious side effects of the medication can include seizures (in less than 10% of patients) and hypotension. In general, the medication is tolerated well. Patients can initially have some sedation or GI upset. No laboratory monitoring is needed with this medication.

Baclofen is started at 5 mg three times per day. The maximum dose is 80 mg/day in divided dosing. Patients may benefit from higher dosing at certain parts of the day if they have a specific timing of pain flares.

Lamotrigine

Lamotrigine was initially shown to be effective for the treatment of trigeminal neuralgia in a double-blinded placebo-controlled crossover trial containing 13 patients with disease refractory to carbamazepine, phenytoin, or a combination of the two.

About 85% of patients preferred lamotrigine to placebo, with seven reporting "much better" pain control [7].

Lamotrigine is an anticonvulsant that inhibits glutamate release by blocking voltage-gated sodium channel which stabilizes neuronal membranes. It also antagonizes certain voltage-gated calcium channels (N- and P/Q/R-types). Lamotrigine is metabolized via glucuronidation in the liver and is excreted primarily in the urine. Concentration peaks between 1 and 5 h depending on the concomitant use of other medications. If a patient is on phenytoin or carbamazepine in addition to lamotrigine, the half-life decreases by 50% from an average of 30–14 h. If the patient is on valproate and lamotrigine, half-life doubles. Both liver and renal impairment require decreased doses due to prolonged half-life.

Stevens–Johnson Syndrome and toxic epidermoid necrolysis are rare but have serious side effects. The skin side effects are more likely if the patient is on both valproate and lamotrigine. The risk is less likely if patients start at a low dose of medication and titrate slowly to a therapeutic dose over 6–8 weeks. These reactions are most common with the initiation of the medication but can also occur at any time on lamotrigine. Patients should be counseled that if they develop a rash on the medication, they should stop it immediately and contact the prescriber for further instructions. Patients are also at risk if they stop the medication and restart at a higher dose. Given these risks, patients must be selected carefully for good compliance. Other side effects of lamotrigine can include nausea and sedation.

Lamotrigine is usually started at 25 mg daily and the dose is increased by 25–50 mg each week to a goal of at least 100 mg twice a day. Because this medication is being used for pain control, however, the dose is targeted to symptom relief, not blood level. Blood levels can be checked to determine if there is room to continue to escalate a dose if, for example, a patient is not receiving pain relief at higher doses.

Pimozide

In a double-blind crossover trial, pimozide was compared to carbamazepine in patients with trigeminal neuralgia that was refractory to medical therapy (baclofen, benzodiazepines, phenytoin, and carbamazepine). All patients receiving pimozide had improvement in their pain, compared with 58% of patients on carbamazepine. Overall, patients on pimozide had a 78.4% decrease in pain versus 49.7% decreased in pain on carbamazepine ($p < 0.001$) [8].

Pimozide is an antipsychotic that antagonizes dopamine and serotonin receptors. It is metabolized by the liver and is a major substrate of CYP3A4 and CYP2D6 with a significant first-pass effect. It is excreted in the urine. It peaks in the serum at 6–8 h but does take up to 6 weeks to reach maximum effectiveness. Use with caution in patients with renal and hepatic impairment.

While pimozide has good evidence for effectiveness for the treatment of trigeminal neuralgia, it is seldom used due to its side effect profile. Commonly, it can cause dry mouth, sedation, and constipation. More significant adverse effects include QT prolongation, Parkinsonism, neuroleptic malignant syndrome, and hemolytic anemia.

Dosing for trigeminal neuralgia is recommended at 4 to 12 mg daily divided bid. Monitoring is extensive and requires periodic ECGs, fasting glucose and lipids, CBC, CMP, monitoring for extrapyramidal symptoms on exam, and ocular exams at least every other year.

Third-Line Treatments

Levetiracetam

Levetiracetam has preliminary evidence as an effective treatment for trigeminal neuralgia with few side effects. Four out of ten patients had "a significant tendency towards improvement in pain severity" at high doses from 3000 to 5000 mg daily [9]. In another open-label, uncontrolled trial, levetiracetam 3000 to 4000 mg/day was added to previously partially effective medication regimens [10]. It was shown over 16 weeks to decrease the mean daily attack frequency from an average of 9.9 to 3.3 (62.4%, p < 0.001). The number of days per week that patients experienced attacks went from 6.3 to 3.5 ($p < 0.001$).

Levetiracetam is an anticonvulsant that binds to SV2A, a synaptic vesicle glycoprotein, and is thought to inhibit presynaptic calcium channels and decrease neuronal excitability [11]. It is metabolized primarily through enzymatic hydrolysis in the blood and excreted in the urine. The medication is renally excreted. Peak doses are seen in about 1 h, with a half-life of 6–8 h. Renal impairment requires decreased doses.

This medication is tolerated very well with few side effects. Use cautiously in patients with a history of severe depression because of concern of worsening depression and suicidal ideation. Patients can also experience agitation. Levetiracetam interacts with few medications but it may increase the toxic effects of carbamazepine.

Levetiracetam can be started as low as 250 mg twice a day and increased relatively quickly up to 1500 mg twice a day. No laboratory monitoring is necessary for this medication.

Gabapentin

There is little evidence for or against using gabapentin for trigeminal neuralgia pain as far as randomized controlled trial data [12]. One trial demonstrated the efficacy of gabapentin alone in newly diagnosed trigeminal neuralgia patients to be 50–60%, but inferior to treatment with oxcarbazepine [13]. Another showed that patients receiving gabapentin in combination with ropivicaine block had a significantly lower number of pain days than with one of the treatments alone [14]. In a retrospective study of patients with paroxysmal trigeminal neuralgia, many of who were refractory to surgical intervention and multiple medications, gabapentin was shown to have at least a partial reduction in pain in 47%. Average dosing was 930 mg divided into three times per day dosing, with time of onset of pain reduction between 1 and 3 weeks [15].

Gabapentin is an anticonvulsant that inhibits the $\alpha_2\delta$ subunit of some voltage-gated calcium channels. It is not metabolized and is excreted unchanged in the urine. Time to peak is 2–4 h, with an elimination half-life of 5–7 h. Dosing must be adjusted downward in patients with renal impairment.

Typical side effects of gabapentin include sedation, dizziness, and foggy thinking. Occasionally patients can develop lower extremity edema on this medication. Patients may also develop weight gain. Laboratory monitoring is not necessary. Gabapentin can be started as low as 100 mg three times per day, but typically patients start with 300 mg tid and increase to a maximum of 1200 mg tid.

Pregabalin

Pregabalin has been studied as an adjuvant treatment to carbamazepine in the setting of refractory trigeminal neuralgia. As a salvage treatment before patients underwent surgery, the addition of pregabalin improved pain in 48.5% of patients. Older age appeared to positively correlate to treatment response and an average dose of 166.7 mg was all that was needed [16]. Patients using pregabalin or lamotrigine in addition to carbamazepine had equal improvement in pain control; however, patients on pregabalin had fewer side effects [17].

Pregabalin, a GABA analog similar to gabapentin, is an anticonvulsant that inhibits the $\alpha_2\delta$ subunit of some voltage-gated calcium channels. It is excreted in the urine after negligible metabolism. It peaks within 1.5 h (peak twice as long when taken with food) and the half-life is 6 h. Decrease dose in patients with renal impairment.

Side effects are similar to those of gabapentin, with patients slightly more likely to develop lower extremity edema. The most common side effects include sedation and dizziness which typically improve as the patient adjusts to the medication. No specific laboratory monitoring is necessary, although in rare cases patients have been seen to develop thrombocytopenia. Monitor platelets if clinically indicated.

Pregabalin is initiated at 25 mg daily and can be increased up to 300–600 mg daily divided in bid dosing. Doses can be increased weekly by 150 mg.

Additional Medication Options

Clonazepam

Clonazepam was trialed in patients that were refractory to carbamazepine when it was released in 1975. In this small study of 30 patients, 40% had complete control of neuralgia and 23.3% were significantly helped by the drug. Dosing however averaged 6–8 mg per day, and 80–88% of patients experience somnolence and unsteady gait. Half of the patients related these side effects as severe [18].

Clonazepam is an anticonvulsant that enhances the inhibitory effect of GABA in the central nervous system. It is metabolized in the liver by CYP3A4 and excreted in the urine. The drug concentration peaks at 1–4 h and has a variable half-life from

17 to 60 h. Use with caution in patients with renal impairment as the drug could build up inappropriately. Clonazepam is contraindicated in patients with hepatic failure.

Side effects of clonazepam include sedation, ataxia, memory impairment, and risk for dementia with long-term use. Patients can also experience a paradoxical reaction and become agitated and behave aggressively; use with caution in the elderly population. As with all antiepileptic medications, there is a risk for suicidal ideation so monitor patients for changes in mood.

Clonazepam is usually initiated at 0.25–0.5 mg at night and increased slowly; however, as mentioned, large doses are usually needed for pain control, up to 6 to 8 mg divided in two or three times per day dosing. Given side effects, it may be prudent to use this medication instead as an adjuvant treatment after failing many other treatments in patients that are having significant difficulty sleeping due to pain.

Valproate

There is minimal evidence that valproate is effective in the treatment of trigeminal neuralgia, but for refractory patients not responding to the above medications it may be an option. In one trial of 20 patients using this medication, six were pain-free for 6–18 months, while three more had a pain reduction by 50% [19].

Valproate is an anticonvulsant that is thought to block voltage-gated sodium channels and increase GABA in the brain. It is metabolized extensively in the liver and excreted in the urine; it is not recommended in patients with hepatic impairment and in renal impairment, it should be monitored by monitoring free valproate levels due to decreased protein binding in this condition. In healthy patients, 80–90% of the drug is protein bound. This medication comes in both delayed-release (bid dosing) and extended-release (qhs dosing), with a time to peak dose from four to 17 h and half-life of nine to 19 h.

In the United States, valproate contains black box warnings for hepatotoxicity, pancreatitis, and fetal malformations. Most commonly people experience weight gain, hair loss, and nausea. Patients may also develop thrombocytopenia. Laboratory monitoring should include total valproate level, free valproate level, liver function tests, and CBC. If patients develop mental status changes or lethargy, check ammonia levels. Patients should also be screened for suicidal ideation.

Depending on the ease of dosing and patient coverage, Depakote can be started at 250 mg once or twice a day. As with headache treatment, recommend a maximum dose of 1500 mg/day.

Phenytoin and Fosphenytoin

Some patients with trigeminal neuralgia can develop pain crises, with pain limiting their ability to talk, eat, and sleep, leading to dehydration and exhaustion. In this setting, a visit to the emergency department for hydration and loading of intravenous phenytoin or fosphenytoin may be necessary. In case studies of three refractory pain patients, IV fosphenytoin produced pain relief within a few hours. Unfortunately, pain relief only lasted 1–2 days. Maintenance medications were adjusted during this time of pain relief, but unfortunately, all patients had to undergo surgical intervention for sustained relief [20]. A randomized double-blinded placebo-controlled cross-over study loading patients with phenytoin for general neuropathic pain, including radiculopathies, polyneuropathies, and neuritis, demonstrated a 30% pain reduction compared with no pain reduction with placebo ($p < 0.05$). On average, patients experience 1 day of pain improvement following the infusion [21].

Phenytoin and fosphenytoin (better tolerated for IV loading due to decreased risk for hypotension, cardiac arrhythmias, and local skin reaction) are anticonvulsants that blocks voltage-gated sodium channels. Patients are loaded intravenously at a dose of 10–15 mg/kg. Because this medication is largely an ineffective maintenance medication, the dose is not usually continued orally, and thus no laboratory monitoring is necessary.

Special Considerations

As previously discussed, trigeminal nerve pain can occur in multiple forms and be due to multiple etiologies. Given the above evidence for the treatment of classic trigeminal neuralgia, it is recommended to try these treatments first if a patient has no contraindications.

There has been research in the setting of trigeminal neuralgia in the setting of multiple sclerosis. These patients were found to have increased difficulty tolerating sodium channel blockers such as carbamazepine and oxcarbazepine, with side effects that mimic disease exacerbation. This has led to earlier surgical intervention, as well as trials that have found combinations of pregabalin and lamotrigine, single use of topiramate, and use of misoprostol to be somewhat effective in treatment [22].

Painful trigeminal neuropathy encompasses conditions such as postherpetic neuralgia, painful post-traumatic trigeminal neuropathy, and trigeminal trophic syndrome. These syndromes may be more refractory to medical management but are also unlikely to be amenable to surgery. In postherpetic neuralgia, gabapentin, or tricyclic antidepressants such as amitriptyline are often trialed first [23]. In a meta-analysis of multiple randomized controlled trials, patients receiving gabapentin had a statistically significant reduction in pain intensity by at least 50% when compared with placebo [24]. If these medications are ineffective or not tolerated, can consider low dose opioids. Tramadol 100–400 mg daily had a higher percentage of pain relief and lower rescue medication use after 6 weeks (level I evidence) [25]. Mean maintenance doses of morphine 91 mg or methadone 15 mg and nortriptyline 89 mg or desipramine 63 mg were more effective than placebo and did not have significant cognitive side effects; the difference between pain control with opioids or tricyclic antidepressants were not statistically significant [26].

Painful post-traumatic trigeminal neuropathy is treated with medications similar to classic trigeminal neuralgia, including carbamazepine, gabapentin, and pregabalin. Patients can also be treated with tricyclic antidepressants. Trigeminal trophic syndrome, with its ulcerations in addition to pain, may respond to both oral medications, custom compound creams, and behavior modification.

Burning mouth syndrome is thought to be caused by trigeminal small-fiber sensory neuropathy [27], although other studies have demonstrated increased unoccupied dopamine receptors in the putamen [28] and one case report has shown success with treatment of the condition with pramipexole [29]. Otherwise, trials of medications successful for the treatment of classic trigeminal neuralgia are recommended.

Atypical facial pain, or persistent idiopathic facial pain, can also be responsive to amitriptyline [30] in addition to previously discussed anticonvulsants. A case report also showed benefit from topiramate [31]. This intractable pain is not usually amenable to surgery, and other treatments such as botulinum toxin, nerve blocks, and infusions may need to be explored.

References

1. Campbell FG, Graham JG, Zilkha KJ. Clinical trial of carbamazepine (Tegretol) in trigeminal neuralgia. J Neurol Neurosurg Psychiatry. 1996;29:265–7.
2. Cruccu G, Gronseth G, Alksne J, Argoff C, Brainin M, Burchiel K, et al. AAN-EFNS guidelines on trigeminal neuralgia management. Eur J Neurol. 2008;15:1013–28.
3. Gomez-Arguelles JM, Dorado R, Sepulveda A, Herrera FG, Arrojo E, Aragón CR, Huete C, Terrón B, Anciones B. Oxcarbazepine monotherapy incarbamazepine-unresponsive trigeminalneuralgia. J Clin Neurosci. 2008;15(5):516–9.
4. Beydoun A. Clinical use of tricyclic anticonvulsants in painful neuropathies and bipolar disorders. Epilepsy Behav. 2002;3S(3):S18–22.
5. Fromm GH, Chattha AS, Terrence CF, Glass JD. Role of inhibitory mechanisms in trigeminal neuralgia. Neurology. 1981;31(6):683–7.
6. Fromm GH, Terrence CF, Chattha AS. Baclofen in the treatment of trigeminal neuralgia: double-blind study and long-term follow-up. Ann Neurol. 1984;15(3):240–4.
7. Zakrzewska JM, Chaudry Z, Nurmikko TJ, Patton DW, Mullens EL. Lamotrigine (Lamictal) in refractory trigeminal neuralgia: results from a double blind placebo controlled crossover trial. Pain. 1997;73(2):223–30.
8. Lechin F, van der Dijs B, Lechin ME, Amat J, Lechin AE, Cabrera A, et al. Pimozide therapy for trigeminal neuralgia. Arch Neurol. 1989;46(9):960–3.
9. Jorns TP, Johnston A, Zakrsewska JM. Pilot study to evaluate the efficacy and tolerability of levetiracetam (Keppra) in treatment of patients with trigeminal neuralgia. J Neurol. 2009;16(6):740–4.
10. Mitsikostas DD, Pantes GV, Avramidis TG, Karageorgiou KE, Gatzonis SD, Stathis PG, et al. An observational trial to investigate the efficacy and tolerability of levetiracetam in trigeminal neuralgia. Headache. 2010;50(8):1371–7.
11. Vogl C, Mochida S, Wolff C, Whalley B, Stephens G. The synaptic vesicle glycoprotein SA ligand levetiracetam inhibits presynaptic Ca^{2+} channels through an intracellular pathway. Mol Pharmacol. 2012;82(2):199–208.
12. Ta PCP, Dinh HQ, Nguyen K, Lin S, Ong YL, Ariyawardana A. Efficacy of gabapentin in the treatment of trigeminal neuralgia: a systemic review of randomized controlled trials. J Investig Clin Dent. 2019;10(4):e12448.

13. Debta FM, Ghom AG, Shah JS, Debta P. A comparative study between oxcarbazepine and gabapentin regarding therapeutic efficiency and tolerability in the treatment of trigeminal neuralgia. J Indian Acad Oral Med Radiol. 2010;22(1):10–7.
14. Lemos L, Flores S, Oliveira P, Almeida A. Gabapentin supplemented with ropivacaine block of trigger points improves pain control and quality of life in trigeminal neuralgia patients when compared with gabapentin alone. Clin J Pain. 2008;24(1):64–75.
15. Cheshire WP. Defining the role for gabapentin in the treatment of trigeminal neuralgia: a retrospective study. J Pain. 2002;3(2):137–42.
16. Hamasaki T, Yano S, Nakamura K, Yamada K. Pregabalin as a salvage preoperative treatment for refractory trigeminal neuralgia. J Clin Neurosci. 2018;47:240–4.
17. Rustagi A, Roychoudhury A, Bhutia O, Trikha A, Srivastava MV. Lamotrigine versus pregabalin in the management of refractory trigeminal neuralgia: a randomized open label crossover trial. J Maxillofac Oral Surg. 2014;13(4):409–18.
18. Court JE, Kase CS. Treatment of tic douloureux with a new anticonvulsant (clonazepam). J Neurol Neurosurg Psychiatry. 1976;39(3):297–9.
19. Peiris JB, Perera GL, Devendra SV, Lionel ND. Sodium valproate in trigeminal neuralgia. Med J Aust. 1980;2(5):278.
20. Cheshire WP. Fosphenytoin: an intravenous option for the management of acute trigeminal neuralgia crisis. J Pain Symptom Manag. 2001;21(6):506–10.
21. McCleane GJ. Intravenous infusion of phenytoin relieves neuropathic pain: a randomized, double blinded, placebo-controlled, crossover study. Anesth Analg. 1999;89(4):985–8.
22. Di Stefano G, Maarbjerg S, Truini A. Trigeminal neuralgia secondary to multiple sclerosis: from the clinical picture to the treatment options. J Headache Pain. 2019;20(1):20.
23. Hadley GR, Gayle JA, Ripoll J, Jones MR, Argoff CE, Kaye RJ, et al. Post-herpetic neuralgia: a review. Curr Pain Headache Rep. 2016;20(3):17.
24. Zhang M, Gao CX, Ma KT, Li L, Dai ZG, Wang S, et al. A meta-analysis of therapeutic efficacy and safety of gabapentin in the treatment of postherpetic neuralgia from randomized controlled trials. Biomed Res Int. 2018; https://doi.org/10.1155/2018/7474207.
25. Boureau F, Legallicier P, Kabir-Ahmadi M. Tramadol in post-herpetic neuralgia: a randomized, double-blind, placebo-controlled trial. Pain. 2003;104(1–2):323–31.
26. Raja SN, Haythornthwaite JA, Pappagallo M, Clark MR, Travison TG, Sabeen S, et al. Opioids versus antidepressants in postherpetic neuralgia: a randomized, placebo-controlled trial. Neurology. 2002;59(7):1015–21.
27. Lauria G, Majorana A, Borgna M, Lombardi R, Penza P, Padovani A, et al. Trigeminal small-fiber sensory neuropathy causes burning mouth syndrome. Pain. 2005;115(3):332–7.
28. Wood PB. Role of central dopamine in pain and analgesia. Expert Rev Neurother. 2008;8(5):781–97.
29. Stuginski-Barbosa J, Rodrigues GGR, Bigal ME, Speciali JG. Burning mouth syndrome responsive to pramipexol. J Headache Pain. 2008;9(1):43–5.
30. Cornelissen P, van Kleef M, Mekhail N, Day M, van Zundert J. Evidence-based interventional pain medicine according to clinical diagnoses. 3. Persistent idiopathic facial pain. Pain Pract. 2009;9(6):443–8.
31. Volcy M, Rapoport AM, Tepper SJ, Sheftell FD, Bigal ME. Persistent idiopathic facial pain responsive to topiramate. Cephalalgia. 2006;26(4):489–91.

Nerve Blocks for the Trigeminal Nerve and Branches

9

Chen Cui and Michelle Poliak-Tunis

Indications for Trigeminal Nerve Blocks

Medical management, including carbamazepine and other antiepileptic drugs, continues to be the first-line management of trigeminal neuralgia [1, 2]. However, some patients do not experience symptomatic control with medications alone. Between 25% and 50% of patients will experience insufficient pain control with pharmacological management [2–5]. The dose titration necessary for symptom relief with the medications of choice is usually limited by the onset of intolerable side effects including sedation and ataxia [1, 2].

If symptoms are incompletely controlled with pharmacologic management alone, further interventions can be pursued which include peripheral nerve blocks, chemodenervation, neuromodulation, and surgeries. Nerve blocks have been shown to provide acute pain relief, sometimes extending to weeks or even months [2, 6, 7]. They can also provide diagnostic value to confirm the etiology of the symptoms before more invasive interventions are pursued including chemodenervation, radiofrequency ablation, and surgery [7]. Additionally, nerve blocks are an invaluable option to patients who are either poor surgical candidates or uninterested in surgery [8].

Type of Injectate

In general, there are no formalized guidelines for types of injectate. The agents used are largely dependent on expert consensus as well as provider preference [9]. This is likely due to the paucity of data comparing the efficacies of

C. Cui (✉) · M. Poliak-Tunis
Department of Orthopedics and Rehabilitation, University of Wisconsin School of Medicine, Madison, WI, USA
e-mail: poliak@rehab.wisc.edu

A. Abd-Elsayed (ed.), *Trigeminal Nerve Pain*,
https://doi.org/10.1007/978-3-030-60687-9_9

different injectates. Given the relative rarity of trigeminal neuralgia, there are no large randomized studies investigating patient response to different injectates [2]. The natural time course of trigeminal neuralgia—marked by periods of spontaneous resolution—also limits precise characterization of treatment efficacy [2, 10, 11].

Local anesthetics are the primary agents used for peripheral nerve blocks. They block painful nerve signals by inhibiting voltage-gated sodium channels [12]. The most commonly used medications are lidocaine 1–2% and bupivacaine 0.25–0.5% [6, 9]. For pregnant patients, lidocaine (FDA Category B) should be used instead of bupivacaine (FDA Category C) due to the potential risk of teratogenicity [6]. In general, smaller volumes (0.5–3.0 mL) are used for superficial blocks while larger volumes (3.0–5.0 mL) are used for deeper blocks [12–16]. The frequency of injection largely depends on clinical response but can be performed as frequently as every 2–4 weeks [6]. Rapid pain relief with local anesthetics has been well documented with variable degrees of long-term pain relief, sometimes lasting a year and only limited by the duration of the study [2, 5, 11, 17, 18].

In these studies, the duration of pain relief is often longer than expected based on the local anesthetic's duration of action. While the mechanism for this is not exactly known, the reason for this phenomenon is likely multifactorial. Even though trigeminal nerve blocks are considered when patients fail medications, these medications are usually still continued and may work well with local anesthetics due to complementary mechanisms of action [5, 17, 18]. Local blockade may also reset the cycle of triggers that cause the painful paroxysms found in trigeminal neuralgia [17] and consequently prevent recurrence of the symptoms. Alternatively, the patients in the studies may have experienced a natural abatement of symptoms that is expected in the usual time course of the disease.

Steroids can also be used as an adjunct with local anesthetics in blocks of the trigeminal nerve; however, they are not universally used. These medications modulate pain through multiple mechanisms including decreasing inflammation, membrane stabilization, and reversible inhibition of C-fiber transmission [9]. For headache disorders, triamcinolone 40–60 mg or an equivalent dose of other steroids may be effective when used with a local anesthetic [6]. For pregnant patients, betamethasone and dexamethasone should be avoided due to the possibility of accelerating fetal lung development [6]. Care should be taken to space out injections with steroids in order to minimize systemic side effects such as hyperglycemia, decreased bone mineral density, and immunosuppression [9]. Special consideration should also be taken when using steroids for trigeminal nerve blocks as the injection sites are located on the face. Adverse events like alopecia and fat atrophy have been observed in other nerve blocks for headache disorders when steroids were added [19]. Some recommendations have suggested avoiding corticosteroids entirely for peripheral blocks of the trigeminal nerve due to these potential adverse events occurring on patients' faces [6].

Selection of Nerve Blocks

The selection of nerves for blockade can follow a stepwise approach starting with superficial targets before moving to deeper targets. Ultimately, the procedure performed should be tailored to the particular clinical scenario. If patients have symptoms isolated to a specific terminal branch of the trigeminal nerve, it is prudent to start with each respective superficial nerve block. Alternatively, if patients have symptoms that cover all sensory territories of the trigeminal nerve, it would be reasonable to attempt blockade of all the terminal branches. These procedures are generally well tolerated and can be performed in clinic with or without imaging guidance. Superficial trigeminal nerve blocks may be preferred over targeting deeper structures like the Gasserian ganglion due to the increased technical difficulty and risk of complications associated with targeting these deeper structures [20].

Blockade of deeper structures can be pursued if superficial trigeminal nerve blocks provide insufficient pain relief. The maxillary nerve can be targeted for symptoms in the V2 territory while the mandibular nerve can be targeted for symptoms in the V3 distribution. The ophthalmic nerve travels in the cavernous sinus before its terminal branches enter the orbit [21], and it cannot be individually targeted for blockade. While the mandibular and maxillary nerves can be targeted with anatomic localization alone, imaging guidance can improve accuracy and is generally recommended.

The deepest structure available for blockade is the Gasserian (trigeminal) ganglion. It can be targeted for symptoms that encompass all sensory territories of the trigeminal nerve as the Gasserian ganglion contains the cell bodies of the afferent sensory fibers of the nerve [21–23]. Given its location, blockade of the Gasserian ganglion is associated with serious complications [20] that necessitate imaging guidance when performing the procedure.

Techniques for Nerve Blocks

Nerve blocks can be performed in a variety of settings—anatomic and ultrasound-guided injections can be performed in the office while fluoroscopic and CT-guided injections require more specialized equipment. Although specifics may vary by provider and institution, superficial injections can usually be performed with a 25-gauge 1.5-inch needle and deep injections can usually be performed with a 22-gauge 3-inch spinal needle [13].

Landmark-Guided Nerve Blocks of Superficial Branches

The terminal and superficial branches of the trigeminal nerve can be targeted with landmark-guided nerve blocks. Each of these superficial nerves exits the skull via their respective foramen which are located along a para-sagittal mid-pupillary line

[12, 24]. These foramina can usually be located using a combination of anatomical knowledge and palpation of the foramina [24]. The goal of the injections should be placement of medication next to the nerve as it exits the foramen and not advancement of the needle through the foramen which could cause unintended neurovascular injury [14]. Aspiration should always be performed before the medication is injected to prevent intravascular entry. Other possible complications include infection, hematoma, swelling, paresthesias, and damage to vital structures like the eye [12, 15]. Prior to any injection, the skin should be sterilely prepped and topical analgesia can be provided with infiltration using local anesthetic or in the case of mucosal membranes, a gauze soaked in viscous lidocaine can be applied [15].

Targets of the V1 branch of the trigeminal nerve include the supraorbital and supratrochlear nerves. The supraorbital nerve exits the skull via the supraorbital foramen (notch) which is located approximately at the junction of the middle third and lateral two-thirds of the superior orbital rim [12] (Fig. 9.1a). The needle is introduced just below the inferior edge of the eyebrow (the inferior aspect of the corrugator muscle at the mid-pupillary line can be used as an anatomic landmark [6]) and directed at the foramen [6, 12, 15]. Just medial to this location, the supratrochlear nerve exits underneath the superior orbital rim (Fig. 9.1b). The supratrochlear nerve can be targeted by redirecting the needle positioned for a supraorbital nerve block approximately 1 cm toward the midline [12, 14] or the nerve can be directly targeted by inserting the needle at the inferomedial aspect of the corrugator muscle [6].

For the V2 branch of the trigeminal nerve, the infraorbital nerve can be targeted via intraoral and extraoral routes. The infraorbital foramen can be found below the inferior orbital rim along the mid-pupillary line at the level of the alae nasi [12] (Fig. 9.1c). For the intraoral approach, the cheek is retracted and the needle is inserted in the buccal mucosa above the second upper premolar and directed upwards toward the infraorbital foramen [12, 15]. A finger is generally placed over the infraorbital foramen to confirm needle placement [12, 15]. Alternatively, the extraoral approach can be used with the needle inserted from a lateral-to-medial approach aimed at the infraorbital foramen [12, 14, 15]. Gently massaging the area after injection and putting a finger beneath the lower eyelid can help with swelling and limit the cranial spread of the medication [15].

Blockade of the V3 branch of the trigeminal nerve includes injections of the mental nerve as well as the auriculotemporal nerve. The mental foramen is located approximately 1 cm below the second lower premolar along the mid-pupillary line [12, 15] (Fig. 9.1d). Similar to the infraorbital nerve, the infraorbital nerve can be blocked via an intraoral or extraoral approach. During the intraoral approach, the needle is advanced caudally through the buccal mucosa toward the foramen [15]. For the extraoral approach, the infraorbital foramen is approached with a slightly lateral to medial approach before medication is injected around the foramen [12, 14]. The auriculotemporal nerve exits superficially behind the temporomandibular joint [6] and can be palpated in the preauricular region [9] (Fig. 9.1e). The temporal artery is used for anatomic localization as it runs anterior to the tragus and the

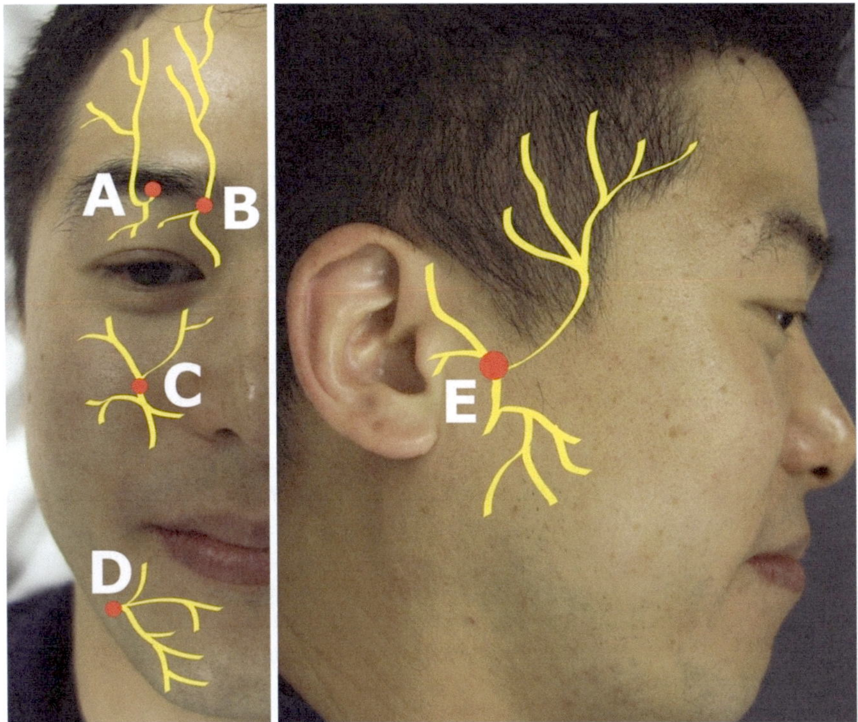

Fig. 9.1 Targets for superficial trigeminal nerve blocks. (**A**) Supraorbital nerve traveling out of the supraorbital foramen. (**B**) Supratrochlear nerve traveling underneath the superior orbital rim. (**C**) Infraorbital nerve traveling out of the infraorbital foramen. (**D**) Mental nerve traveling out of the mental foramen. (**E**) Auriculotemporal nerve traveling in the preauricular area

needle is inserted just anterior to the artery in order to block the auriculotemporal nerve [6]. The facial nerve travels close to the tragus and temporary facial nerve palsy is a possible complication [25].

Landmark-Guided Nerve Blocks of Deep Branches

Blockade of more proximal aspects of the trigeminal nerve can be performed, especially if symptoms involve the sensory territories of the maxillary or mandibular nerves [16]. Precautions similar to the superficial nerve blocks should be taken regarding sterile skin preparation and negative aspiration prior to injection. The possible complications are similar as well though the increased depth puts the needle in closer proximity to major neurovascular and other vital structures [26, 27]. Given the nearby vascular structures during these injections, intermittent aspiration is recommended during needle advancement [14] which also allows for deposition of local anesthetic to provide procedural pain relief [16]. Patients may experience paresthesias in the distribution of the maxillary or mandibular nerves which can help confirm correct needle placement [14, 28]. Neurostimulation during needle advancement can also be utilized to assist with placement [12].

The maxillary nerve exits the skull via the foramen rotundum [16] and it can be targeted in the pterygopalatine fossa with multiple approaches, including the suprazygomatic or infrazygomatic approaches [12, 14, 16]. With landmark-guided injections, the suprazygomatic approach is recommended as the infrazygomatic approach has increased risk of inadvertent puncture into the orbit, maxillary artery, and posterior pharyngeal wall [26, 27]. In the suprazygomatic approach, the needle enters the skin at the point bordered by the zygomatic arch caudally and the posterior orbital rim ventrally where it is advanced perpendicularly to the skin for about 1 to 1.5 cm until it contacts the sphenoid bone [12] (Fig. 9.2a). The needle is then redirected caudally and ventrally before being advanced another 3.5–4.5 cm toward the pterygopalatine fossa where the medication can be injected after aspiration [12]. This same area can be targeted with an infrazygomatic approach. The needle is introduced perpendicularly to the skin at the inferior margin of the zygomatic arch approximately at the center of the mandibular arch [14] (Fig. 9.2b). The needle is advanced approximately 4–5 cm until it contacts the lateral pterygoid plate and at this depth, the maxillary nerve can be individually blocked [14].

Blockade of the mandibular nerve occurs as it exits the skull at the foramen ovale [16] and it is usually targeted via the infrazygomatic approach [29]. The needle

Fig. 9.2 Sites of needle entry for mandibular and maxillary nerve blocks. (**A**) Suprazygomatic approach. (**B**) Infrazygomatic approach

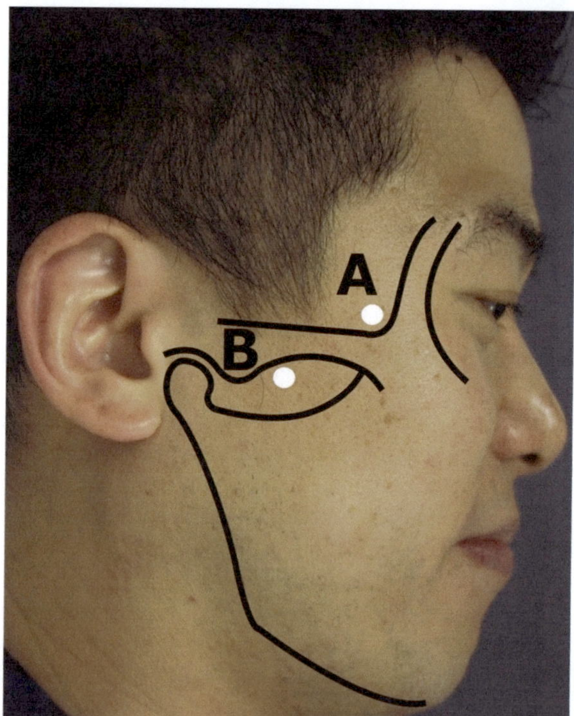

enters perpendicularly through the skin in the space between the zygomatic arch and the center of the mandibular notch [12, 16] (Fig. 9.2b). To minimize arterial injury, the needle should be as close to the inferior border of the zygomatic arch as possible [12, 16]. The needle is advanced until it contacts the lateral pterygoid plate after which it is redirected dorsally and caudally, further advancing approximately 1 cm while it passes the inferior aspect of the plate [14]. Medication can then be injected at this location after aspiration.

Ultrasound-Guided Nerve Blocks

Ultrasound technology provides clinicians with the ability to perform real-time and dynamic evaluations in the clinic setting. Continuous improvements in technology have provided the resolution necessary to evaluate soft tissues, nerves, vasculature, and bones. Cadaveric [8] and clinical [13, 24, 30–33] studies have demonstrated the utility of ultrasound guidance in blocks of the trigeminal nerve. The images referenced in this section were acquired using a 5–18 MHz hockey stick probe paired with the GE Logiq e ultrasound system (GE Healthcare. Chicago, IL, USA).

For nerve blocks of the superficial branches, the foramina are identified as hypoechoic breaks in the cortex of the bone [24] with the ultrasound probe placed in the same locations as the landmark-guided injections (Fig. 9.1). An in-plane or out-of-plane approach can be used for these superficial injections with similar accuracy [8]. Given the superficial location of these terminal branches, multiple approaches other than the ones described here are reasonable and the choice of approach largely depends on provider preference. Evaluation with color doppler and confirmation of negative aspiration is recommended before all injections. A hockey stick or linear probe can be used to identify these superficial structures.

The supraorbital foramen can be identified with the probe placed in the axial plane on the superior orbital rim with the center approximately at the mid-pupillary line [8, 13, 24] (Fig. 9.3). During nerve blocks, the needle is advanced using an in-plane approach with the needle traveling lateral to medial [13].

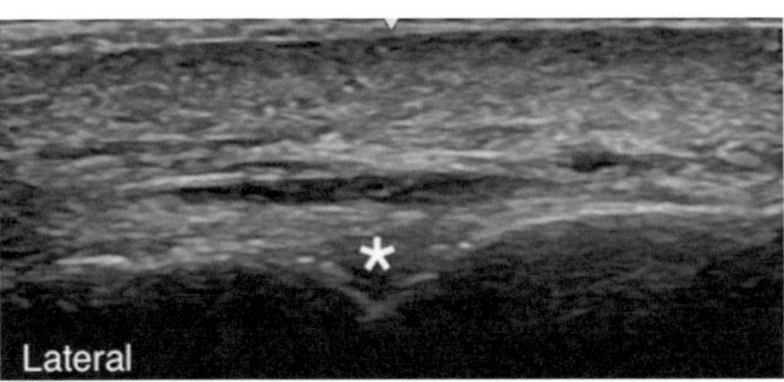

Fig. 9.3 Ultrasound of the Supraorbital Foramen. Probe placed in the axial plane and centered on the supraorbital foramen which is located along the superior orbital rim of the frontal bone as shown in Fig. 9.1a. The supraorbital foramen is visualized as a break in the cortex, marked with (*)

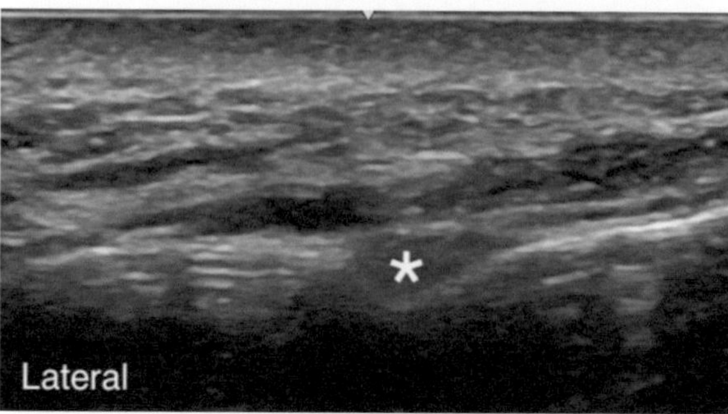

Fig. 9.4 Ultrasound of the Infraorbital Foramen. Probe placed in the axial plane and centered on the infraorbital foramen which is located on the maxilla below the inferior orbital rim as shown in Fig. 9.1c. The infraorbital foramen is visualized as a break in the cortex, marked with (*)

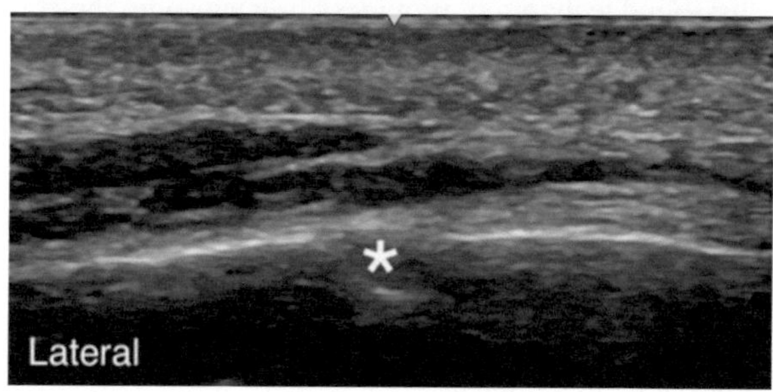

Fig. 9.5 Ultrasound of the Mental Foramen. Probe placed in the axial plane and centered on the mental foramen which is located on the mandible as shown in Fig. 9.1d. The mental foramen is visualized as a break in the cortex, marked with (*)

Evaluation of the infraorbital foramen can be accomplished with the probe placed in the axial plane on the maxilla at the level of the nostril with the center of the probe at the mid-pupillary line [13, 28] (Fig. 9.4). Injections can be performed lateral to medial using an in-plane approach [13] or caudal to cephalad using an out-of-plane approach [28].

Moving more caudally, the mental foramen can be identified with the probe placed in the axial plane at the inferior angle of the mandible [13, 24] and centered approximately at the second lower premolar [8] (Fig. 9.5). Once the foramen is located, the needle can be advanced lateral to medial using the in-plane approach [13].

The auriculotemporal nerve can be localized on ultrasound in front of the ear. The ultrasound probe is placed in the axial plane along the posterior aspect of the zygomatic arch by the tragus and the superficial temporal artery is identified with doppler [13, 25]. The auriculotemporal nerve travels closely with the superficial temporal artery [34] and the needle can target the nerve with a posterior to anterior in-plane approach [13].

Ultrasound-Guided Nerve Blocks of Deep Branches

Ultrasound guidance can help significantly with needle localization while performing injections of the deeper branches. This is generally accomplished with a linear probe, but evaluation with a curvilinear probe may help as well [13, 30]. The deeper branches include the maxillary nerve, mandibular nerve, and Gasserian (trigeminal) ganglion.

While volumes of 3–5 mL of local anesthetic can be used to individually block each deep branch, larger volumes up to 10 mL injected into the pterygopalatine fossa have been shown to block both the maxillary and mandibular nerves [14, 33] due to their proximity. Previous reports have also demonstrated that due to the small volume of the pterygopalatine fossa, injections into the fossa will generate retrograde flow causing medication to travel to the Gasserian ganglion [31, 32].

The mandibular and maxillary nerves are usually evaluated and blocked using an infrazygomatic approach. With the affected side facing upward, the ultrasound probe is placed in the axial plane just inferior to the zygomatic arch with the anterior aspect of the probe over the maxilla and posterior aspect in front of the mandibular condyle [12, 13, 31]. The probe may need to be directed 45 degrees anterior in the axial plane and 45 degrees caudally in the frontal plane [12]. This position allows visualization of the pterygopalatine fossa, bordered anteriorly by the maxilla and posteriorly by the lateral pterygoid plate of the sphenoid bone [35]. Doppler allows visualization of the maxillary artery within the fossa [12, 13, 31]. The maxillary nerve can be targeted by advancing the needle to the area anterior to the lateral pterygoid plate while the mandibular nerve can be targeted in the area posterior to the lateral pterygoid plate [13]. Given the depth of these structures, an in-plane approach is recommended and the needle can be introduced from a posterior to anterior direction.

A suprazygomatic approach has been described as well. The probe is placed just superior to the zygomatic arch and tilted until the pterygoid fossa comes into view [33]. Instead of targeting the fossa itself, the needle is introduced via an in-plane approach from posterior to anterior and advanced until the maxilla is contacted [33]. This approach can be used to minimize vascular injury and injection of 10 mL of local anesthetic caused maxillary as well as mandibular nerve blockade [33].

Fluoroscopic-Guided Nerve Blocks

Prior to the wide adoption of ultrasound, physicians used fluoroscopy in order to perform deeper blocks of the trigeminal nerve including the Gasserian ganglion, mandibular nerve, and maxillary nerve [7]. Fluoroscopy allows continuous visualization of osseous structures and confirmation of intravascular injection if it occurs, though the evaluation of soft-tissue structures is limited.

The Gasserian ganglion is the sensory ganglion of the trigeminal nerve [23], and it is located within a fold of dura called Meckel's cave, contained in the middle cranial fossa [14, 22]. The ganglion can be targeted via an injection through the foramen ovale. The patient is positioned supine with the neck extended and the fluoroscope in the anteroposterior position. After confirming anatomic landmarks in the anteroposterior position, the C-arm is obliqued toward the ipsilateral side and tilted

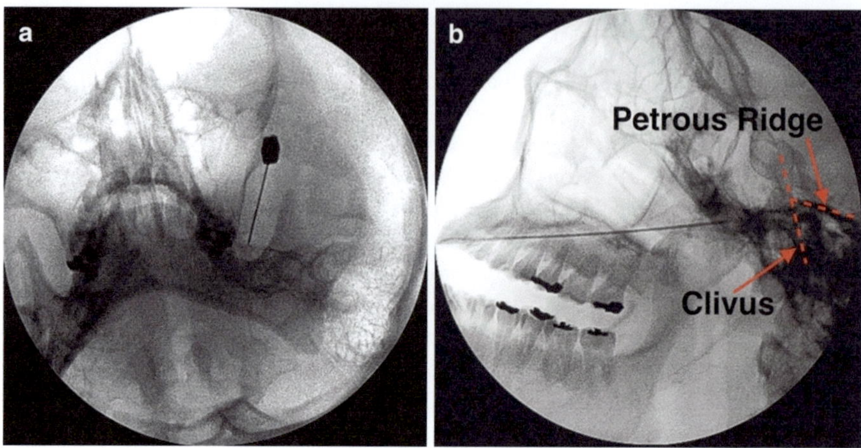

Fig. 9.6 Fluoroscopic-guided Injection of the Gasserian Ganglion. (**a**) Shows the anteroposterior fluoroscopic view with the needle directed toward the foramen ovale. (**b**) Shows the lateral fluoroscopic view with the needle directed toward the foramen ovale. The intersection of the clivus and petrous ridge is highlighted with the dashed line. Adapted from "Uncommon cause of trigeminal neuralgia: tentorial ossification over trigeminal notch," by Bang et al. (2015), *Case reports in Anesthesiology.* CC BY

caudally to reveal the foramen ovale [14] (Fig. 9.6a). The needles enter the skin just lateral to the ipsilateral side of the mouth where it is at the mid-pupillary line and underneath the zygoma [14]. When the needle appears close to the foramen, a lateral view should be obtained to confirm the depth and the needle should advance until the tip is at the intersection of the clivus and the petrous ridge of the temporal bone [14] (Fig. 9.6b). If the needle enters Meckel's cave, there will be a return of cerebrospinal fluid and contrast should be injected to confirm that the needle is not intravascular or in the subarachnoid space [14]. For nerve blocks, a total of 0.4–0.5 mL of anesthetic can be injected in 0.1 mL increments [14]. Given the location of the ganglion, the procedure is associated with a myriad of complications. Vascular injury could cause hematoma in the face and orbit while inadvertent injections could cause spinal anesthesia or unintended motor blockade of the trigeminal and facial nerves [20].

If desired, the maxillary and mandibular nerves can be individually targeted with fluoroscopic guidance. In a process similar to anatomic-guided injections of these deep branches, the needle can be introduced via the infrazygomatic approach, centered at the mandibular arch [14]. After the needle is advanced to the lateral pterygoid plate, the maxillary nerve can be individually blocked, but if the needle is withdrawn approximately 2 cm and a sufficient volume of local anesthetic is used (5–10 mL), both maxillary and mandibular nerves can be blocked [14]. To specifically target the mandibular nerve, the needle can be redirected approximately 1 cm caudally and dorsally after contacting the lateral pterygoid plate [14].

CT-Guided Nerve Blocks

In certain cases, computed tomography (CT)-guidance may be necessary to perform accurate blocks of the deep branches of the trigeminal nerve. CT-guidance provides excellent visualization of bony structures while also providing definition of soft tissue structures and advancements in CT-fluoroscopy have added real-time visualization of these structures as well [7]. This advanced form of imaging guidance does have its limitations including increased radiation exposure and costs related to the specialized equipment [7]. Consequently, CT-guidance should be reserved for situations where anatomic variability in the patient makes it difficult to localize landmarks like the foramen ovale, foramen rotundum, and pterygopalatine fossa with imaging modalities like fluoroscopy [26, 29, 36]. The Gasserian ganglion can be targeted with CT-guidance in a procedure that is similar to fluoroscopic-guided injections. The needle pierces the skin just below the zygoma along the mid-pupillary line and is advanced in a cranial-medial direction toward the foramen ovale (Fig. 9.7a, b) [37]. CT-guidance allows for the measurement of distance between the entry site and the foramen ovale (Fig. 9.8a) which can assist with safe needle placement into the foramen ovale while avoiding inadvertent entry into the subarachnoid space (Fig. 9.8b) [37]. Reports have also outlined how CT-guidance can be utilized to target the maxillary nerve in the pterygopalatine fossa [26] and the mandibular nerve at the foramen ovale [29]. In these cases, the usage of CT-guidance

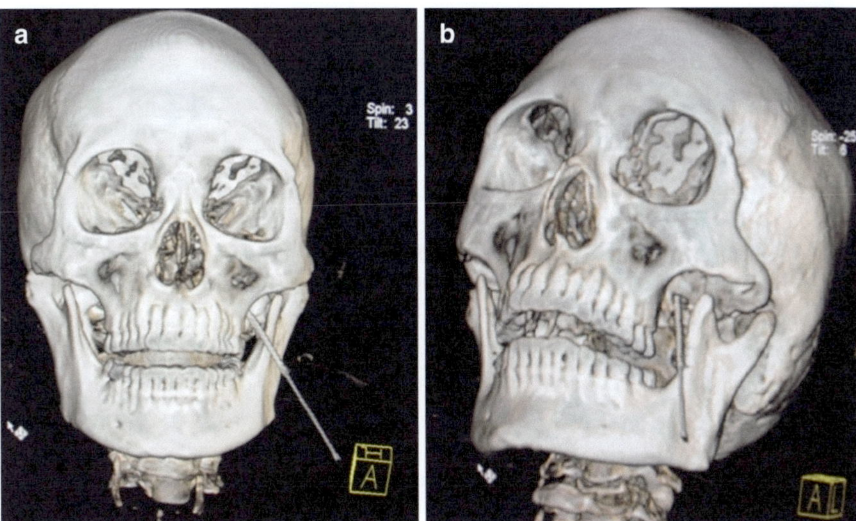

Fig. 9.7 3D CT Reconstruction of Needle Trajectory. Reconstructed CT image demonstrates the needle trajectory as it travels underneath the zygomatic arch to target the foramen ovale. (**a**) Presents a frontal view while (**b**) presents an oblique view. From "Computed tomography-guided percutaneous ozone injection of the Gasserian ganglion for the treatment of trigeminal neuralgia," by An et al. (2018), Journal of Pain Research, 11, pp 255–263, Copyright 2018 by Dove Medical Press. Reprinted and adapted with permission

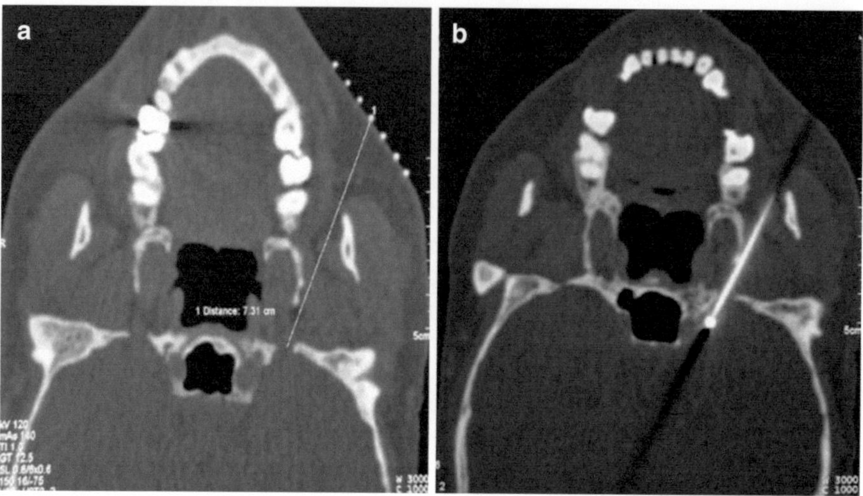

Fig. 9.8 CT-guided Injection of the Gasserian Ganglion. With CT-guidance, the needle is visualized targeting the Gasserian Ganglion via the foramen ovale. (**a**) illustrates the needle just prior to entry into the foramen ovale and a distance measurement from the entry site to the foramen ovale (7.31 cm in this case). (**b**) illustrates the needle within the foramen ovale. From "Computed tomography-guided percutaneous ozone injection of the Gasserian ganglion for the treatment of trigeminal neuralgia," by An et al. (2018), Journal of Pain Research, 11, pp 255–263, Copyright 2018 by Dove Medical Press. Reprinted and adapted with permission

allowed accurate needle placement when anatomic variability prevented the ideal positioning of the patient and identification of osseous landmarks with conventional means.

In conclusion, nerve blocks are an invaluable tool for physicians in the management of trigeminal neuralgia. They can provide acute relief of symptoms while acting as an adjunct to oral medications. Injections may also provide needed relief to patients who are not surgical candidates. In addition to their therapeutic benefit, nerve blocks may also provide diagnostic information before patients undergo more invasive procedures. The trigeminal nerve has many targets for blockade which can be sequentially targeted based on the patients' symptoms, availability of equipment, and expertise of the practitioner. Superficial structures can be targeted in the office setting while more advanced imaging can aid with localization, especially of the deeper structures.

Acknowledgments The authors would like to thank Donald Kasitinon, MD for acting as a model.

References

1. Joffroy A, Levivier M, Massager N. Trigeminal neuralgia. Pathophysiology and treatment. Acta Neurol Belg. 2001;101(1):20–5.
2. Moore D, et al. A systematic review of rescue analgesic strategies in acute exacerbations of primary trigeminal neuralgia. Br J Anaesth. 2019;123(2):e385–96.

3. Dalessio DJ. Trigeminal neuralgia. A practical approach to treatment. Drugs. 1982;24(3):248–55.
4. Haridas A, Mathewson C, Eljamel S. Long-term results of 405 refractory trigeminal neuralgia surgeries in 256 patients. Zentralbl Neurochir. 2008;69(4):170–4.
5. Stani FD, et al. Combination of pharmacotherapy and lidocaine analgesic block of the peripheral trigeminal branches for trigeminal neuralgia: a pilot study. Arq Neuropsiquiatr. 2015;73(8):660–4.
6. Blumenfeld A, et al. Expert consensus recommendations for the performance of peripheral nerve blocks for headaches—a narrative review. Headache. 2013;53(3):437–46.
7. Koizuka S, Nakajima K, Mieda R. CT-guided nerve block: a review of the features of CT fluoroscopic guidance for nerve blocks. J Anesth. 2014;28(1):94–101.
8. Spinner D, Kirschner JS. Accuracy of ultrasound-guided superficial trigeminal nerve blocks using methylene blue in cadavers. Pain Med. 2012;13(11):1469–73.
9. Dach F, et al. Nerve block for the treatment of headaches and cranial neuralgias – a practical approach. Headache J Head Face Pain. 2015;55(S1):59–71.
10. Arnold M. Headache classification committee of the international headache society (IHS) the international classification of headache disorders. Cephalalgia. 2018;38(1):1–211.
11. Han K, et al. Efficacy and safety of high concentration lidocaine for trigeminal nerve block in patients with trigeminal neuralgia. Int J Clin Pract. 2008;62(2):248–54.
12. Gropper MA, Miller RD. Miller's anesthesia. New York: Elsevier; 2020.
13. Allam AE-S, et al. Ultrasound-guided intervention for treatment of trigeminal neuralgia: an updated review of anatomy and techniques. Pain Res Manag. 2018;2018:5480728.
14. Benzon HT. Practical management of pain. Philadelphia, PA: Elsevier/Saunders; 2014.
15. Roberts JR, Custalow CB, Thomsen TW. Roberts and Hedges' clinical procedures in emergency medicine and acute care. Philadelphia, PA: Elsevier/Saunders; 2019.
16. Stajčič Z, Todorović L. Blocks of the foramen rotundum and the oval foramen: a reappraisal of extraoral maxillary and mandibular nerve injections. Br J Oral Maxillofac Surg. 1997;35(5):328–33.
17. Baykal M, Kaplan M. Effects of oral carbamazepine with 2% lidocaine on maxillary and mandibular nerve blocks in trigeminal neuralgia. Duzce Med J. 2010;12(3):19–23.
18. Lemos L, et al. Gabapentin supplemented with ropivacain block of trigger points improves pain control and quality of life in trigeminal neuralgia patients when compared with gabapentin alone. Clin J Pain. 2008;24(1):64–75.
19. Shields KG, Levy MJ, Goadsby PJ. Alopecia and cutaneous atrophy after greater occipital nerve infiltration with corticosteroid. Neurology. 2004;63(11):2193–4.
20. Benzon HT. Complications associated with neurolytic blocks. Philadelphia, PA: Elsevier/Saunders; 2007. p. 273–85.
21. Joo W, et al. Microsurgical anatomy of the trigeminal nerve. Clin Anat. 2014;27(1):61–88.
22. Davis AR, et al. Gasserian Ganglion (Semilunar/Trigeminal Ganglion). In: Schmidt-Erfurth U, Kohnen T, editors. Encyclopedia of ophthalmology. Heidelberg: Springer; 2016. p. 1–1.
23. Kim J, et al. Cranial nerve V (trigeminal nerve). In: Schmidt-Erfurth U, Kohnen T, editors. Encyclopedia of ophthalmology. Heidelberg: Springer; 2016. p. 1–2.
24. Tsui BC. Ultrasound imaging to localize foramina for superficial trigeminal nerve block. Can J Anesth. 2009;56(9):704–6.
25. Trescot AM. Peripheral nerve entrapments: clinical diagnosis and management. Berlin: Springer; 2018.
26. Okuda Y, et al. Use of computed tomography for maxillary nerve block in the treatment of trigeminal neuralgia. Reg Anesth Pain Med. 2000;25(4):417–9.
27. Singh B, Srivastava S, Dang R. Anatomic considerations in relation to the maxillary nerve block. Reg Anesth Pain Med. 2001;26(6):507–11.
28. Takechi K, et al. Real-time ultrasound-guided infraorbital nerve block to treat trigeminal neuralgia using a high concentration of tetracaine dissolved in bupivacaine. Scand J Pain. 2015;6(1):51–4.

29. Okuda Y, et al. Use of computed tomography for mandibular nerve block in the treatment of trigeminal neuralgia. Reg Anesth Pain Med. 2001;26(4):382.
30. Chang K-V, et al. Recognition of the lateral pterygoid muscle and plate during ultrasound-guided trigeminal nerve block. J Clin Diagn Res. 2017;11(5):UL01.
31. Nader A, et al. Ultrasound-guided trigeminal nerve block via the pterygopalatine fossa: an effective treatment for trigeminal neuralgia and atypical facial pain. Pain Physician. 2013;16(5):E537–45.
32. Nader A, Schittek H, Kendall MC. Lateral pterygoid muscle and maxillary artery are key anatomical landmarks for ultrasound-guided trigeminal nerve block. Anesthesiology. 2013;118(4):957.
33. Zou F, et al. A novel approach for performing ultrasound-guided trigeminal nerve block: above the zygomatic arch. J Clin Anesth. 2019;60:36.
34. Janis JE, et al. Anatomy of the auriculotemporal nerve: variations in its relationship to the superficial temporal artery and implications for the treatment of migraine headaches. Plast Reconstr Surg. 2010;125(5):1422–8.
35. Daniels DL, et al. Osseous anatomy of the pterygopalatine fossa. Am J Neuroradiol. 1998;19(8):1423–32.
36. Horiguchi J, et al. Multiplanar reformat and volume rendering of a multidetector CT scan for path planning a fluoroscopic procedure on Gasserian ganglion block—a preliminary report. Eur J Radiol. 2005;53(2):189–91.
37. An J-X, et al. Computed tomography-guided percutaneous ozone injection of the Gasserian ganglion for the treatment of trigeminal neuralgia. J Pain Res. 2018;11:255.

Radiofrequency Ablation

10

Priyanka Singla, Alaa Abd-Elsayed, and Lynn R. Kohan

Introduction

Trigeminal neuralgia (TN) can be treated by a number of different treatment modalities ranging from non-pharmacological management to microvascular decompression. Pharmacological therapy is generally the first line of treatment [1, 2] and is discussed in Chap. 8. However, it can be either ineffective or associated with significant and intolerable side effects [3]. Percutaneous procedures such as balloon compression (BC), glycerol rhizotomy (GR), and radiofrequency thermocoagulation (RF) offer a minimally invasive approach for the treatment of trigeminal neuralgia [1, 4]. All three techniques provide effective pain relief via the creation of a partial destructive lesion in the preganglionic trigeminal rootlets but differ in selectivity of trigeminal divisions and type of injury inflicted [3, 4]. Glycerol rhizotomy is discussed in Chap. 11 and balloon compression in Chap. 16. RF involves the destruction of trigeminal ganglion or roots using radiofrequency [1]. This technique is the most selective of the three techniques and allows for a greater degree of dermatomal mapping before inflicting injury to trigeminal nerve fibers [4, 5].

P. Singla
Department of Anesthesiology, University of Virginia, Charlottesville, VA, USA
e-mail: PS7EY@hscmail.mcc.virginia.edu

A. Abd-Elsayed
Department of Anesthesiology, University of Wisconsin School of Medicine and Public Health, Madison, WI, USA
e-mail: abdelsayed@wisc.edu

L. R. Kohan (✉)
Department of Anesthesiology, University of Virginia, Charlottesville, VA, USA

Pain Management Center, Fontaine Research Park, Charlottesville, VA, USA
e-mail: LRK9G@hscmail.mcc.virginia.edu

© The Author(s), under exclusive license to Springer Nature Switzerland AG 2021
A. Abd-Elsayed (ed.), *Trigeminal Nerve Pain*,
https://doi.org/10.1007/978-3-030-60687-9_10

History

Electrocoagulation to target the trigeminal nerve rootlets was first developed in 1913 by Réthi [4, 5]. Early use of this technique was associated with serious complications, including death [3, 4, 6]. Sweet and Wepsic in the 1970s made several improvements in both equipment and technique that resulted in fewer complications and better patient outcomes [6]. These include the use of temperature monitoring, use of short-acting anesthetic agents, and electric stimulation with awake-patient feedback [4, 6]. Since then, further advancements in the electrode such as the use of a smaller [7] or curved [4, 8, 9] electrode have led to a low incidence of sensory complications.

Criteria for Patient Selection

Criteria for patient selection involves multiple components and involves a detailed discussion with the patient about the risks and benefits of all the possible techniques for treatment of TN [2, 4]. The first step includes patient preference and expectations from the procedure [4, 10]. Expectations include tolerance for side effects such as numbness and dysesthesia [4]. The pathophysiology of TN, including the presence of vascular compression of nerve root [10] and associated patient comorbidities, should be taken into account [4]. Other factors that guide decision-making include which division of the trigeminal nerve is affected, the presence of typical versus atypical pain, and the success of prior treatments [2, 4, 11].

Appropriate patient selection is important for successful treatment. Patients who receive a short duration of good to excellent pain relief with a diagnostic trigeminal ganglion block benefit most from this intervention [1]. However, in patients in whom the first branch of the trigeminal nerve is involved, microvascular decompression is recommended [2].

Patients who have refractory or incompletely controlled symptoms are good candidates for surgical or percutaneous interventions [3]. In this group, particularly older patients with significant comorbidities benefit from radiofrequency ablation as it can be done under sedation without the need for general anesthesia and at the same time avoid craniotomy [3]. Therefore, it is not an appropriate choice for patients who cannot tolerate an awake procedure or who are unable to cooperate with localization [5].

Procedure

The procedure is generally accomplished under monitored anesthesia care to facilitate patient cooperation during the stimulation phase [4]. This is critical for the localization of lesion [4]. Short-acting anesthetic agents such as propofol or alfentanil or remifentanil are used for sedation [2]. The patient is placed supine with a neck roll to achieve 15 degrees of extension [4, 5]. Patients should be monitored with continuous pulse oximetry, electrocardiogram, and blood pressure monitoring [1].

C-arm fluoroscopy is used to assist in the proper needle placement in the foramen ovale [4, 5]. Some authors have described the use of computerized tomography [4, 12] and neuronavigation [4, 13] for accurate placement of the electrode. Hartel's anatomic landmarks guide the needle placement [5]. The three points that are plotted include the initial skin insertion point which is 2.5 cm lateral to the corner of the mouth on the side of the intervention [4, 5], a second point 3 cm anterior to the external auditory canal, and the third one inferior to the medial aspect of the ipsilateral pupil [5]. After adequate depth of sedation is achieved, a needle with an obturator is inserted and advanced along the target trajectory to the foramen ovale [4, 5]. Care should be taken that the needle remains medial to the mandible and does not enter the oral cavity [5]. The needle is advanced in a trajectory that bisects a triangle between the insertion point, the mid pupillary line, and the marking 3 cm anterior to the external auditory meatus [5] (Fig. 10.1). Once, the needle is at the skull base, a submental view is obtained and is used to guide the needle to foramen ovale [4, 5] (Fig. 10.2a) [14]. Entry of the needle in foramen ovale may elicit the trigeminal depressor response, causing contraction of the masseter and pterygoid muscles [4, 5]. Trigeminal depressor response is characterized by transient but significant hypotension and bradycardia, which may require anticholinergic medications such as atropine or transcutaneous pacing [4]. 0.4 mg atropine can be given intramuscularly before the procedure to prevent bradycardia [5]. The trigeminal depressor response occurs less commonly with RF as compared to BC [5]. The position of the needle is confirmed via lateral view fluoroscopy [4, 5] (Fig. 10.2b) [14]. The obturator is removed, and the electrode is introduced [5]. The electrode should not be placed beyond 10 mm of the profile of the clivus to avoid the trochlear and abducens nerve [5]. The patient is awakened, and sensory and motor responses are tested [4, 5]. Optimal location is determined by detailed mapping to provide maximum pain relief while minimizing dysesthesia and motor weakness [4, 5]. Electric stimulation is typically achieved at 0.2–1 V (50 Hz for 0.2 ms) [4]. The electrode is then replaced with the thermocouple, and lesions are made at a maximum of 0.5 V at 5 and 75 cycles per second at 55 °C to 80 °C for 30–120 s [4, 5]. The electrode and cannula are removed [4, 5]. Pressure is applied to the puncture site [4, 5]. Patients can be discharged home the same day after a short observation period.

Ultrasound-Guided Technique Via the Pterygopalatine Fossa

An alternative approach is through the pterygopalatine fossa. The pterygopalatine fossa is bordered posteriorly by the palatine plates, medially and anteromedially by the palatine bone, and anteriorly by the maxillary bone (Fig. 10.3a) [15].

The patient is placed in the lateral decubitus position. The ultrasound should be positioned on the opposite side of the table. Standard ASA monitors should be applied.

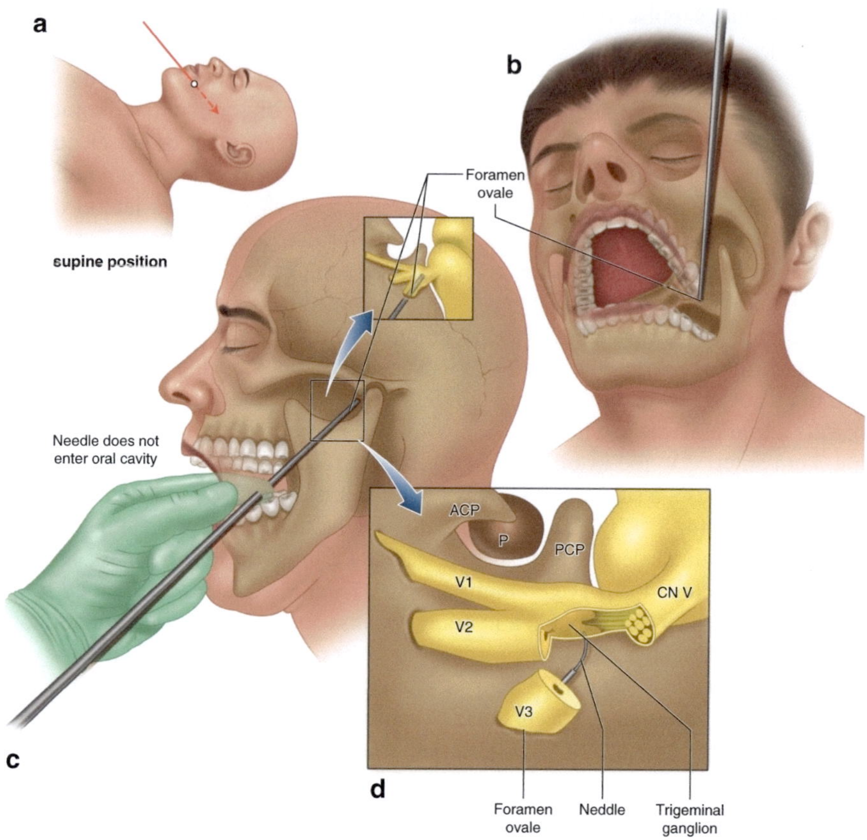

Fig. 10.1 Artist's illustration depicting needle insertion into the foramen ovale for radiofrequency thermocoagulation. (**a**) Patient position and needle trajectory. Three-dimensional paramedian (**b**) and lateral (**c**) views of the needle trajectory through the buccal tissue to reach the foramen ovale. Care is taken not to enter the oral cavity. (**d**) Final needle position at the trigeminal ganglion. Careful manipulation allows selective lesioning of individual trigeminal divisions. *ACP* anterior clinoid process; *CN* cranial nerve; *P* pituitary; *PCP* posterior clinoid process

A high-frequency linear transducer probe should be positioned longitudinally on the side of the face immediately below the zygomatic bone, superior to the mandibular notch, and anterior to the mandibular condyle (Figs. 10.3, and 10.4a, b) [15, 16]. The lateral pterygoid muscle and maxillary artery can be identified. The needle should be advanced below the lateral pterygoid muscle anterior to the lateral pterygoid plate into the pterygoid palatine fossa (Fig. 10.4c) [16]. The needle should be advanced from a lateral to medial and posterior to anterior direction toward the pterygoid fossa using an in-plane approach.

Radiofrequency ablation needles can be advanced using this approach using ultrasound as described or fluoroscopy to ablate the V2 and V3 branches as they emerge from the foramen ovale. More than one needle is usually needed to target both branches. Sensory and motor testing should be performed to ensure the

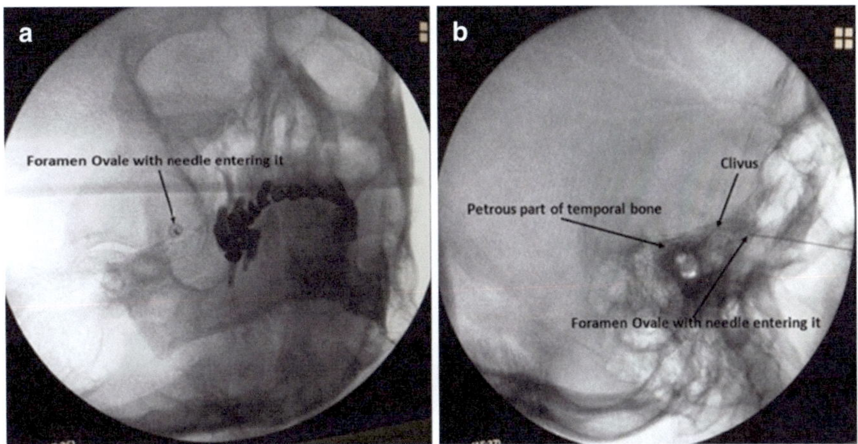

Fig. 10.2 (**a**) Submental view of the foramen ovale and (**b**) lateral view to confirm the depth of the needle insertion. Used with permission from Akbas, M., Salem, H.H., Emara, T.H. et al. Radiofrequency thermocoagulation in cases of atypical trigeminal neuralgia: a retrospective study. Egypt J Neurol Psychiatry Neurosurg 55, 46 (2019)

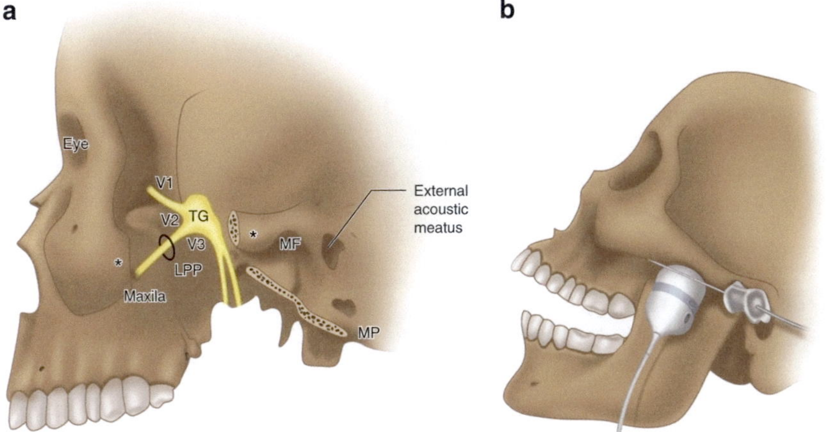

Fig. 10.3 (**a**) Anatomical drawing showing the trigeminal ganglion (Gasserian ganglion) and its corresponding branches V1 ophthalmic, V2 maxillary, and V3 mandibular divisions. The pterygopalatine fossa is bound posteriorly by the palatine plates, medially and anteromedially by the palatine bone, and anteriorly by the maxillary bone. The pterygopalatine fossa is a very compact space and an injection into the space places it close to the foramen rotundum allowing the injectate to reach all branches of the trigeminal nerve. (**b**) A skull model showing the ultrasound probe positioned longitudinally just below the zgyomatic bone, superior to the mandibular notch and anterior to the mandibular condyle. Using the in-plane approach, the needle is advanced from a lateral to medial and posterior to anterior direction toward the pterygopalatine fossa. * zygomatic process (removed); *TG* trigeminal ganglion; *LPP* lateral pterygoid plate; *MF* mandibular fossa; *MP* mastoid process, dashed circle = target area

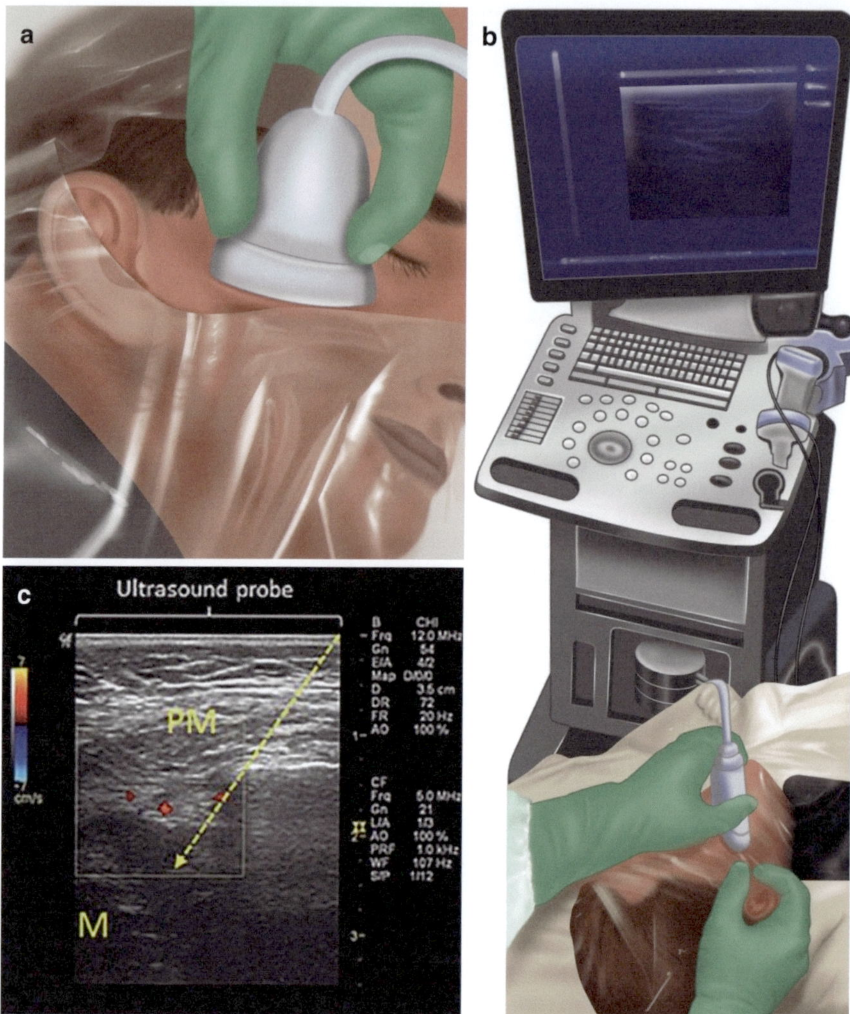

Fig. 10.4 (**a**) The ultrasound probe is positioned caudad to the zygomatic arch with cephalad angulation facilitating visualization of the target area below the zygoma. (**b**) The needle is placed in-line with the transducer. (**c**) The ultrasound image represents a transverse view with the top of the image displaying the ultrasound probe position. Dashed line = needle trajectory, *PM* lateral pterygoid muscle; *M* maxilla. Maxillary artery detected by color flow Doppler

appropriate location of the needles. Same radiofrequency settings as described before can be used at this location.

Complications After RF

Complications after RF such as recurrence of pain and dysesthesia can be bothersome to patients and impact their quality of life negatively. Catastrophic complications such as carotid-cavernous fistula and aseptic meningitis are very rare [17]. In a series of 1600 patients, around 0.13% of the patients developed permanent abducens nerve paralysis and cerebrospinal fluid leak [17].

1. Dysthesia—Dysthesia develops in 3.7% of patients on average [4]. The incidence of dysesthesia has been shown to be correlated with the intensity of loss of touch perception [8]. Dense hypalgesia, defined as loss of more than 75% pain sensation without loss of touch perception, is the optimum lesion as it has a similar long-term pain recurrence rate to analgesia but half the risk of dysesthesia [8]. Anesthesia dolorosa developed in less than <1% of patients in one of the studies [17].
2. Ocular complications—ocular complications range from the development of impaired corneal reflex to keratitis. On an average, about 10% of the patients suffer from corneal numbness [4].
3. Trigeminal motor weakness—In a study of 154 patients, 22 patients developed trigeminal motor weakness [8].
4. Recurrence—various authors have reported a 25–50% incidence of recurrence [2, 8, 10, 17]. In one series, 15% required retreatment [8, 10]. Recurrence timing varied according to the degree of sensory loss [8]. Patients with less severe sensory loss had higher and earlier recurrence [8]. Recurrence of trigeminal neuralgia can be treated with a repeat percutaneous procedure, but repetition can cause an increased risk of numbness and dysesthesia [3].

Efficacy

The goal for optimum lesion in RF is to provide long-term pain relief with minimal sensory loss [5, 8]. RF has a high success rate with 97–99% patients reporting initial pain relief [8, 17]. In a study of 1600 patients, Kaplan–Meier analysis 57.7% and 42.2% of patients showed complete pain relief at 60 and 180 months, respectively, after one intervention [4, 17]. However, both those rates increased to more than 90% of the patients when patients treated multiple times with RF were included [4, 17].

Character of pain is a predictor for long-term treatment success [4]. Patients with atypical pain symptoms (no defined trigger points, intermittent or persistent pain, with concurrent sensory abnormalities or with other comorbidities such as multiple sclerosis) [4] reported lower satisfaction and more postoperative problems than those with typical pain symptoms [11].

Concomitant use of navigation for the procedure has been shown to improve needle localization and therefore improve efficacy and decrease the rate of recurrence and complications after RF [4, 13].

A combination of pulsed and conventional RF has shown promising results in two randomized control trials [18, 19]. However, when used alone, conventional or thermal RF as described in the procedure above has shown to be superior to pulsed radiofrequency in terms of efficacy [18]. However, there have been individual case reports of pulsed radiofrequency being used successfully for the treatment of TN [20].

In conclusion, RF is a safe and effective modality for the treatment of TN in appropriately selected patients. The procedure is generally well-tolerated; however, side effects can occur. Risks and benefits should be discussed with patients prior to proceeding.

References

1. Emril DR, Ho KY. Treatment of trigeminal neuralgia: role of radiofrequency ablation. J Pain Res. 2010;3:249–54.
2. Tronnier VM, Rasche D, Hamer J, Kienle AL, Kunze S. Treatment of idiopathic trigeminal neuralgia: comparison of long-term outcome after radiofrequency rhizotomy and microvascular decompression. Neurosurgery. 2001 Jun;48(6):1261–7.
3. Liu JK, Apfelbaum RI. Treatment of trigeminal neuralgia. Neurosurg Clin N Am. 2004 Jul;15(3):319–34.
4. Cheng JS, Lim DA, Chang EF, Barbaro NM. A review of percutaneous treatments for trigeminal neuralgia. Neurosurgery. 2014 Mar;10(Suppl 1):25–33.
5. Wang JY, Bender MT, Bettegowda C. Percutaneous procedures for the treatment of trigeminal neuralgia. Neurosurg Clin N Am. 2016 Jul;27(3):277–95.
6. Sweet WH, Wepsic JG. Controlled thermocoagulation of trigeminal ganglion and rootlets for differential destruction of pain fibers. J Neurosurg. 1974;40:143–56.
7. Nugent GR. Radiofrequency treatment of trigeminal neuralgia using a cordotomy-type electrode. A method. Neurosurg Clin N Am. 1997 Jan;8(1):41–52.
8. Taha JM, Tew JM Jr, Buncher CR. A prospective 15-year follow up of 154 consecutive patients with trigeminal neuralgia treated by percutaneous stereotactic radiofrequency thermal rhizotomy. J Neurosurg. 1995 Dec;83(6):989–93.
9. Tobler WD, Tew JM Jr, Cosman E, Keller JT, Quallen B. Improved outcome in the treatment of trigeminal neuralgia by percutaneous stereotactic rhizotomy with a new, curved tip electrode. Neurosurgery. 1983 Mar;12(3):313–7.
10. Sanchez-Mejia RO, Limbo M, Cheng JS, Camara J, Ward MM, Barbaro NM. Recurrent or refractory trigeminal neuralgia after microvascular decompression, radiofrequency ablation, or radiosurgery. Neurosurg Focus. 2005;18(5):1–6.
11. Zakrzewska JM, Jassim S, Bulman JS. A prospective, longitudinal study on patients with trigeminal neuralgia who underwent radiofrequency thermocoagulation of the Gasserian ganglion. Pain. 1999 Jan;79(1):51–8.
12. Gusmão S, Oliveira M, Tazinaffo U, Honey CR. Percutaneous trigeminal nerve radiofrequency rhizotomy guided by computerized tomography fluoroscopy. Technical note. J Neurosurg. 2003 Oct;99(4):785–6.
13. Xu SJ, Zhang WH, Chen T, Wu CY, Zhou MD. Neuronavigator-guided percutaneous radiofrequency thermocoagulation in the treatment of intractable trigeminal neuralgia. Chin Med J (Engl). 2006 Sep 20;119(18):1528–35.
14. Akbas M, Salem HH, Emara TH, et al. Radiofrequency thermocoagulation in cases of atypical trigeminal neuralgia: a retrospective study. Egypt J Neurol Psychiatry Neurosurg. 2019;55:46.
15. Nader A, Kendall M, De Oliveira G, et al. Ultrasound-guided trigeminal nerve block via the pterygopalatine fossa: an effective treatment for trigeminal neuralgia and atypical facial pain. Pain Physician. 2013;16:E537–45.
16. Nader A, Bendok B, Prine J, Kendall M. Ultrasound-guided pulsed radiofrequency application via the pterygopalantine fossa: a practical approach to treat refractory trigeminal neuralgia. Pain Physician. 2015;18:E411–5.
17. Kanpolat Y, Savas A, Bekar A, Berk C. Percutaneous controlled radiofrequency trigeminal rhizotomy for the treatment of idiopathic trigeminal neuralgia: 25-year experience with 1,600 patients. Neurosurgery. 2001 Mar;48(3):524–32.
18. Elawamy A, Abdalla EEM, Shehata GA. Effects of pulsed versus conventional versus combined radiofrequency for the treatment of trigeminal neuralgia: a prospective study. Pain Physician. 2017 Sep;20(6):E873–81.
19. Abdel-Rahman KA, Elawamy AM, Mostafa MF, Hasan WS, Herdan R, Osman NM, Ibrahim AS, Aly MG, Ali AS, Abodahab GM. Combined pulsed and thermal radiofrequency versus thermal radiofrequency alone in the treatment of recurrent trigeminal neuralgia after microvascular decompression: a double blinded comparative study. Eur J Pain. 2020 Feb;24(2):338–45.
20. Thapa D, Ahuja V, Dass C, Verma P. Management of refractory trigeminal neuralgia using extended duration pulsed radiofrequency application. Pain Physician. 2015 May–Jun;18(3):E433–5.

Chemodenervation of Trigeminal Nerve

Akshat Gargya and Rany T. Abdallah

Introduction

Chemodenervation has been in use as a treatment modality for trigeminal neuralgia since the early nineteenth century when Dr. Wilfred Harris successfully injected alcohol into the Gasserian ganglion of three patients and reported sustained pain relief from Trigeminal neuralgia [1]. Chemical neurolysis is the technique for destruction of neural tissue by application of a chemical agent to inhibit nerve conduction. Agents commonly used for the process include alcohol and glycerol. Elderly and medically debilitated patients with trigeminal nerve disorders can greatly benefit from chemodenervation of trigeminal nerve. These types of patients are generally unfit for surgical management and have failed multiple other treatment modalities including pharmacological management. The patient selection criteria, procedural technique, risks, complications, and use of different agents including phenol, alcohol,and glycerol are discussed in this chapter.

Patient Selection

Following patients suffering from painful sensations in the distribution of the trigeminal nerve branches can be considered for chemical denervation procedure. These patients typically have insufficient pain control, suffer from unacceptable side effects from medication, are elderly and have underlying medical conditions which make them unsuitable candidates for anesthesia requiring surgery. Patient

A. Gargya
Weill Cornell Medical Center, New York Presbyterian Hospital, New York, NY, USA

R. T. Abdallah (✉)
Center for Interventional Pain and Spine, Milford, DE, USA
e-mail: ranyabdallah@centerisp.com

A. Abd-Elsayed (ed.), *Trigeminal Nerve Pain*,
https://doi.org/10.1007/978-3-030-60687-9_11

preference also plays a role when deciding which procedure to use. Below is a list of trigeminal nerve disorders for which chemodenervation procedure may potentially be beneficial:

- Refractory Typical or type 1 Trigeminal neuralgia (characterized by intermittent episodic pain), or atypical or type 2 TN (characterized by continuous pain).
- Chronic trigeminal neuropathy due to herpes zoster.
- Post-traumatic trigeminal neuralgia.
- Paratrigeminal Oculosympathetic Syndrome.
- Trigeminal pain in the context of underlying medical conditions, like multiple sclerosis or connective tissue disorders.

Procedural Technique

Various techniques can be utilized for injection of a chemical into the trigeminal cistern to cause chemodenervation of the trigeminal nerve ganglion. Trigeminal cistern is the subarachnoid space that envelops the gasserian/trigeminal ganglion. This ganglion is composed of sensory cell bodies of all three branches of the trigeminal nerve namely the ophthalmic, mandibular, and maxillary branch.

Hakanson in 1981 described the use of glycerol injection for relief of trigeminal neuralgia and his procedural technique [2]. The technique was later modified by Bergenheim and associates [3].

Most of these patients are elderly and frail and hence proper anesthetic equipment should be available in case of emergency. Fluoroscopy is required for major part of the procedure and proper radiation protective gear is recommended.

In this technique, patient is kept awake and is placed in supine position with head slightly bent. 1% Lidocaine is administered around 2–3 cm lateral to the corner of the mouth. It is recommended to inject lidocaine 2 cm lateral to the corner of mouth for V2 distribution and 3 cm to cover more of V3 distribution. Hartel percutaneous route is used to locate the foramen ovale (refer to other chapters for fluoroscopic imaging for location of foramen ovale).

Once the entry point is ascertained, a 20G spinal rhizotomy needle can then be inserted aiming toward the intersection point of medial canthus and around 3 cm anterior to the internal auditory meatus (Fig. 11.1). Systolic blood pressure should be monitored continuously as inadequate pain relief during this stage may lead to hypertension. Care must also be taken to avoid sudden vagal response and hypotensive episodes in younger population. Oxygen, ECG, and BP monitoring should be done throughout the procedure.

Care must be taken to avoid accidental needle penetration into the oral cavity. This can be prevented by using one gloved hand as a guide inside the mouth. There are several variations of foraminal anatomy seen in different patients and hence prior imaging and procedure records, especially MRI of the skull, can be of great help in certain patients.

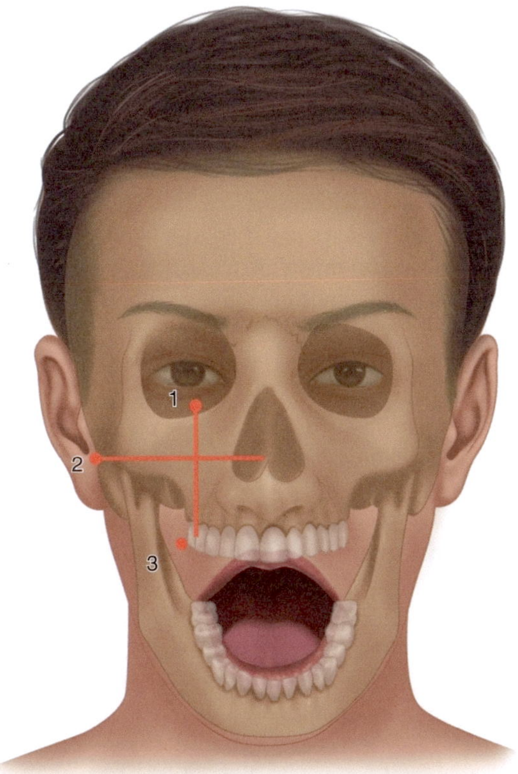

Fig. 11.1 Diagram of skull with intersection point of medial canthus and around 3-cm anterior to the internal auditory meatus

Under fluoroscopic guidance, the needle should be pointed toward the petrous bone and clivus. On the lateral view, the needle should be around 10-mm posterior to the dorsum sella. Care must be taken to avoid needle depth extension beyond clival line to avoid inadvertent injury to adjacent vascular structures like internal carotid artery and jugular vein.

Fluoroscopy can then be directed parallel to the needle to identify the location of the needle tip in relation to foramen ovale. This can be achieved by turning the patient's head contralaterally to about 30° and extending the neck. Submental X-ray view can also be taken to visualize the needle at the medial border of foramen ovale.

Needle can now be further inserted and directed to fall inside the foramen. Sometimes a sudden give or loss of resistance may also be seen. Patients at this point might reflexly produce jaw contraction, which further will verify the correct placement of the needle. This usually happens due to irritation of motor branches of the trigeminal nerve.

In some cases, entry into the ganglion (Meckel's cave) may also be suggested by CSF flow coming through the needle when stylet is withdrawn. However, lack of CSF flow should not be used as a criterion for unsuccessful placement of needle, especially when patients may have undergone prior microvascular decompression surgeries.

Once the position of the needle is confirmed 0.1 ml of omnipaque contrast should be injected under live fluoroscopy for further confirmation. Digital subtraction may be used to rule out vascular uptake of contrast.

At this point, around 0.25–3 cc of 99.9% glycerol or 70% alcohol can be injected, and needle can be withdrawn slowly. Care must be taken to remove any air bubbles from the tuberculin syringe used to inject the chemical agent.

After successful injection, needle and syringe may now be removed and patient can now be taken to postoperative care unit.

It is recommended to carefully monitor for CSF leak or other complications by close neurological monitoring during the following hours. It is advised to keep the patient in sitting position with head slightly flexed to decrease the chances of headaches. The patient should experience pain relief within hours from procedure conclusion and can be discharged home on the same procedure day.

Risks and Complications

Postoperative facial hyperesthesia, hypoalgesia, and dysesthesia remain the most common complications seen in patients with percutaneous glycerol trigeminal rhizotomy. When compared with percutaneous balloon compression trigeminal rhizotomy, patients who underwent percutaneous glycerol rhizotomy have higher rates of dysesthesia [4].

Other complications include decreased corneal sensitivity and herpetiform rashes. Mild hearing loss has also been reported by some patients, which can be due to trauma to tensor tympani motor fibers [5]. There is also small but significant risk of bacterial and chemical meningitis and hence proper aseptic technique is needed. Early postoperative headaches lasting up to several hours have also been reported in some patients [6].

Cadaveric models have shown the distance between the foramen ovale and the trigeminal ganglion to be around 6 mm. Insertion of needle beyond 10-mm carries the risk of internal carotid artery and nerve injury, especially cranial nerve 6, which lies on the medial side of petrolingual ligament [7].

Advantages

Chemodenervation of trigeminal ganglion with injection of Glycerol or Alcohol has various advantages:

- Procedure is minimally invasive and can be done in outpatient settings. Usual procedure time is anywhere from 30 min to an hour.
- Patients do not need to be anesthetized and thus have relatively short post procedure recovery time.

- Procedure has a short learning curve for the providers.
- It requires fewer resources when compared with percutaneous balloon compression trigeminal rhizotomy.
- Subjective patient feedback of successful needle placement is not required in comparison to radiofrequency ablation procedure of trigeminal nerve.
- Chemical neurolysis with glycerol only produces mild injury to nerve. Facial numbness is rarely seen and thus few paresthesia's are seen during follow up.

Disadvantages

Some of the drawbacks of gasserian ganglion chemodernervation are:

- This procedure is nonselective and hence cannot be utilized in patients who have pain in the distribution of single branch of trigeminal nerve.
- Recurrence of pain is common after some years and hence repeat injection/rhizotomy may be needed at that time.
- Procedure can sometimes get technically more demanding since patients are awake when compared with percutaneous balloon compression trigeminal rhizotomy where patients are usually sedated.
- Injury to adjacent structures like internal carotid artery and Cranial Nerve VI can lead to disastrous compilations in some patients.

Mechanism of Pain Relief from Chemodenervation

Although the exact mechanism is unknown, some studies have suggested that chemical neurolysis causes normalization of temporal summation which leads to pain reduction [8]. Prior works on animal studies have also hypothesized that pain relief may be due to selective lysis of axonal sheath in damaged myelinated nerve fibers [8–11].

Alcohol and Phenol have shown in various models to cause protein denaturation and dehydration of protoplasm. This causes interference with nerve conduction and muscle innervation [12]. Neuropraxia and Wallerian degeneration can also be seen at higher concentrations. However, alcohol and phenol do not affect the central core of the nerve fibers [13–15].

When used in concentration of 45% or greater, alcohol has also shown to cause inflammatory reaction in the muscles, muscle fiber damage, and necrosis [14]. We recommend the use of alcohol in 50–100% concentration and phenol at concentrations between 5 and 7%.

In various studies, the amount of glycerol did not influence the degree of sensory disturbance. However, the use of 99.5% pure glycerol preparation has been proven to be a significant factor, which governs the surgical outcome of retro-gasserian glycerol rhizotomy [3, 16, 17].

Types of Injectant

Glycerol

Glycerol when used as the neurolytic agent can be especially useful in treating trigeminal neuralgia. Pure glycerol in concentrations above 99% is highly hypertonic and hence can cause nerve damage by fragmentation of myelin [2, 18]. It can also directly penetrate the perineurium [19]. Glycerol has been shown to help patients with trigeminal neuralgia even when injected locally around the trigeminal nerve and not specifically inside the cistern [11, 20]. Advantages of using glycerol include low cost and easy accessibility, especially in developing countries. On the other hand, diffusion of glycerol outside Meckel cavity can cause various complications [5].

Phenol and Alcohol

Phenol is a derivative of benzene and in concentrations less than 6.7% is soluble in water and glycerine at room temperature [21]. Alcohol is used at 70% concentration or higher. Both are nonselective chemodenervating agents and affects both motor and sensory nerves [22]. They act via causing Wallerian degeneration of nerve fiber [13–15]. These agents act immediately and their effects usually last 6–12 months in most patients. A significant advantage of using phenol or alcohol is the agents' lack of antigenicity. Use of these agents may require sedation since alcohol can cause pain at the time of injection. Adverse effects include paresthesia, pain, vagal reaction, and damage to surrounding tissue. In patients with insufficient pain relief after phenol and alcohol chemodenervation, titration of additional doses has not been shown to have any additional benefit.

A combined mixture of 5% phenol and glycerol has been used historically in sympathetic blocks and cancer pain treatment, but its use in treating trigeminal neuralgia has not been reported [23, 24].

In conclusion, percutaneous chemodenervation is a technique used to treat trigeminal neuralgia pain. In patients who have failed medication management and cannot safely undergo general anesthesia, percutaneous chemodenervation is a safe procedure to consider. While there are chances of reoccurrence of trigeminal nerve pain symptoms, most of the patients do achieve early pain relief. When compared with percutaneous balloon compression trigeminal rhizotomy, percutaneous chemodeneravation procedures do have slightly higher incidence of dysthesia and rate of recurrence of symptoms [4, 6]. Although its role in current pain practice is limited, chemodenervation can still be an effective treatment modality in appropriate patients.

References

1. Harris W. Three cases of alcohol injection of the gasserian ganglion for trigeminal neuralgia. Proc R Soc Med. 1912;5(clin sect):115–9.
2. Hakanson S. Trigeminal neuralgia treated by the injection of glycerol into the trigeminal cistern. Neurosurgery. 1981;9:638–46.

3. Bergenheim A, Hariz M. Influence of previous treatment on outcome after glycerol rhizotomy for trigeminal neuralgia. Neurosurgery. 1995;36(2):303–10.
4. Kouzounias K, Lind G, Schechtmann G, et al. Comparison of percutaneous balloon compression and glycerol rhizotomy for the treatment of trigeminal neuralgia. J Neurosurg. 2010;113(3):486–92.
5. Sindou M, Tatli M. Traitement de la névralgie trigéminale par injection de glycérol au niveau du ganglion de Gasser. Neurochirurgie. 2009;55(2):211–2.
6. Asplund P, Blomstedt P, Bergenheim A. Percutaneous balloon compression vs percutaneous retrogasserian glycerol rhizotomy for the primary treatment of trigeminal neuralgia. Neurosurgery. 2015;78(3):421–8.
7. Kaplan M, Erol F, Ozveren M, Topsakal C, Sam B, Tekdemir I. Review of complications due to foramen ovale puncture. J Clin Neurosci. 2007;14(6):563–8.
8. Jho H, Lunsford L. Percutaneous retrogasserian glycerol rhizotomy. Neurosurg Clin N Am. 1997;8(1):63–74.
9. Eide P, Stubhaug A. Sensory perception in patients with trigeminal neuralgia: effects of percutaneous retrogasserian glycerol rhizotomy. Stereotact Funct Neurosurg. 1997;68(1–4):207–11.
10. Eide P, Stubhaug A. Relief of trigeminal neuralgia after percutaneous retrogasserian glycerol rhizolysis is dependent on normalization of abnormal temporal summation of pain, without general impairment of sensory perception. Neurosurgery. 1998;43(3):462–72.
11. Lunsford LD, Bennett MH, Martinez AJ. Experimental trigeminal glycerol injection: electrophysiological and morphological effects. Arch Neurol. 1985;42(2):146–9.
12. Taylor JJ, Woolsey RM. Dilute ethyl alcohol: effect on the sciatic nerve of the mouse. Arch Phys Med Rehabil. 1976;57:233–7.
13. Carpenter EB, Seitz DG. Intramuscular alcohol as an aid in management of spastic cerebral palsy. Dev Med Child Neurol. 1980;22:497–501.
14. Gordon A. Experimental study of intraneural injections of alcohol. J Nerv Ment Dis. 1914;41:81–95.
15. Zafonte RD, Munin MC. Phenol and alcohol blocks for the treatment of spasticity. Phys Med Rehabil Clin North Am. 2001;12:817–32.
16. Sweet WH, Poletti CE. Problems with retrogasserian glycerol in the treatment of trigeminal neuralgia. Appl Neurophysiol. 1985;48:252–7.
17. Bergenheim AT, Hariz MI, Laitinen LV, Olivecrona M, Rabow L. Relation between sensory disturbance and outcome after retrogasserian glycerol rhizotomy. Acta Neurochir. 1991;111:114–8.
18. King JS, Jewett DL, Sundberg HR. Differential blockade of cat dorsal root C-fibers by various chloride solutions. J Neurosurg. 1972;36:569.
19. Dulhunty AF, Gage PW. Differential effects of glycerol treatment on membrane capacity and excitation-contraction coupling in toad sartorius fibres. J Physiol. 1973;234(2):373–408.1.
20. North RB, Kidd DH, Piantadosi S, Carson BS. Percutaneous retrogasserian glycerol rhizotomy. Predictors of success and failure in treatment of trigeminal neuralgia. J Neurosurg. 1990;72:851.
21. Brashear A, Elovic E, editors. Spasticity, chapter 9. Diagnosis and management. 2nd ed. New York: Demos Medical.
22. Nathan PW, Sears TA, Smith MC. Effects of phenol solution on the nerve roots of the cat. J Neurol Sci. 1965;2(1):7–29.
23. Kirvelä O, Svedström E, Lundbom N. Ultrasonic guidance of lumbar sympathetic and celiac plexus block: a new technique. Pain. 1992;17:43–6.
24. Westerlund T, Vuorinen V, Röyttä M. The effect of combined neurolytic blocking agent 5% phenol-glycerol in rat sciatic nerve. Acta Neuropathol. 2003;106:261–70. https://doi.org/10.1007/s00401-003-0730-1.

Cryotherapy of the Trigeminal Nerve

12

Nicholas Mata, Travis Cleland, and Chong Kim

Introduction

Applying cold temperatures to reduce pain has been used for millennia. In ancient times, cold therapy was rudimentary, performed with the simple placement of ice, snow, or cold water on the skin to dull pain. Even today, the most common methods of cold therapy, also known as cryotherapy, involve cold baths or frozen bags of ice or vegetables. But despite its basic use for thousands of years, many do not realize that more innovative methods of cryotherapy dates as far back as the 1800s. In 1819, James Arnott published his findings in the *Treatment of Cancer by the Regulated Application of an Anaesthetic Temperature*. This early report documented the application of a device that combined a mixture of ice and salt through a specialized machine for the palliative treatment of cancer [1].

Since that time, the field of cryotherapy has become significantly more sophisticated. In 1852, a landmark paper demonstrated that if insulated liquids in a high-pressure environment crossed a valve and expanded into an area of low pressure, the liquid and its surrounding environment would decrease in temperature. This became known as the Joule–Thomson effect [2]. Unfortunately, this effect was not effectively utilized for cryotherapy until the 1900s when refrigerants such as liquid nitrogen became readily available commodities. By the early to mid-1900s, scientists and physicians applied these two tools to create specialized devices that used refrigerants and applied the Joule–Thomson effect to create extremely cold temperatures at specifically targeted tissues.

As with all sensory input, pain signals are carried from peripheral nerves to the brain. The application of cold temperatures to mitigate this signal is a

N. Mata · T. Cleland · C. Kim (✉)
Case Western Reserve University School of Medicine, MetroHealth, Cleveland, OH, USA
e-mail: nmata@metrohealth.org; tcleland@metrohealth.org; ckim3@metrohealth.org

A. Abd-Elsayed (ed.), *Trigeminal Nerve Pain*,
https://doi.org/10.1007/978-3-030-60687-9_12

topic that has been well studied and established physiologic mechanisms. As nerves are cooled below physiologic temperature, the speed at which they are able to transmit action potentials is slowed. The primary mechanism for this slowing is decreased speed of salutatory conduction due to the delayed inactivation of sodium channels, which prolongs the time of depolarization [3]. Animal studies have shown that as nerves are cooled even further, they undergo a nerve-injury classified as "axonotmesis" [4, 5]. Axonotmesis, as first described by Sydney Sunderland in 1951, is an injury of the nerve axon such that it is physically disrupted and undergoes Wallerian degeneration; yet the connective tissues surrounding the axon (the endoneurium, perineurium, and epineurium) remain unaffected [6]. This continuity of the neural connective tissue has the benefits of an increased likelihood of successful axon regeneration to the appropriate anatomic location and a decreased risk of neuroma formation. The overall physiologic effect of this induced axonotmesis is a prolonged decrease in pain sensation in the dermatome of the targeted nerve. Based on this knowledge, some may logically conclude that "the colder, the better," but further study would show that there is a limit for which the benefits outweigh the risk.

Early on, not much data existed to show outcome differences or anatomical changes for nerves undergoing cryotherapy for varying durations or extremes in cooling. In 1995, a new study started to define some of the parameters for cryotherapy. In his study, Zhou recommended the ideal temperatures for inducing axonotmesis were between -60 and -140 °C, with lower temperature treatments leading to delayed times of nerve regeneration. There have been studies showing that bones, major blood vessels, and most connective tissue are much more resilient to freezing [7]. In fact, one study on the heart showed that thrombus formation is much more likely in radiofrequency ablations than in cryoablations [8]. However, there is evidence that freezing nerves at temperatures below -140 °C led to nerve necrosis and destruction of nerve connective tissues [9]. While both axonotmesis and total nerve destruction can lead to the alleviation of pain, axonotmesis allows for the likely return of sensation through nerve regeneration whereas total nerve destruction does not. In 1996, another study showed that the total duration of freeze time was directly related to the number of nerve fibers injured and the magnitude of Wallerian degeneration. However, it showed that if cryotherapy did not result in a complete injury to the axons in a nerve, then there was an increased risk of hyperalgesia [10]. The data on total duration of freezing was then supported by another study of perineal pain wherein patients who had a longer total duration of freeze (greater than 8 min) had a higher likelihood of pain relief compared to shorter total duration [11]. Then, in 2003, Andrea Trescot wrote that individual cycles of freezing (as opposed to the total duration of freezing) longer than 3 min at a time provided no additional benefit to the cryolesion [12]. However, there are no guidelines for target temperatures for cryoneurolysis. As stated above, temperatures should be below -60 °C and above -140 °C. The intrinsic properties of the commonly used refrigerants (carbon dioxide and nitrous oxide) will limit freezing temperatures to -90 °C, which provides a natural barrier to causing the nerve destruction that can be seen at colder temperatures. Until further evidence or guidelines are published, these authors recommend a target temperature of −70 to −90° with three cycles of 2-min freezes separated by 30 s of thawing. Based on current evidence, this can help optimize pain relief while minimizing risks of neuroma formation, hyperalgesia, and permanent loss of sensation.

Cryotherapy for blocking of peripheral nerves was first described in 1976 by J. W Lloyd [13]. At the time, nerve blocks were performed mostly with local anesthetic agents, which would only last hours at a time. Some providers used alcohol or phenol to destroy nerves for longer term analgesia, but if nerve destruction was incomplete patients were at risk of painful neuritis. In his chapter, Lloyd introduced a new device (the Spembly-Lloyd nerve blocking unit) and a generalized technique for using it. Like most cryotherapy units, this nerve blocking unit applied the Joule–Thomson effect with nitrous oxide through a cryosurgical probe to create an iceball at −60 °C. The main differentiator of this probe was the addition of a nerve stimulator that allowed for precise neurolocalization and a thermistor to record temperature around a probe and ensure iceball formation when direct target visualization was not possible.

Lloyd described a few methods of using this new device. After briefly discussing an open surgical approach, wherein a patient under general anesthesia undergoes surgical exposure of the nerve followed by cryotherapy of that nerve under direct visualization, he then went into more detail about a generalized technique for a closed procedure. Here, briefly, nerves are first localized via anatomic landmarks or imaging modalities. Then, superficial tissues are numbed with local anesthetics so that a cryoprobe (via an introducer) can be inserted in close proximity to the nerve. The nerve stimulator is then used to localize the nerve until a sensory response can be reproduced with minimal current. Finally, the cryoprobe creates an iceball (Fig. 12.1), which is confirmed via temperature recording with the thermistor. For both the open and the closed techniques, two cycles of freezing at −60 °C, separated by a brief cycle of returning the tissue to 0 °C, are performed [13].

In addition to describing a new technique, Lloyd also published the first results from this procedure. There were multiple target sites in this first data set, but overall, 52/64 patients had pain relief. The median duration of relief was only 11 days, but some patients achieved relief for up to 224 days. More importantly, he studied a group of patients who underwent cryotherapy for facial pain. Amongst this group, all 6 of whom underwent open cryotherapy for differing branches of the trigeminal nerve demonstrated pain relief for a median of 21 days [13].

Fig. 12.1 Iceball formation at the tip of a cryoprobe

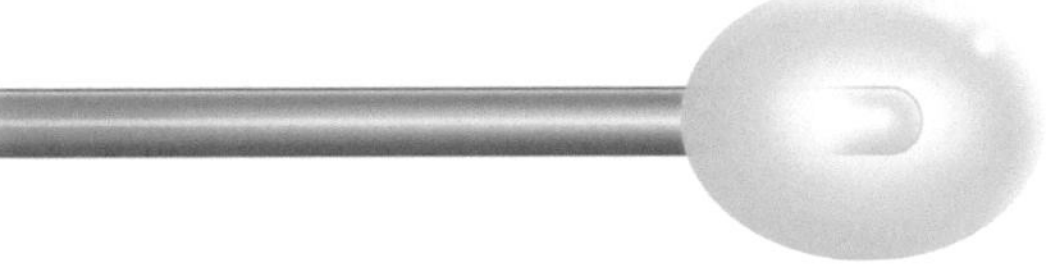

Description of Cryo Procedure

Since Lloyd's first article, multiple cryoprobes have been developed and implemented for targeting peripheral nerves. As with Lloyd's probe, all others have a nerve stimulator to help localize the nerve, a thermistor to measure temperature at the tip of the probe, and a pressurized gas release system that allows the probe to rapidly drop the temperature of the surrounding tissues. While the basics of the probe and the technique were described in the introduction, this next section will provide a much more detailed description.

As referenced earlier, the cryoprobe forms an iceball by allowing highly pressurizing liquid gas to expand as it passes through a valve to move into a low-pressure environment, which results in cooling of the surrounding environment (i.e., the Joule–Thomson effect) (Fig. 12.2) [2]. To achieve this, the cryoprobe consists of a sealed tube within which resides a smaller tube that has a valve at the end. When activated, liquid gas is passed from a pressurized gas container through the small tube, then through the valve into the low-pressure, larger tube. As the gas passes into the larger tube, the temperature drops in the surrounding area, which is located at the tip of the probe. The tip of the probe is in contact with the target tissue, leading to the formation of an iceball. To retain the now depressurized gas, the large tube then funnels the gas back to the storage unit where it can become pressurized once again [12]. Most probes use compressed carbon dioxide or nitrous oxide for this effect [14].

Though the overall concept is straightforward, there are many specific settings and requirements to ensure that cryotherapy is successful. There are many different versions of these devices which including handheld options. All available units are able to create iceballs of appropriate size to create a cryolesion on a nerve. The machine itself must be precisely calibrated for the gas to flow at a specific rate. Gas

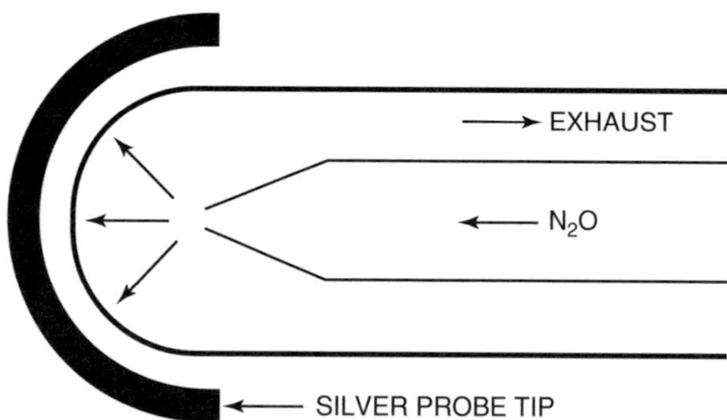

Fig. 12.2 Provided with permission from EPIMED. A schematic representation of the cryoprobe. High-pressure gas (N_2O in this figure) is passed through the small inner-tube. It expands as it exits the inner-tube's valve (demonstrated in this figure by the group of three, fanning arrows) into the larger tube. It is here, at the point of expansion at the probe tip, that temperature cools. The gas is then rerouted to the storage unit (demonstrated in this figure by "Exhaust," pointing to the right) where it can be repressured for continuation of cooling

flow that is too slow will not reduce temperature enough to form an iceball [15]. Gas flow that is too fast could lead to a less precise freeze along the probe, which could result in potential skin burn [15]. The diameter of the probe itself is also very specific. The diameter range is typically between 1.4 and 2.0 mm, with a corresponding variation in iceball size from 3.5 to 5.5 mm, respectively [12]. Many providers also choose to use an introducer before inserting the cryoprobe. The four main reasons for doing this are: ease of maneuvering through tissue, insurance that stimulation and freezing remain at the tip of the probe, and ability to provide local anesthetic while maneuvering through patient tissue [12].

Accuracy is of the utmost importance to ensure that a nerve undergoes an appropriate freeze. In order to achieve accurate localization of the nerve, anatomic landmarks, fluoroscopy, or ultrasound imaging are used prior to final target acquisition by the probe's nerve stimulator. The nerve stimulator is calibrated for sensory and motor responses [12]. For sensory nerves, longer duration pulses are used at diminishing voltage as the probe comes closer to its target [16]. The target nerve is considered to be close enough to the probe for cryotherapy when a sensory response can be consistently stimulated at 0.5 V or less [14]. Once this is achieved, the stimulator is switched to its motor setting, which consists of short duration pulses. The voltage is then maximized while observing for motor responses. If no motor responses are observed, this is determined that the risk for performing cryotherapy on a motor nerve is minimized [12, 14]. It should be noted though that an animal study of cryotherapy on mixed, motor-sensory nerves showed only showed small effects on motor function for 14 days, which were resolved by 30 days [17].

This procedure is indicated for patients with an appropriate diagnosis for facial pain who have been refractory to conservative care including pharmacologic treatments, have undergone a differential diagnostic neural blockade when targeting a specific nerve, and are a candidate for percutaneous interventions. If largely beneficial to the patient, the procedure can be repeated when symptoms return. However, if the response is short-lived or provides poor pain relief, repeating the procedure is unlikely to provide benefit.

Relative contraindications for cryoneurolysis are not established but follow a similar pattern for radiofrequency ablation. These include patient refusal, local infection, sepsis, coagulopathy, increased intracranial pressure, behavioral abnormalities, allergy to local anesthetics, lack of patient cooperation, and anticoagulation status. The most important contraindication to general cryotherapy overall is bleeding diathesis into areas that may go unnoticed by providers, such as in the pelvis or thorax. However, due to the location of the trigeminal nerve and its branches, this risk is not pertinent for the pathology covered in this book. There have not been specific studies looking at complication rates of cryoneuroablation of the trigeminal nerve, but general complications to cryotherapy include skin pigmentation changes, alopecia (especially of the eyebrows), and frostbite of the skin if the cryotherapy is performed superficially. Radiofrequency ablation of specifically the trigeminal nerve can lead to early or late pain recurrence, diminished corneal reflex, masseter weakness and paralysis, and keratitis. Though many cryotherapy sites for the trigeminal nerve are performed through the oral mucosa, there are several percutaneous procedures. So the warnings listed above should be provided based on the specific procedure to be performed. Regardless of procedure site, patients must be warned that in addition to pain relief, a temporary or chronic numbness may ensue follow the procedure. Many patients may not mind this, but loss of sensation may be bothersome, especially in the face.

In the following section, the general procedure for cryotherapy will be described. Due to the fact that most applications of cryotherapy for trigeminal neuralgia target specific branches of the trigeminal nerve (as opposed to the base of the nerve itself), there will be subsequent discussion on specific approaches for branches of the trigeminal nerve.

The first step to cryotherapy is to localize the correct target. A highly accurate diagnostic block with a low dose of a local anesthetic should be performed. The method of the block depends upon the target, and may include use of a nerve stimulator, fluoroscopy, ultrasound, or direct visualization. If the block is successful, the provider can consider cryotherapy. Prior to commencement of the procedure, the patient is consented and placed in the proper position. For most, little to no sedation is recommended because the patient needs to provide input about sensory responses to stimulation while trying to localize the nerve. The rest of the procedure should be carried out under an aseptic technique. The nerve is first localized via fluoroscopy, anatomic landmarks, or palpation. Local anesthetic is then injected at the target site before the introducer is placed. Some providers then inject epinephrine diluted with saline into the subcutaneous tissue to cause local vasoconstriction which creates both hemostasis and decreases the temperature surrounding the target. Next, a small incision is made to advance a larger introducer towards the target. More local anesthetic is provided as needed. After the introducer has reached the target area, the cryoprobe is inserted through the introducer in such a way that only the tip of the probe is exposed.

Next, the nerve stimulator is used to bring the probe as close as possible to the nerve. Starting at the sensory setting, high voltage charges are emitted through the probe to elicit a dermatomal sensory paresthesia. Patient feedback is needed to correlate the stimulation with a sensory response. If there is no response, the probe is repositioned and another stimulation at the same voltage is emitted. This cycle is repeated until the patient experiences paresthesia in an appropriate dermatomal pattern. Once this occurs, the provider adjusts the probe and attempts to obtain the same paresthesia response with a lower voltage. This process repeats until the provider is able to consistently achieve the same dermatomal paresthesia at stimulation intensities of 0.5 V or lower. Next, the provider needs to screen the surrounding area for motor nerves. The stimulator on the cryoprobe is switched to its motor settings. A high voltage stimulation is then emitted with the provider observing for a muscle twitch. If none is observed, the provider can be assured that the risk of ablating a motor nerve is as low as possible. If a muscle twitch is observed, the provider should consider the risks and benefits of performing the procedure at that location, and consider targeting a different location along the nerve.

When using the stimulator to localize the nerve, there are two different problems to avoid. First, simple movement of the probe itself can cause paresthesia, which may confound the paresthesia caused by stimulation. Thus, certainty that the paresthesia response is related to the stimulation, not probe movement, is paramount. Second, the stimulator should not continuously emit stimulations. Once the patient feels the stimulation, the probe should promptly be shut off. Failure to do so could lead to overstimulation of the nerve, which potentially leads to poor, or no-response to subsequent stimulations [12].

After nerve localization, the cryoprobe is used to create an iceball. Gas flow is turned on for 2–3 min, then turned off for 30 s. This cycle is repeated 2–3 times to ensure proper iceball formation and freezing. The temperature needs to be at least −60 °C, but no colder than −140 °C. After the rounds of freezing have been completed, ample time is given for the iceball to completely thaw before removing the probe. Removing the probe too quickly after a freeze can lead to blunt trauma to the nerve and surrounding tissues. Last, the introducer is removed and the patient is appropriately cleaned and bandaged. Of note, patients typically experience discomfort for the first 30 s of the freeze, but are generally pain free for the remainder of the procedure [12].

As mentioned earlier, most providers target specific branches, not the base of the trigeminal nerve. The most common nerves targeted are the supraorbital nerve (from the ophthalmic branch), the infraorbital nerve (from the maxillary branch), the base of the mandibular branch, the mental nerve (from the mandibular branch), and the auriculotemporal nerve (from the mandibular branch). Some providers target the trigeminal nerve itself as it exits the foramen ovale, but there are risks of hypoesthesia of the eye due to blocking the entirety of the ophthalmic division (Fig. 12.3).

The following will be more specific technical aspects about the common target branches for trigeminal neuralgia interpreted mostly from Andrea Trescot's article on cryotherapy [12]. If an open technique exists, it will be mentioned; but more focus will be given for the closed technique of each target.

Fig. 12.3 Image of cryoneurolysis of the trigeminal nerve. (SpringerLink)

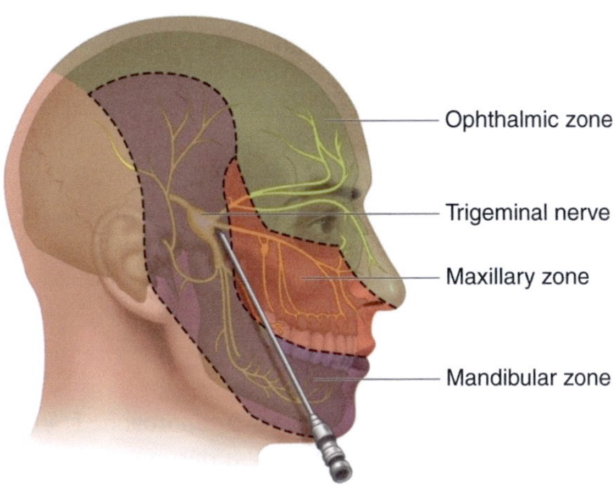

The maxillary nerve can be approached via two landmark techniques or through an ultrasound-guided technique. Under ultrasound, the transducer is placed inferior to the zygomatic arch over the maxilla in order to evaluate the pterygopalatine fossa. Needle is advanced in short axis. Landmark guided approach superior to the zygomatic arch requires the patient to be supine, with the head being neutral. Insert needle superior to the zygomatic arch, posterior to the orbital rim. Needle is inserted perpendicular to the skin until bony landmark contact at 1.0 cm. The needle is then reoriented caudal and posterior and advanced 3.5–4.5 cm to the pterygopalatine fossa [16].

Irritation of the supraorbital nerve typically occurs at the supraorbital notch, making it the typical target site. There is an open surgical approach with direct visualization and a closed technique. The closed technique is typically performed with the smaller, 1.4 mm probe and the smaller, 14-gauge introducer. The skin around the eye is particularly sensitive, so care must be taken with this procedure. Cryotherapy should be performed above or below the eyebrow (to minimize the risks of alopecia), aiming at the supraorbital notch. Patients should be warned of skin pigmentation changes that can last for a few months or longer [12].

The infraorbital nerve is typically irritated at the infraorbital foramen. Again, an open surgical approach with direct visualization can be used. There are also two closed techniques. One is percutaneously at the infraorbital foramen using the 1.4-mm probe and 14-gauge catheter. The other technique is intraoral, with insertion of the probe at the superior mucobuccal fold at the first premolar, aiming toward the infraorbital notch. This approach uses the larger 2.0 mm probe with a 12-gauge catheter [18].

The mandibular nerve has been targeted in three areas: the base of the mandibular nerve, the mental nerve branch, and auriculotemporal nerve branch.

For the base of the mandibular nerve, an open surgical approach with direct visualization can be used. Conversely, closed intraoral and extraoral techniques can be performed. For the extraoral technique, the probe is inserted posterior to the coronoid process of the mandible until it sits between the temporalis and lateral pterygoid muscles (which is identified as the second of two tactile "pops" as the probe moves into the appropriate fascial plane). The intraoral approach entails placing the probe at the mandibular foramen, which sits at the medial-superior border of the lingula of the mandible [12]. A landmark guided technique can be performed in which the needle is inserted below the zygomatic arch, posterior to the mandibular notch below the tragus of the ear. It is important that the needle remains as superior as possible in the space to avoid arterial puncture. Advance the needle perpendicular to the skin 2–4 cm, then posteriorly and inferiorly, stopping when noting mandibular twitch. After negative aspiration, medication or freezing can occur [16].

The mental nerve is typically approached with a closed technique, using the 14-mm probe. Either percutaneous or intraoral approach at the mental foramen is performed.

The auriculotemporal nerve is approached with a closed technique. Trescot describes localization of the distal portion of the nerve by targeting the apex of an equilateral triangle with base its at a line between the corner of the eye and the anterior tragus. This approach typically uses the larger 2.0 mm probe. Conversely, the proximal aspect of the auriculotemporal nerve can be targeted using a closed, extraoral technique with the target site just anterior to the temporomandibular joint. The smaller probe is used to help avoid hitting the facial nerve, which resides close to the target area [12].

Approach of the trigeminal ganglion itself is not a common target. The approach requires the patient to be supine with the neck in extension. Submental and lateral views are used to identify the foramen ovale. Needle placement starts 2.5 cm lateral to the corner of the mouth. The needle is directed cephalad, aiming toward the auditory meatus. Needle trajectory is in a plane that is perpendicular to the pupil of the eye. Needle is advanced until contact is made with the base of the skull. Then, step-down technique is used to walk the needle to the foramen ovale. Aspiration is important at this point to ensure that there is no CSF or blood return prior to any injections. There is increased risk of hematoma or loss of consciousness compared to targeting other nerves due to relatively close location to CSF and the internal carotid artery [12, 16].

Literature Review of Efficacy of Cryotherapy for Paroxysmal Trigeminal Neuralgia

Because the majority of patients with paroxysmal trigeminal neuralgia are controlled on oral medications, there are only limited data available studying the effect of cryotherapy. Furthermore, of the data that does exist, there are limitations of which studies are applicable to the overall population of trigeminal neuralgia because most of the studies show effect on patients with symptoms refractory to traditional treatment. As mentioned above, the trigeminal nerve consists of three main branches (ophthalmic, maxillary, and mandibular) with many terminal nerves from each of these branches. Because patients may be experiencing symptoms on only discreet portions of the trigeminal nerve, providers tend to target discreet sections of the trigeminal nerve for cryotherapy. This is beneficial for study subjects, but diminishes the generalizability of studies to patients because not all of the studies target the same branches at the same rate. Thus, it is important when reviewing the literature to note which nerves are targeted.

One of the first studies to publish data on cryotherapy success was the original article introducing the new probe for cryoneuroablation, but only consisted of six patients defined as having facial pain, not specifically trigeminal neuralgia [13]. All of the patients obtained pain relief for a median of 21 days. Nearly all patients underwent ablation of the infraorbital nerve, with one patient undergoing treatment on the mental nerve. Open surgical technique was used, which theoretically allowed the researchers to have accurate localization of the nerve. The short duration of freeze length (two, 2-min cycles) and the relatively high temperature ($-60\,^\circ$C) may be the reason for the short duration of pain relief.

Another study assessed 42 patients with paroxysmal trigeminal neuralgia. In these 42 patients, 55 nerves were treated after prior localization via local anesthetic injection. The primary nerves targeted were the mental, infraorbital, and long buccal nerves. An intraoral, open, surgical technique with direct visualization was used. There was no uniformity in duration of the freeze or number of freezes, and the temperature was −45 °C. Authors report that 54 of the 55 nerves had no return of pain, but tie of follow up was not well defined. However, this was one of the earlier observations of pain migration, wherein 16 patients experienced migration of the pain to a different area of the trigeminal nerve. In some of these patients, repeat procedure was done, but for 2 min at −100 °C. This relieved the recurrent pain, which led the authors to conclude that freezing at −100 °C for three, 2-min cycles with 5 min between each cycle would give a better chance of success [19].

In 1987, Zakrzewska published his first set of data for cryotherapy for paroxysmal trigeminal neuralgia. A retrospective look of 29 patients who had undergone cryotherapy 5 years prior. An intraoral, open, surgical technique with direct visualization was used. Test blocks with local anesthetics were used to identify the target nerves (mainly the mental, infraorbital, and long buccal nerves). They performed three cycles of 2-min freezes with 5 min thaws at −120 °C. 85% of the patients had immediate relief of pain. However, only 41% of patients had pain relief for longer than 1 year. These authors were the first to report individual nerve success, noting that despite the relatively low proportion of patients who were pain free, 63% of individual nerve distributions were pain free for longer than 1 year. They did not delineate well which results were from repeat procedures versus the original procedure, which is important because the 29 patients underwent a total of 83 sessions of cryotherapy in the 5-year observation period [20].

The next year, Zakrzewska published a second set of data in a prospective case series of 145 patients. Length of follow up was extremely variable, ranging from 1 month to 6 years. The procedure followed the same technique as his prior article, but decreased the freezing temperature to −140 °C. Patients were also again allowed to get repeat procedures if the pain recurred during the observation period. Only 27% of patients were pain free at 1 year and the mean time to recurrence was 10 months. However, instead of solely looking at the subjects' control of overall facial pain, the authors again looked at the results for individual nerves, which provided even more promising results. The mean time for recurrence of the infraorbital and mental nerves was significantly longer than overall pain at 20 months and 17 months respectively. The buccal nerve had the shortest time to recurrence at 13 months. In all of these patients, sensory function returned at 2–3 months and the rate of migration of pain amongst patients after cryoanalgesia was 38%. They did note a high rate of patients who had facial pain after the procedure and a local infection rate of 4% [21]. In 1991, a cross-sectional survey was sent to previously studied patients. Overall, it was found that 52% of patients had recurrence (much higher than that of other treatments studied by the authors). Though this may seem like a high number, it is not unexpected considering the pathophysiology of cryotherapy. Because freezing of nerves between −60 and −140 °C causes axonotmesis, it is expected that axons will likely regrow through their preserved endoneurium with time, thus likely resulting in recurrence of pain. This is especially true considering the duration of time from the procedure to completion of the survey. Fortunately, 74% of patients stated they would be willing to undergo the procedure again: an optimistic number for the ease and efficacy of the procedure [22].

A small case series was published around the same time in Belgium. Only 10 patients were observed, and the follow-up time was variable. As with the other studies, a test block was used before using an open surgical procedure to directly visualize the nerve and perform cryotherapy. There was variability in number of freezes depending on which nerve was targeted, but did use −70 °C for all freezes. Overall 9 of 10 had immediate relief and 7 of 10 had relief until the follow-up period (varied between 3 and 13 months). Sensation loss recovered in 6–12 weeks and they did not observe the migration that was seen in other studies [23].

In 2002, a new cryoprobe was introduced with a small case series. Authors claimed it allowed for a quicker freeze and slower thaw as well as potentially making closed procedures easier. In contrast to the majority of the previous research, this study used a closed technique. Like all other studies, a test block was used. Two cycles of 90-s freezes were completed, though temperature was not noted. All patients achieved pain relief in the short term, which lasted for at least 6–12 months [24].

The studies conducted thus far appear promising and do have some aspects of uniformity. All patients received diagnostic blocks before choosing the target peripheral nerve. This technique appears to help with patient outcome, since the vast majority of patients achieve at least short-term pain relief after the diagnostic block. This high proportion of patients achieving some success with cryotherapy after one diagnostic block suggests that paired diagnostic blocks would likely provide little value. Though it should be noted that no studies attempted to perform cryotherapy without any prior diagnostic block. While the vast majority of patients achieved pain relief in the short term after the procedure, the length of pain relief varied widely. On average, most responders experienced at least 6 months of relief across the studies, with some being pain free for 5 years or more. Though pain recurred in most patients, there appears to be data that the open surgical technique is quite effective for select nerves, without recurrence for many over 1.5 years for the infraorbital and mental nerves. A few of the studies have noted migration of pain to other peripheral branches of the trigeminal nerve, though it is not uniform and the mechanism for this is unknown. Most studies seem to agree that the loss of facial sensation in responders seems to return within a few months, though the cross-sectional survey by Zakrzweska seems to suggest this could be a longer and more bothersome effect than noted. Despite this, data also seems to suggest that the patient-burden of this procedure is low: most patients are satisfied with the procedure and willing to have it performed multiple times as necessary.

Now, though this data is promising, it is important to understand the limitations of these studies. Most importantly, it is worth reiterating that all but one of these studies used an open surgical technique. The interventionalist had direct visualization of the nerve they were performing cryotherapy on. Data for closed technique for the trigeminal nerve is lacking, with only a small case series. So though possible with strong anatomical knowledge, more research needs to be published to validate success of this technique. There is a lack of data concerning the temperature of freeze and duration of freeze for nerves, which are localized by nerve stimulator. There are limited data comparing closed to open surgical techniques. This brings up another limitation of the available data: all of the studies are essentially case series. There are no trials with a comparison group let alone a randomized control trial with a robust placebo group. With some patients achieving pain control for longer than 5 years, there is potential for a procedure like this to possibly become standard or care with less side effects than an anti-seizure medication. But without robust data, this is can never be determined. Another limitation is the relative lack of data for specific target branches. Though a couple of studies did report data for specific nerve responses in addition to overall patient pain, there are no studies dedicated to these nerves. Furthermore, the majority of patients had treatment on the buccal, mental, and infraorbital nerve, with little to no data presented on a large number of other target sites for the trigeminal nerve. These differences make it difficult to standardize a treatment recommendation for providers or for the medical community to easily compare data and results of these studies. More work on these aspects will continue to strengthen the case for cryotherapy as a treatment for paroxysmal trigeminal neuralgia.

In conclusion, Cryotherapy for trigeminal neuralgia, despite the lack of robust randomized control trials, appears to be beneficial for paroxysmal trigeminal neuralgia. There are well-documented physiologic and anatomic mechanisms explaining how cryotherapy affects peripheral nerves. Additionally, the procedure provides little risk to patients.

At this time, the best recommendation for this treatment in paroxysmal trigeminal neuralgia patients is for use in those who have pain refractory to oral medications. Though they should be warned that sensation loss in the face is likely to last up to a couple of months and that the likelihood of recurrence of the pain is high, some patients have success for longer than 5 years and most patients tolerate the procedure very well.

References

1. Arnott J. Treatment of cancer by the regulated application of an anaesthetic temperature. London: Churchill; 1852.
2. Weisend J. Cryogenic Society of America [online]. Available: https://cryogenicsociety.org/resources/defining_cryogenics/joule-thomson_effect/. Accessed 11 Mar 2020.
3. Shapiro BE. Artifacts and technical factors. In: Electromyography and neuromuscular disorders. Philadelphia, PA: Elsevier; 2013.
4. Moorjani N, et al. Effects of cryoanalgesia on post-thoracotomy pain and on the structure of intercostal nerves: a human prospective randomized trial and histological study. Eur J Cardiothorac Surgery. 2001;20(3):502–7.
5. Saueressig F, et al. Morphofunctional Analysis of sciatic nerve and motor performance of rats after cryotherapy with liquid nitrogen. Oral Surg Oral Med Oral Pathol Oral Radiol. 2012;113(3):319–26.
6. Sunderland S. A classification of peripheral nerve injuries producing loss of function. Brain. 1951;74(4):491–516.

7. Gage AA, Baust JM, Baust JG. Experimental cryosurgery investigations in vivo. Cryobiology. 2009;59(3):229–43.
8. Khairy P, Chauvet P, Lehmann J, Lambert J, Macle L, Tanguay J-F, Sirois MG, Santoianni D, Dubuc M. Lower incidence of thrombus formation with cryoenergy versus radiofrequency catheter. Circulation. 2003;107(15):2045–50.
9. Zhou L, et al. Mechanism research of cryoanalgesia. Neurol Res. 1995;17(4):307–11.
10. Myers RR, Heckman HM, Powell HC. Axonal viability and persistence of therapeutic hyperalgesia after partial freeze lesions of nerve. J Neurol Sci. 1996;139:28–38.
11. Evans PJ, Lloyd JW, Jack TM. Cryoanalgesia for intractable perineal pain. J R Soc Med. 1981;74:804–9.
12. Trescot A. Cryoanalgesia in interventional pain management. Pain Physician. 2003;6:345–60.
13. Lloyd J, Barnard JD, Glynn CJ. Cryoanalgesia: a new approach to pain relief. Lancet. 1976;2(7992):932–4.
14. Law L, Rayi A, Derian A. Cryoanalgesia. [Updated 2020 Aug 30]. In: StatPearls [Internet]. Treasure Island (FL): StatPearls Publishing; 2020 Jan-. Available from: https://www.ncbi.nlm.nih.gov/books/NBK482123/.
15. Garamy G . Engineering aspects of cryosurgery. In: Rand RW , Rinfret A , von Leden H (eds). Cryosurgery. 1968.
16. NYSORA. Electrical nerve stimulators and localization of peripheral nerves. New York School of Regional Anesthesia [online]. Available: https://www.nysora.com/foundations-of-regional-anesthesia/equipment/electrical-nerve-stimulators-localization-peripheral-nerves/. Accessed 11 Mar 2020.
17. Shah SB. Does cryoneurolysis result in persistent motor deficits? A controlled study using rat peronel nerve injury model. Reg Anesth Pain Med. 2020;45:287–92.
18. NYSORA. Oral & maxillofacial regional anesthesia [online]. Available.: https://www.nysora.com/regional-anesthesia-for-specific-surgical-procedures/head-and-neck/maxillofacial/oral-maxillofacial-regional-anesthesia/. Accessed 17 Mar 2020.
19. Nally F. A 22-year study of paroxysmal trigeminal neuralgia in 211 patients with a 3-year appraisal of the role of cryotherapy. Oral Surg. 1984;58(1):17–23.
20. Zakrzewska J. Cryotherapy in the management of paroxysmal trigeminal neuralgia. J Neurol Neurosurg Psychiatry. 1987;50:485–7. Chapter: Cryotherapy.
21. Zakrzweska J. The role of cryotherapy (cryoanalgesia) in the management of paroxysmal trigeminal neuralgia: a six year experience. Br J Oral Maxillofac Surg. 1988;26:18–25.
22. Zakrzewska J. Cryotherapy for trigeminal neuralgia: a 10 year audit. Br J Oral Maxillofac Surg. 1991;29:1–4.
23. Politis C, Adriaensen H, Bossuyt M, Fossion E. The management of trigeminal neuralgia with cryotherapy. Acta Stomatol Belg. 1988;85(3):197–205.
24. Pradel W. Cryosurgical treatment of genuine trigeminal neuralgia. Br J Oral Maxillofac Surg. 2002;40:244–7.

Botox Injections

13

Greta Nemergut

Background

Botulinum toxin (BoNT) is a toxin produced by anaerobic bacterium, *Clostridium botulinum*. There are seven neurotoxins (A–G) that exist, with types A and B utilized for therapeutic use in humans. Type A is the most commonly used. Botulinum toxin works by binding to the acceptor at the motor and autonomic nerve terminals, inhibiting acetylcholine, resulting in neuromuscular transmission being blocked. The binding of acetylcholine to its receptor is needed for muscle contraction. Acetylcholine is inhibited when BoNT cleaves the synaptosomal associated protein-25 kDa (SNAP-25), a protein needed to allow acetylcysteine to be released within the nerve endings [1]. When BoNT is injected into the muscle, it causes partial chemical denervation, resulting in less muscle activity, and reversible paralysis within the locally injected muscles. When administered intradermally, it results in lack of nerve supply of the sweat glands, reducing sweating [2].

Mechanism of Action

The mechanism of how BoNT aids in the relief of neuropathic pain is not fully understood. Ongoing study of the use of BoNT in various pain conditions has suggested that the pain relief achieved by BoNT is not solely related to muscle relaxation but has other mechanisms that result in an analgesic effect.

There are four main mechanisms BoNT is thought to work through in the treatment of neuropathic pain. It is believed to block the release of pain mediators,

G. Nemergut (✉)
Pharmacy Program, Department of Pharmacy, University of Wisconsin Hospital and Clinics, Madison, WI, USA
e-mail: gnemergut@uwhealth.org

A. Abd-Elsayed (ed.), *Trigeminal Nerve Pain*,
https://doi.org/10.1007/978-3-030-60687-9_13

including substance P and calcitonin related protein (CGRP), at nerve endings and dorsal root ganglions; reduce inflammation around nerve endings; deactivate sodium channels; and exhibit axonal transport [1]. These areas have been evaluated in animal models. The cleavage at the SNAP-25 results in downregulation of transient receptor potential vallinoid 1 (TRPV1) and ankyrin 1 (TRPA1), channels on peripheral nerves that are involved in the sensation of pain, in turn reducing pain [1, 3]. Botulinum toxin has also been shown to block the release of neuropeptides, like CGRP, from the trigeminal ganglion [1]. This same reduction in neurotransmitters (CGRP and substance P) is believed to result in local anti-inflammatory effects, due to these transmitters playing a role in the sensory aspect of inflammation. In a study by Lucioni A et al., use of BoNT in the bladder of a rat that was induced into an inflammatory response, resulted in reduced amounts of neurotransmitters [4]. Reduction of inflammation locally at the nerve terminals was evaluated, finding that BoNT demonstrated reduced inflammation at the site without any corresponding muscle weakness. Not all studies assessing BoNT role in anti-inflammatory responses demonstrated positive reductions in inflammatory markers, indicating additional investigation needs to be completed to confirm the overall efficacy and extent of potential use of BoNT in inflammation. Botulinum toxin has also been found to deactivate sodium channels resulting in a reduction of neuropathic pain. It is believed to work differently than traditional antiepileptic drugs that block sodium channels in that is changes the sodium current of the excitable membrane. Lastly, there is some belief that BoNT shows axonal transport from the peripheral to central nervous system to exert activity. There are some data to suggest cleavage at SNAP-25 occurs centrally when the drug is administered in facial and trigeminal nerves. The effects of BoNT have been seen bilaterally, even when administered unilaterally, supporting this believed mechanism. However, this theory has not been confirmed and other trials have demonstrated via radio-labeled drug that the BoNT stays at the local site of injection [1]. While the full and exact mechanism of action of BoNT for the treatment of neuropathic pain is not fully understood, it has shown benefit in migraine headaches and small clinical trials for various pain disorders, including TN.

Migraines

Several factors, including genetics and hormones, and various pain pathways all contribute to migraine headaches. One pathway is the trigeminovascular system, which is the sensory innervation of the cerebral vessels with cell bodies on the trigeminal ganglion. The neuron on the trigeminal ganglion submits a signal to the neuron at the trigeminal nucleus caudalis and then on to the thalamus and results in extracranial hypersensitivity. The dura mater vessels are also innervated from nerves through the trigeminal ganglion that have similar aspects as the TRPV1 and other neurotransmitters. The ophthalmic division of the trigeminal nerve has peripheral fibers that are involved in producing pain in the cranial vessels and dura matter and supports the pain experienced in the ophthalmic territory during migraine. Additionally, pain felt in the back of the head is related to where the trigeminal and

Table 13.1 PREEMPT 1 and 2 primary efficacy analysis

	PREEMPT 1		PREEMPT 2	
Reduction in HA days	BoNT	Placebo	BoNT	Placebo
	−5.2	−5.3	−9.0	−6.7

cervical afferents converge at the trigeminocervical complex [5]. Use of BoNT in the prevention of migraine headaches is not only related to the effect on the trigeminal nerve system but this mechanism does contribute to the efficacy of the drug. The PREEMPT trials were the major clinical trials that demonstrated the efficacy of BoNT type A in the prevention of chronic migraine and resulted in an FDA approval of the drug for this indication.

PREEMPT 1 and 2 were randomized, controlled trials demonstrating the safety and efficacy of BoNT in the prevention of migraine headaches in adults [6, 7]. In PREEMPT 1, the primary efficacy endpoint of reduction in headache days was not different between the BoNT and placebo groups. The authors suggest that this outcome was affected by the fact patients in the BoNT arm experienced more headaches and longer duration of headaches that the placebo group at baseline [6]. PREEMPT 2 did show a benefit with the use of BoNT, reducing headache days (primary endpoint) to a greater extent than placebo (Table 13.1). Both trials were designed in the same fashion and efficacy results were evaluated at 24 weeks, after two BoNT injections, 12 weeks apart. Baseline mean of headache days were similar at around 20 days per month and doses of BoNT used were 155–195 U. Injections are administered at several muscle locations and the recommended procedure is as follows (all are bilaterally given, except the procerus muscle): 5 U corrugator, 10 U frontalis, 20 U temporalis, 15 U occipitalis, 10 U cervical paraspinal, and 15 U trapezious (Fig. 13.1) [2].

There are very limited data for use of BoNT in children with migraine (Table 13.2). Two retrospective reviews were completed; one with 10 patients and a second with 30 patients [8, 9]. Both utilized BoNT in a similar manner to the PREEMPT trials. The first review included patients age 8–18 years, with the majority (12 patients) between the ages of 16 and 18 years. The mean age in the second trial was 16.5 ± 1.83 years of age. In both trials, patients experienced a reduction in headaches and the drug was tolerated. Further prospective randomized trials should be completed to confirm the efficacy and safety of BoNT in children and adolescents.

Trigeminal Neuralgia

There were for main randomized trials describing the efficacy of BoNT in TN. These are accompanied by several case reports of use and efficacy of the drug. Meta-analyses and systematic reviews were also completed reporting on the use of BoNT in TN; however, the same randomized trials were used for each of the reviews. All the trials utilized BoNT type A, with varying doses, administration sites, and administration techniques.

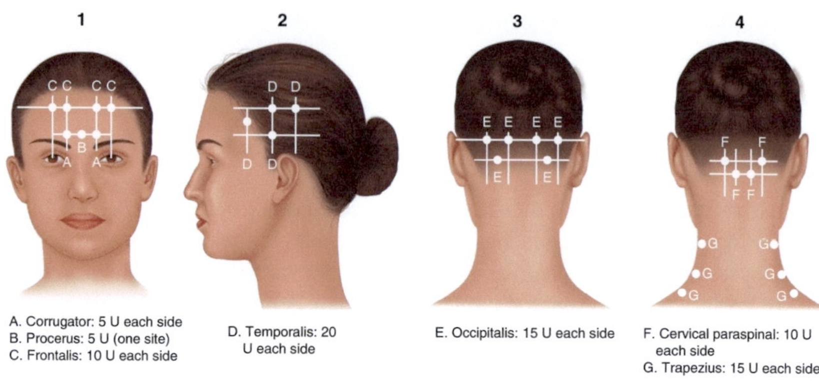

Fig. 13.1 Botulinum injection regimen for migraines [2]

Table 13.2 Reduction in headache days in pediatric BoNT retrospective reviews

	Headache days at baseline	Headache days posttreatment
Shah et al. [8] (10 patients)	15 (8, 29)	4 (2, 10)
Ali et al. [9] (30 patients)	24.4 ± 7.49	14.8 ± 12.52

Wu et al. complete a randomized, placebo-controlled trial evaluating the efficacy of BoNT type A in patient with TN [10]. A total of 42 patients were randomized to receive either BoNT type A 75 U ($n = 22$) or saline ($n = 20$). The trial lasted 13 weeks. Patients were an average of 58 years old and most were on other drug treatment for TN. Primary endpoints were pain severity, using the 11-point Visual Analogue Scale (VAS) and reduction of pain attacks per day. Percent of responders was also assessed, with a 50% reduction in pain considered a response to therapy. Drug was administered at 15 sites, 5 U at each site, intradermally and submucosally, as determined by the pain identified by the patient. Saline was given in the same manner (Fig. 13.2).

Patients receiving BoNT type A had a greater reduction in pain, less pain attacks, and responded more frequently than those receiving saline (Table 13.3)

Zhang et al. completed a very similar trial [11]. The main difference was the treatment groups. The study included three groups, using two different doses of BoNT and placebo: BoNT type A 25 U ($n = 27$), 75 U ($n = 29$), and placebo ($n = 28$). This study was only 8 weeks in duration. Drug was given intradermally or submucosally in 20 different locations depending on the patient's description of the pain. Patients receiving BoNT type A had a significantly better response than those receiving placebo; however, there was no difference in response between the two BoNT doses. The response rates of a pain reduction of at least 50% were as follows: BoNT 25 U, 70.4%; BoNT 75 U, 86.2%; and placebo 32.1%; $p < 0.017$ between treatment and placebo groups and $p > 0.05$ (not significant) between the two BoNT groups.

In the trial by Shehata et al. 20 patients were randomized to receive BoNT Type A ($n = 10$) or placebo ($n = 10$) [12]. Patients in the BoNT group received between 40 and 60 U, doses were given subcutaneously based on location of pain and follow-up assessment was at 12 weeks. The primary endpoint was the reduction of pain

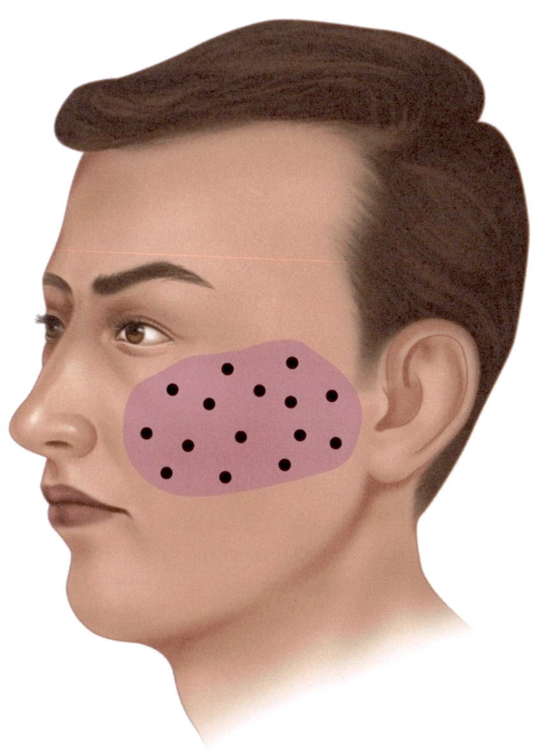

Fig. 13.2 Injection sites for botulinum and placebo in area of trigeminal neuralgia pain [10]

Table 13.3 Efficacy endpoints

	BoNT Type A	Saline	p value
VAS score at week 12	1.5	5.5	<0.05
Mean pain attacks per day at week 12	1	19	<0.05
Responders (≥50 reduction in pain)	68.18%	15.00%	<0.01

based on VAS. The patients treated with BoNT had a significantly greater reduction than those patients receiving placebo. Baseline pain scores were 8.3 in the BoNT group and 8.5 in the placebo group. Final pain scores at week 12 were 1.8 in the BoNT group and 8.2 in the placebo group ($p < 0.0001$).

Zuniga et al. demonstrated similar results as the above three trials [13]. In this trial, BoNT type A 50 U ($n = 20$) was used and compared to placebo ($n = 16$). The drug was given subcutaneously and the change in pain score was assessed at 12 weeks. A significant difference in pain reduction was seen between groups, BoNT, 4.75; placebo 6.94, $p = 0.01$.

Side effects in the trials were not severe and were typical of BoNT adverse events, with facial asymmetry occurring in several patients in each trial [14].

In the meta-analysis completed by Morra ME et al. combined the results of these studies in order to group the smaller studies and evaluate the overall efficacy seen with BoNT for the treatment of TN [14]. In the analysis, all outcomes favored BoNT, despite the varying doses and methods used for administration. All of the data suggest that BoNT improved VAS pain ratings and has an effect that lasts at least 12 weeks in many cases. However, since the trials did not evaluate response past 12 weeks, it cannot be known if repeated injections are needed or how often repeated injections may be needed based on the available data. The dose was not standardized between trials. The trial by Zhang et al. did determine that a higher dose (75 U) did not produce a significantly better response than a lower dose (25 U), suggesting higher doses are not needed to elicit a response [11]. There also was an open-label trial that demonstrated efficacy at doses as low as 6.45–9.11 U [13].

Boru et al. completed an open-label trial to assess the long-term effects of BoNT in the treatment of TN in 27 patients [15]. Patients were given BoNT type A, 50 U injected into the maxillary root and mandibular root, respectively (Fig. 13.3).

The VAS pain scale, attack frequency, and percent of responders were assessed at week 1, month 2, and month 6. If patients' pain returned, they were given another injection in the same manner as the first (Table 13.4).

Fifteen patients (55.5%) required a second dose of BoNT at 2 months and seven of those 15 (47%) required a third dose within the 6-month period. Twelve patients (44.4%) were pain free at 6 months. One patient did not get any pain relief despite getting three injections over the 6-month period. The trial is ongoing and two

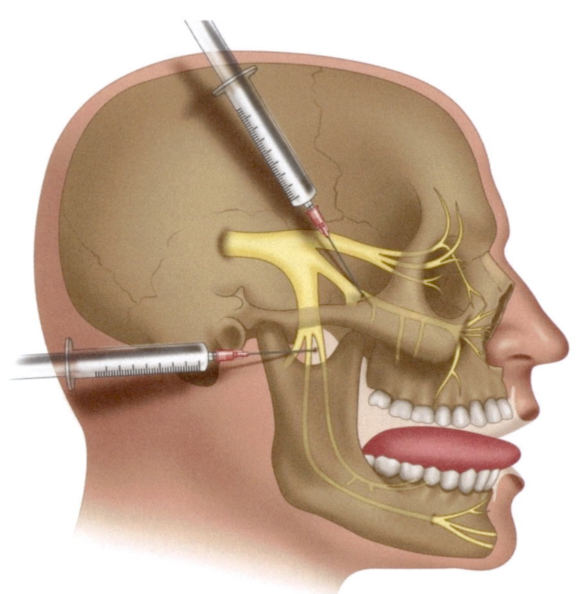

Fig. 13.3 Botulinum injection into maxillary and mandibular root [15]

Table 13.4 Efficacy outcomes baseline vs. 6 months

VAS		Pain attacks per day		% Responders at 6 months
9.7 ± 0.6	1.6 ± 2.4	217.7 ± 331.5	55.15 ± 196.2	88.9%

patients are still pain free at 2 years; however, it is not reported what the frequency or quantity of injections are for the ongoing trial. The injection method used in this trial differed from the randomized controlled trials. The trial did demonstrate efficacy of BoNT in TN and suggested results could last over time; potentially with regularly repeated injections. However, it was an open-label design with no control group, so more data are needed to understand ongoing efficacy.

In a review of adverse events reported from clinical trials of myofascial pain and TN, it was concluded that BoNT is safe without any major adverse events [16]. The most commonly reported events in the TN trials were weakness at the injection site, short-term facial asymmetry and edema, itching, and pain at the injection sites. The majority of events resolved spontaneously. Liu et al. completed a trial to assess safety and efficacy in patients 80 years old and older [17]. A total of 43 patients were enrolled in the trial, 14 patients 80 years and older, and 29 patients under 60 years of age. The doses of BoNT type A was 91.3 ± 25.6 U in the older group and 71.8 ± 33.1 U in the younger group (no difference, $p = 0.061$). Both groups had reductions in VAS score and there was no difference between the age groups. In the 80 and over group, VAS score at baseline was 8.5 and reduced to 4.5 at 1 month. In the younger group, VAS score decreased from 8.0 to 5.0. Two patients in each group experienced minor side effects that resolved on their own.

All of the available data for use of BoNT in TN is limited by trial size or design. The dose and injection techniques vary from trial to trial, so a standardized dose and method of treatment are not determined. It is not known how long the effects of BoNT last for patients with TN or how often a repeat injection would be needed. However, all of the data suggest positive results when BoNT is used to treat TN that is not responding adequately to traditional first-line therapies and could serve as a treatment regimen before surgical intervention is pursued.

The European Academy of Neurology guideline on trigeminal neuralgia that was developed in 2019 suggests BoNT can be considered as add-on treatment [18]. This recommendation was based on the data from the clinical trials reviewed here.

Botulinum toxin has become a standard treatment in patients with chronic migraine who have not responded adequately to other preventive measures. Not all patients respond to therapy, but a significant portion has at least some reduction in headache frequency or severity, which often occurs after multiple injections of BoNT given every 12 weeks. The drug is not considered standard treatment for TN due to limited high-quality data; however, can be considered for use as part of the treatment plan in patients who fail to respond or lose response to standard therapy. More data are needed to confirm what an adequate dosing regimen would be in the treatment of TN. Available information suggests low doses given at 12 week or longer increments could be beneficial but no set dosing regimen is defined.

References

1. Park J, Park HJ. Botulinum toxin for the treatment of neuropathic pain. Toxins. 2017;9:260. https://doi.org/10.3390/toxins9090260.
2. Botox. Package insert. Allergan; 2019.

3. Nugent M, Yusef YR, Meng J, Wang J, Dolly JO. A SNAP-25 cleaving chimera of botulinum neurotoxin /A and /E prevents TNFα-induced elevation of the activities of native TRP channels on early postnatal rat dorsal root ganglion neurons. Neuropharmacology. 2018;138:257–66.

4. Lucioni A, Bales GT, Lotan TL, McGehee DS, Cook SP, Rapp DE. Botulinum toxin type A inhibits sensory neuropeptide release in rat bladder models of acute injury and chronic inflammation. BJU Int. 2008;101:366–70.

5. Dima L, Balan A, Moga MA, Dinu CG, Dimienescu OG, Varga I, et al. Botulinum toxin a valuable prophylactic agent for migraines and a possible future option for prevention of hormonal variations-triggered migraines. Toxins. 2019;11:465. https://doi.org/10.3390/toxins11080465.

6. Aurora SK, Dodick DW, Turkel CC, DeGryse RE, Silbertstein SD, Lipton RB, et al. OnabotulinumtoxinA for treatment of chronic migraine: results from the double-blind, randomized, placebo-controlled phase of the PREEMPT I trial. Cephalalgia. 2010;30:793–803. https://doi.org/10.1177/0333102410364676.

7. Deiner HC, Dodick DW, Aurora SK, Turkel CC, DeGryse RE, Lipton RB, et al. OnabotulinumtoxinA for the treatment of chronic migraine:results from the double-blind, randomized, placebo-controlled phase of the PREEMPT 2 trial. Cephalagia. 2010;30:804–14. https://doi.org/10.1177/0333102410364677.

8. Shah S, Calderon MD, Wu WD, Grant J, Rinehart J. Onabotulinumtoxin A (Botox) for the prophylactic treatment of pediatric migraine:a retrospective longitudinal analysis. J Child Neurol. 2018;33:580–6.

9. Ali SS, Bragin I, Rende E, Mejico L, Werner KE. Further evidence that onabotulinum toxin is a viable treatment option for pediatric chronic migraine patients. Cureus. 2019;11:e4343. https://doi.org/10.7759/cureus.4343.

10. Wu CJ, Lian YJ, Zheng YK, Zhang HF, Chen Y, Xie NC, et al. Botulinum toxin type A for the treatment of trigeminal neuralgia:results from a randomized, double-blind, placebo-controlled trial. Cephalagia. 2012;32:443–50. https://doi.org/10.1177/0333102412441721.

11. Zhang H, Lian Y, Ma Y, Chen Y, He C, Xie N, et al. Two doses of botulinum toxin type A for the treatment of trigeminal neuralgia:observation of therapeutic effect from randomized, double-blind, placebo-controlled trial. J Headache Pain. 2014;15:65. http://www.thejournalof-headacheandpain.com/content/15/1/65

12. Shehata HS, El-Tamawy MS, Shalaby NM, Ramzy G. Botulinum toxin-type A: could it be an effective treatment option in intractable trigeminal neuralgia? J Headache Pain. 2013;14:92. http://www.thejournalofheadacheandpain.com/content/14/1/92

13. Zuniga C, Piedimonte F, Diaz S, Micheli F. Acute treatment of trigeminal neuralgia with onabotulinum toxin A. Clin Neuropharamcol. 2013;36(5):146–50.

14. Morra ME, Elgebaly A, Elmaraezy A, Khalil AM, Altibi AM, Vu TLH, et al. Therapeutic efficacy and safety of botulinum toxin A therapy in trigeminal neuralgia: a systematic review and meta-analysis of randomized controlled trials. J Headache Pain. 2016;17:63. https://doi.org/10.1186/s10194-016-0651-8.

15. Boru UT, Duman A, Boluk C, Duman SC, Tasdemir M. Botulinum toxin in the treatment of trigeminal neuralgia: 6-month follow-up. Medicine. 2017;96:e8133. https://doi.org/10.1097/MD.0000000000008133.

16. De la Torre Canales G, Poluha RL, Lora VM, Ferreira DMAO, Stuginski-Barbosa J, Bonjardim LR, et al. Botulinum toxin type A applications for masticatory myofascial pain and trigeminal neuralgia: what is the evidence regarding adverse events? Clin Oral Investig. 2019;23:3411–21.

17. Liu J, Xu YY, Zhang QL, Luo WF. Efficacy and safety of botulinum toxin type A in treating patients of advanced age with idiopathic trigeminal neuralgia. Pain Res Manag. 2018;2018:7365148. https://doi.org/10.1155/2018/7365148.

18. Bendtsen L, Zakrzewska JM, Abbott J, Braschinsky M, Di Stefano G, Donnet A, et al. European Academy of Neurology guideline in trigeminal neuralgia. Neurology. 2019;26:831–49. https://doi.org/10.1111/ene.13950.

Regenerative Medicine for Trigeminal Nerve Pain

14

Chandni B. Patel, Ankur A. Patel,
and George C. Chang Chien

Introduction

The field of regenerative medicine has exponentially grown over the past two decades. Broadly speaking, regenerative medicine focuses on administering cells or their products to damaged tissues to stimulate the body's innate repair mechanisms to induce healing and restoration of function. Regenerative therapies, including platelet-rich plasma (PRP) and stem cell therapy, have been at the forefront in the treatment of peripheral nerve disorders, such as trigeminal neuralgia (TN) and other trigeminal nerve conditions. The application of regenerative therapies for trigeminal nerve disorders and other peripheral nerve disorders will be the focus of this chapter.

Mechanism of Action

Before the application of regenerative therapies can be discussed, it is important to review the proposed mechanism of action.

C. B. Patel
Department of Physical Medicine and Rehabilitation, Icahn School of Medicine, Mount Sinai Hospital, New York, NY, USA

A. A. Patel (✉)
Department of Physical Medicine and Rehabilitation, New York-Presbyterian Hospital, Columbia University Irving Medical Center and Weill Cornell Medical Center, New York, NY, USA

G. C. Chang Chien
GCC Regenerative Medicine Institute, Irvine, CA, USA

GCC Regenerative Medicine Institute, Newport Beach, CA, USA

A. Abd-Elsayed (ed.), *Trigeminal Nerve Pain*,
https://doi.org/10.1007/978-3-030-60687-9_14

Platelet-Rich Plasma

Platelet-rich plasma is a preparation of autologous plasma containing a concentration of platelets above baseline produced by centrifuging blood [1, 2]. Platelets are anucleate, disc-shaped, and cytoplasmic fragments of megakaryocytes responsible for hemostasis. Platelet activation occurs in the setting of injury to vascular endothelium, leading to platelet adhesion, and aggregation. After activation, signaling pathways are initiated with subsequent secretion of alpha granules releasing a plethora of growth factors and mediators [2, 3].

The clinical application of PRP lies in these growth factors and mediators possessing regenerative properties [4]. Growth factors released include platelet-derived growth factor (PDGF), transforming growth factors (TGF), insulin-like growth factor 1 (IGF-1), epidermal growth factor (EGF), vascular endothelial growth factor (VEGF), and fibroblast growth factor B (FGF-B). Cytokines released include pro- and anti-inflammatory factors.

Platelet-rich plasma is prepared by centrifuging whole blood separating it into three layers: red blood cells (RBCs), platelet-poor plasma (PPP), and "buffy coat" [2, 4]. Platelets are then isolated using various methods and ready for injection into a patient. PRP preparations are categorized into leukocyte-rich PRP (LR-PRP) and leukocyte-poor (LP-PRP), containing neutrophil concentrations above and below baseline, respectively [2]. The elevated neutrophil levels in LR-PRP are associated with pro-inflammatory effects and catabolic cytokines including interleukin-1 beta and tumor necrosis factor-alpha.

Platelet-rich plasma is one of the most common and readily available regenerative medicine therapies [4]. Although PRP deems a promising modality within musculoskeletal medicine, evidence on efficacy is mixed depending on PRP composition and application [2].

Stem Cell Therapy

Stem cells are derived from different tissues and have the potential to differentiate into various cell types. The application of these cells is called stem cell therapy. Specifically, stem cell therapy uses non-embryonic somatic cells or adult cells called mesenchymal stem cells (MSCs) and hematopoietic stem cells (HSCs). Mesenchymal cells have the potential to give rise to osteoblasts, osteocytes, chondrocytes, adipocytes, myocytes, and stromal cells [4]. Clinically, the most common source of MSCs is adipose tissue [4, 5]. Hematopoietic stem cells have the potential to give rise to blood cells including red blood cells, B and T lymphocytes, natural killer cells, neutrophils, basophils, eosinophils, monocytes, and macrophages [4]. Clinically, the most common source of HSCs is bone marrow [4, 6].

Mechanism of Regenerative Therapies on Neuropathic Pain

Neuropathic pain is a sharp and burning sensation caused by damage to the somatosensory nervous system in the form of compression, trauma, infection, or metabolic abnormalities [7].

Specifically, neuropathic pain pathophysiologically stems from molecular and cellular level changes involving chemokines and their receptors modulating neuronal electrical activity leading to increased neurotransmitter release and subsequent activation of pain pathways [8].

The role of regenerative medicine in neuropathic pain management lies in the platelets and stem cells leading to wound healing and re-establishment of normal nerve function. One theorized mechanism of action of the use of regenerative therapies in the treatment of neuropathic pain is axon regeneration and tissue reinnervation mediated by growth factors, IGF-1 and VEGF [9]. Specifically, VEGF promotes Schwann cell proliferation thus facilitating axonal growth and angiogenesis enhancing vascular permeability.

Mesenchymal stem cells have reported anti-inflammatory effect through cytokine release and differentiation into Schwann cells secreting growth factors, nerve growth factor (NGF) and brain-derived neurotrophic factor (BDNF), contributing to nerve healing and regeneration [10, 11]. Together, these factors reduce excitatory nerve activity resulting in neuropathic pain management.

Use in Trigeminal Nerve Conditions

The use of PRP and stem cell therapy have expanded to various musculoskeletal and pain conditions, including neuropathic pain, discogenic pain, osteoarthritis, and musculoskeletal diseases, over the past two decades [12]. Specifically, the use of regenerative therapies for neuropathic pain is a growing area of interest and will be the main focus of this chapter.

Neuropathic pain is one of the most difficult pain conditions to treat. Affecting about 6% of the population, it is poorly managed with over-the-counter analgesics and opioids [12]. Current first-line management includes serotonin and norepinephrine reuptake inhibitors (SNRIs), tricyclic antidepressants (TCAs), and anticonvulsants acting at calcium channels [13].

A common cause of neuropathic pain includes pain within the distribution of the trigeminal nerve. Such conditions include trigeminal neuralgia, secondary trigeminal neuralgia, idiopathic trigeminal neuralgia, trigeminal neuropathy, and postherpetic neuralgia. Of these conditions, TN is the most prevalent. Trigeminal neuralgia is a disease process first documented in the 1600s characterized as episodic, unilateral pain localized to the face in the distribution of the trigeminal nerve [14]. Common descriptors of the pain include sharp, burning, and stabbing. Pain is commonly localized to the maxillary (V2) or mandibular (V3) branches [15].

In the literature, limited studies are discussing the use of regenerative therapies for TN. Stamotoski et al. conducted a prospective pilot study with 29 patients experiencing unspecified trigeminal nerve pain [16]. Patients were injected with PRP a total of five times with each injection being 7 days apart. Pain scores measured by visual analogue scale (VAS) were recorded prior to each injection, and at 2 and 6 months follow up. Prior to the first application, mean VAS was 9.1 and continued to downtrend and was reported to be 0.1 before the fifth application and 0.0 at 6 months follow up.

Vickers et al. conducted a prospective observational study with 10 subjects who underwent lipoaspirate MSCs injection into the center of pain and adjacent pain field of the affected branches of the trigeminal nerve [10]. The patients presented with different etiologies of trigeminal nerve pain. Seven of these patients experienced atypical odontalagia secondary to tooth extractions, dental crowns, or dental implants. Two of the patients had idiopathic facial neuropathic pain. One patient experienced trigeminal nerve pain due to idiopathic trigeminal autonomic cephalgia. Patients were followed up 6 months post injection and revealed a decrease in mean pain score from 7.5 to 4.3 and a reduction in anti-neuropathic pain medications in 5/9 subjects.

Although the studies by Stamotoski et al. and Vickers et al. alluded to promising results for trigeminal nerve pain with the use of respective regenerative therapies, it is important to note that these studies represented a small sample size and were not controlled. Randomized controlled trials are the next step to evaluate the efficacy of these therapies for trigeminal nerve pain and long-term outcomes. However, at the time this chapter was written, there were no on-going clinical trials evaluating the use of regenerative therapies for trigeminal nerve pain listed in the clinicaltrails.gov database.

Use of Regenerative Therapies in Other Peripheral Nerve Diseases

Although there are limited studies evaluating the efficacy of regenerative therapies for trigeminal nerve disorders, there are a number of prospective studies assessing the use of these therapies for other peripheral neuralgias.

One such peripheral nerve disorder targeted by regenerative medicine is pudendal neuralgia. Venturi et al. conducted a prospective, observational study involving 15 patients who received transperineal injections of autologous lipoaspirate MSCs targeting the pudendal nerve [17]. At 12 months follow up, the mean VAS significantly decreased from 8.1 to 3.2. Although the reduction in pain score was significant, there was no control group in this study, and two patients were excluded due to no improvement in pain.

Carpal tunnel syndrome (CTS) is one of the most studied peripheral nerve disorders regarding the application of regenerative therapies, specifically using PRP. Two studies in particular investigated the use of PRP versus control in the setting of mild to moderate idiopathic CTS. The first study by Güven et al. was a prospective, controlled, observational study evaluating 30 patients [18]. In this study, there was improvement in the Boston Carpal Tunnel Questionnaire (BCTQ) scores and cross-sectional area (CSA) of the median nerve (MN) in both the PRP injection and the control groups at 4 weeks follow up. When assessing the distal motor latency and sensory nerve conduction of the MN through electrodiagnostic testing (EDX), the PRP group had significant improvement in both parameters. Similarly, Malahias et al. conducted a prospective, randomized trial consisting of 50 patients with a placebo-controlled group assessing the Quick-Disabilities of the Arm, Shoulder, and Hand (Q-DASH) questionnaire as one of the primary outcome measures [19]. Based on the Q-DASH questionnaire, there was a statistically significant difference in the PRP group compared to the control group (76.9% success versus 33.3% success, respectively).

The initial management of mild CTS consists of applying a static wrist splint to allow for offloading of the MN within the carpal tunnel. Two major studies evaluated the use of PRP versus conservative wrist splint for mild to moderate CTS. A randomized, single-blinded, controlled trial by Wu et al. evaluated 60 subjects at 1-, 3- and 6-month intervals concluded the group that received PRP therapy had a significant reduction in VAS, BCTQ scores, and CSA of median nerve compared to patients who used only a night splint at 6 months post-injection [20]. Comparatively, Raeissadat et al., found the use of a single injection of PRP did not significantly improve outcomes with and without use of nightly wrist splints at 10 months follow up [21].

With corticosteroid injections as a common modality used in the algorithm for CTS poorly responsive to night splinting, Senna et al. and Uzun et al. compared the effectiveness of PRP versus corticosteroid injections. Senna et al. conducted a prospective, randomized study evaluating 96 subjects with mild to moderate CTS [22]. The authors of this study found significant improvement in VAS, BCTQ, EDX parameters, and CSA of MN for both PRP and corticosteroid injection groups; however, PRP injection group was superior in MN conduction velocity and sensory latency and conduction at three months follow up. In contrast, a quasi-experimental study by Uzun et al. evaluating 40 subjects found no significant difference in nerve conduction studies between both PRP and corticosteroid groups [23].

Prolotherapy, a technique involving repeated injections into a structure triggering an inflammatory response subsequently leading to healing and strengthening of the structure, is a therapy used for many pain syndromes. Shen et al. compared the effects of PRP and prolotherapy using dextrose injections for moderate CTS [24]. Results showed that the PRP group had significant reduction in BCTQ scores at 3 months, distal motor latency at 6 months, and CSA at 3 and 6 months.

Extracorporeal shock wave therapy (ECSWT) is a noninvasive treatment option delivering shock waves to injured tissue aimed at promoting healing and pain reduction. Physicians have applied this therapy as a treatment modality for various musculoskeletal and peripheral nerve disorders including, but not limited to, CTS, Achilles tendonitis, and plantar fasciitis. To evaluate the use of ECSWT, Chang et al. conducted a randomized, double-blind, placebo-controlled study comparing the effects of PRP injection versus PRP injection with radial ECSWT [25]. Results indicated that the combination of RPR and radial ECSWT did not show statistically superior outcomes compared to those managed with PRP only. Although there are cases of pain and functional improvements with the use of ECSWT for peripheral nerve disorders, the use of PRP alone seems to be more beneficial in the setting of CTS.

From the studies discussed in this chapter (Table 14.1), it is suggested that regenerative therapies including stem cells and PRP are emerging modalities in the management of neuropathic pain. However, there is limited evidence in its role in managing trigeminal nerve pain, indicating the need for further investigation at this time, specifically evaluating the efficacy of regenerative therapies for various trigeminal nerve conditions previously discussed.

In conclusion, although there is a paucity of literature supporting the use of regenerative medicine in the treatment of trigeminal nerve pain, there is growing interest in its application for such neuropathic conditions. The use of PRP and stem cell-based therapies may serve to be beneficial for these disorders; however, further prospective, randomized, controlled studies are necessary before incorporating the use of such modalities into standard practice. If determined to be efficacious, the use of regenerative medicine would serve as an alternative to pharmacologic therapies, ablative techniques, and surgical decompression.

Table 14.1 Clinical studies on regenerative medicine for peripheral nerve disorders

Authors (year published)	Study title	Regenerative therapy used	Disease	Study design	Number of subjects	Treatment arms	Outcome measures	Length of follow up	Results	Comments
Stamatoski et al. (2017)	Novel perineural approach of platelet-rich plasma application in idiopathic trigeminal neuralgia treatment: a six-month follow-up pilot study	PRP	Trigeminal neuralgia	Prospective, observational	29	PRP administered 5 times in 7 day intervals	VAS	Prior to each PRP administration, 2 and 6 months	Significant pain reduction evaluated by VAS with mean VAS 9.1 before application I; 7.6 before application II; 3.0 before application III; 0.6 before application IV; 0.1 before application V, 0.0 at third month examination and 0.0 and at sixth month examination 0.0	Pilot study with only abstract published, non-randomized, non-controlled
Vickers et al. (2014)	A preliminary report on stem cell therapy for neuropathic pain in humans	Lipoaspirate MSCs	Trigeminal nerve pain	Prospective, observational	10	Injection of lipoaspirate MSCs	Pain intensity measured by NRS and daily dosage requirements of anti-neuropathic pain medication	6 months	Mean pain score decreased from 7.5 to 4.3 at 6 months post-treatment.	Small study, not controlled

(continued)

Table 14.1 (continued)

Authors (year published)	Study title	Regenerative therapy used	Disease	Study design	Number of subjects	Treatment arms	Outcome measures	Length of follow up	Results	Comments
Venturi et al. (2015)	Pudendal neuralgia: a new option for treatment? Preliminary results on feasibility and efficacy	Lipoaspirate MSCs	Pudendal neuralgia	Prospective, observational	15	Transperineal injections of lipoaspirate MSCs	Clinical examination, PNMTL, SF-36, and VAS	7 days through 12 months	VAS score significantly improved (3.2 vs. 8.1) at 12 months	No control group, three patients did not follow up, two patients excluded due to no improvement in pain
Güven et al. (2019)	Short-term effectiveness of platelet-rich plasma in carpal tunnel syndrome: a controlled study	PRP	Mild to moderate idopathic CTS	Prospective, observational	30	Single 1cc perineural PRP injection vs. control	BCTQ, CSA of MN, EDX	4 weeks	Improvement in BCTQ scores in both group; significant improvement in distal motor latency (ms) and sensory nerve conduction velocity (m/s) in the PRP group and significant improvement in CSA in both groups	Small sample size; no randomization or blinding

Malahias et al. (2018)	Platelet-rich plasma ultrasound-guided injection in the treatment of carpal tunnel syndrome: a placebo-controlled clinical study	PRP	Mild to moderate CTS	Prospective, randomized trial	50	Ultrasound Guided PRP injection into carpal tunnel vs. placebo (0.9% NS)	Q-DASH , VAS	0, 4, and 12 weeks	PRP injection group demonstrated a 76.9% success, whereas placebo group demonstrated 33.3% success, which was significantly less than PRP group	Q-DASH obtained pre-injection minus the final Q-DASH obtained after 12 weeks follow-up. Success was defined as a difference more than 25% in Q-DASH
Wu et al. (2017)	Six-month efficacy of platelet-rich plasma for carpal tunnel syndrome: a prospective randomized, single-blind controlled trial	PRP	Unilateral mild to moderate CTS	Randomized, single-blind, control trial	60	One dose 3 ml PRP vs. night splint	BCTQ, CSA of MN, EDX, finger pinch strength, VAS	1, 3, and 6 months	PRP group had significant reduction in VAS, BCTQ score, and CSA of MN compared to the control group at 6 months post-treatment	

(continued)

Table 14.1 (continued)

Authors (year published)	Study title	Regenerative therapy used	Disease	Study design	Number of subjects	Treatment arms	Outcome measures	Length of follow up	Results	Comments
Raeissadat et al. (2018)	Safety and efficacy of platelet-rich plasma in treatment of carpal tunnel syndrome; a randomized controlled trial	PRP	Mild to moderate idopathic CTS	Randomized controlled trial	41	PRP injection with splinting vs. wrist splint only	BCTQ, EDX, VAS	10 weeks	A single injection of PRP does not significantly add to the effects of conservative management with wrist spints at 10 months follow up	Limited interval follow up
Senna et al. (2019)	Platelet-rich plasma in treatment of patients with idiopathic carpal tunnel syndrome	PRP	Mild to moderate idopathic CTS	Prospective, randomized, observational	98	PRP injection vs. corticosteroid injection	BCTQ, CSA of MN, EDX, VAS	1 month and 3 months	Significant improvement in VAS, BCTQ, EDX parameters and CSA of the MN for both groups; however, PRP injection was superior to steroid injection in improvement of MN motor conduction velocity, sensory latency and conduction, particularly at 3 months	Moderate sample size compared to similar studies, shorter follow-up interval

Uzun et al. (2016)	Platelet-rich plasma versus corticosterorid injections for carpal tunnel syndrome	PRP	Mild CTS	Prospective, quasi-experimental	40	PRP injections vs. corticosteroid injections	BCTQ, EDX	3 and 6 months	No significant difference between groups in NCS. In BCTQ, both symptom severity and functional capacity score of PRP group were significantly better than corticosteroid group at 3 months; however, no significant difference at 6 months	Small study, non-randomized, single-blinded study posing potenial bias
Shen et al. (2019)	Comparison of perineural platelet-rich plasma and dextrose injections for moderate carpal tunnel syndrome: a prospective randomized, single-blind, head-to-head comparative trial	PRP	Unilateral, moderate CTS	Prospective, randomized, single-blind	52	Single perineural injection with PRP or D5W	BCTQ, CSA of MN, EDX	1, 3, and 6 months post-injection	PRP group had significant reduction in BCTQ at 3 months, distal motor latency at 6 months, and CSA at 3 and 6 months. A single perineural injection of PRP reduced the CSA of the MN more effectively than D5 injection at 3 and 6 months	Potential bias from single-blinded study commented on per author

(continued)

Table 14.1 (continued)

Authors (year published)	Study title	Regenerative therapy used	Disease	Study design	Number of subjects	Treatment arms	Outcome measures	Length of follow up	Results	Comments
Chang et al. (2019)	The effectiveness of platelet-rich plasma and radial extracorporeal shock wave compared with platelet-rich plasma in the treatment of moderate carpal tunnel syndrome	PRP	Moderate CTS	Randomized, double-blind, placebo-controlled trial	40	PRP injection with radial ECSWT vs. PRP injection only	BCTQ, CSA of MN, EDX	1, 3, and 6 months post-PRP injection	The PRP + ECSWT group did not show statistically significant superior outcomes, except BCTQs at 1 month and distal motor latency at 3 months	No control group

Abbreviations: *BCTQ* Boston Carpal Tunnel Questionnaire, *CSA* cross sectional area, *CTS* carpal tunnel syndrome, *D5W* 5% dexrose in water, *ECSWT* extracorporeal shock-wave therapy, *EDX* electrodiagnostic testing, *MN* median nerve, *MSCs* mesenchymal stem cells, *NRS* Numerical Rating Scale, *NS* normal saline, *PNMTL* Pudendal Nerve Motor Terminal Latency, *PRP* platelet rich plasma, *Q-DASH* Quick Disabilities of the Arm, Shoulder and Hand, *SF-36* Short Form Health Survey, *VAS* Visual Analog Scale

References

1. Marx RE. Platelet-rich plasma (PRP): what is PRP and what is not PRP? Implant Dent. 2001;10(4):225–8. https://doi.org/10.1097/00008505-200110000-00002.
2. Le ADK, Enweze L, DeBaun MR, Dragoo JL. Current clinical recommendations for use of platelet-rich plasma. Curr Rev Musculoskelet Med. 2018;11:624–34.
3. Hosseinzadegan H, Tafti DK. Mechanisms of platelet activation, adhesion and aggregation. Thromb Haemost Res. 2017;1:1008.
4. Chen H, Purita J, Nguyen M. Regenerative medicine for pain management. In: Yong RJ, Nguyen M, Nelson E, Urman RD, editors. Pain Medicine. An essential review. Cham: Springer International; 2017. p. 575–80.
5. Bosetti M, Borrone A, Follenzi A, Messaggio F, Tremolada C, Cannas M. Human lipoaspirate as autologous injectable active scaffold for one-step repair of cartilage defects. Cell Transplant. 2016;25:1043–56.
6. Centeno CJ, Al-Sayegh H, Bashir J, Goodyear SH, D Freeman M. A prospective multi-Site registry study of a specific protocol of autologous bone marrow concentrate for the treatment of shoulder rotator cuff tears and osteoarthritis. J Pain Res. 2015;8:269–76.
7. Kuffler DP. Platelet-rich plasma and the elimination of neuropathic pain. Mol Neurobiol. 2013;48:315–32.
8. Dadon-Nachum M, Sadan O, Srugo I, Melamed E, Offen D. Differentiated mesenchymal stem cells for sciatic nerve injury. Stem Cell Rev Rep. 2011;7:664–71.
9. Takeuchi M, Kamei N, Shinomiya R, Sunagawa T, Suzuki O, Kamoda H, Ohtori S, Ochi M. Human platelet-rich plasma promotes axon growth in brain-spinal cord coculture. Neuroreport. 2012;23:712–6.
10. Vickers ER, Karsten E, Flood J, Lilischkis R. A preliminary report on stem cell therapy for neuropathic pain in humans. J Pain Res. 2014;7:255–63.
11. Wang X, Luo E, Li Y, Hu J. Schwann-like mesenchymal stem cells within vein graft facilitate facial nerve regeneration and remyelination. Brain Res. 2011;1383:71–80.
12. Chakravarthy K, Chen Y, He C, Christo PJ. Stem cell therapy for chronic pain management: review of uses, advances, and adverse effects. Pain Physician. 2017;20:293–305.
13. Fornasari D. Pharmacotherapy for neuropathic pain: a review. Pain Ther. 2017;6:25–33.
14. Patel SK, Liu JK. Overview and history of trigeminal neuralgia. Neurosurg Clin N Am. 2016;27:265–76.
15. Olesen J. Headache Classification Committee of the International Headache Society (IHS) The International Classification of Headache Disorders, 3rd edn. Cephalalgia. 2018;38:1–211.
16. Stamatoski A, Fidoski J. Novel perineural approach of platelet-rich plasma application in idiopathic trigeminal neuralgia treatment: a six-month follow-up pilot study. Int J Oral Maxillofac Surg. 2017; https://doi.org/10.1016/j.ijom.2017.02.1259.
17. Venturi M, Boccasanta P, Lombardi B, Brambilla M, Contessini Avesani E, Vergani C. Pudendal neuralgia: A new option for treatment? Preliminary results on feasibility and efficacy. Pain Med. 2015;16:1475–81.
18. Güven SC, Özçakar L, Kaymak B, Kara M, Akıncı A. Short-term effectiveness of platelet-rich plasma in carpal tunnel syndrome: a controlled study. J Tissue Eng Regen Med. 2019;13:709–14.
19. Malahias MA, Nikolaou VS, Johnson EO, Kaseta MK, Kazas ST, Babis GC. Platelet-rich plasma ultrasound-guided injection in the treatment of carpal tunnel syndrome: a placebo-controlled clinical study. J Tissue Eng Regen Med. 2018;12:e1480–8.
20. Wu YT, Ho TY, Chou YC, Ke MJ, Li TY, Huang GS, Chen LC. Six-month efficacy of platelet-rich plasma for carpal tunnel syndrome: a prospective randomized, singleblind controlled trial. Sci Rep. 2017;7:1–11.
21. Raeissadat SA, Karimzadeh A, Hashemi M, Bagherzadeh L. Safety and efficacy of platelet-rich plasma in treatment of carpal tunnel syndrome: a randomized controlled trial. BMC Musculoskelet Disord. 2018;19:1–6.

22. Senna MK, Shaat RM, Ali AAA. Platelet-rich plasma in treatment of patients with idiopathic carpal tunnel syndrome. Clin Rheumatol. 2019;38:3643–54.
23. Uzun H, Bitik O, Uzun Ö, Ersoy US, Aktaş E. Platelet-rich plasma versus corticosteroid injections for carpal tunnel syndrome. J Plast Surg Hand Surg. 2017;51:301–5.
24. Shen YP, Li TY, Chou YC, Ho TY, Ke MJ, Chen LC, Wu YT. Comparison of perineural platelet-rich plasma and dextrose injections for moderate carpal tunnel syndrome: a prospective randomized, single-blind, head-to-head comparative trial. J Tissue Eng Regen Med. 2019;13:2009–17.
25. Chang C-Y, Chen L-C, Chou Y-C, Li T-Y, Ho T-Y, Wu Y-T. The effectiveness of platelet-rich plasma and radial extracorporeal shock wave compared with platelet-rich plasma in the treatment of moderate carpal tunnel syndrome. Pain Med. 2019;21:1–8.

Neuromodulation for the Trigeminal Nerve

15

Lynn Kohan, Janki Patel, Alaa Abd-Elsayed, and Matthew Riley

Introduction

The International Neuromodulation Society has defined neuromodulation as technology with direct effects on nerves that alters nerve activity by targeted electrical or pharmaceutical agent delivery [1]. Neuromodulation is based on the gate control theory proposed by Malzeck in 1965. He theorized that nociceptive input is perceived in the brain through pain signals transmitted by small-diameter fibers in the dorsal horn of the spinal cord when they overpower the non-nociceptive signals that are carried by large-diameter fibers. In other words, non-nociceptive sensory fiber signals are able to close the "gates" to nociceptive input when stimulated. An example of this would be a painful sensation being relieved when massaging or rubbing the affected area [2].

Neuromodulation in the treatment of trigeminal nerve pain can be divided into two broad categories: intracranial and extracranial treatments. Intracranial treatments include deep brain stimulation (DBS), motor cortex stimulation (MCS), and gasserian ganglion stimulation. Deep brain stimulation has been most commonly used to treat Parkinson's and essential tremors. However, it has also been found to be effective in treating trigeminal autonomic cephalgias such as cluster headache

L. Kohan · J. Patel · M. Riley (✉)
Department of Anesthesiology, University of Virginia, Charlottesville, VA, USA
e-mail: mdr5gx@hscmail.mcc.virginia.edu; Jp9vt@hscmail.mcc.virginia.edu;
Lrk9g@hscmail.mcc.virginia.edu

A. Abd-Elsayed
Department of Anesthesiology, University of Wisconsin School of Medicine and Public Health, Madison, WI, USA
e-mail: abdelsayed@wisc.edu

A. Abd-Elsayed (ed.), *Trigeminal Nerve Pain*,
https://doi.org/10.1007/978-3-030-60687-9_15

and further hypothesized that DBS can be effective in reducing the pain of other trigeminal nerve pathologies [3]. Motor cortex stimulation can be used for thalamic pain and atypical facial pain syndromes. The process involves placing electrodes into the epidural space over the motor cortex through small burr holes. Stimulation of the contralateral motor cortex is postulated to cause corticocortical feedback with inhibition of the active sensory cortex nociceptive neurons. Potential risks of MCS include lead infection, epidural hematoma, or seizures [4]. Intracranial techniques can potentially modulate more nerve signals over larger areas of innervation compared to extracranial techniques but are generally higher risk procedures with more serious complications such as seizures, intracranial bleeding, and intracranial infections.

Extracranial stimulation methods include spinal cord stimulation (SCS), peripheral nerve stimulation (PNS), subcutaneous peripheral nerve field stimulation (PNFS), and transcutaneous electrical nerve stimulation (TENS). Dorsal column stimulation, now known as spinal cord stimulation, targets several different areas of the brainstem and high cervical spine and has shown early promise in the treatment of trigeminal nerve pain. The cervicomedullary junction is a common target for stimulation for the management of general headaches and facial pain syndromes [5]. A more specific target for trigeminal neuralgia is the route of entry to the caudal dorsal nucleus [6]. Stimulation over the second-order neurons in the trigeminocervical complex, which projects from the trigeminal nucleus caudalis in the cervical spine, has potential neuromodulation effects in the trigeminal and occipital distributions of the head. In peripheral nerve stimulation, the leads are placed adjacent to the nerve or within the peripheral nerve's distribution. The branches of the trigeminal nerve, including the ophthalmic, maxillary, and mandibular branches are the most common targets for PNS. However, targeting more distal branches such as the supraorbital, infraorbital, and auriculotemporal nerves may prove to be useful targets as well [7]. Transcutaneous electrical nerve stimulation involves placing padded electrodes on the skin in the areas of pain. This method has the least amount of adverse effects noted of all the techniques discussed above. Possible adverse reactions include skin sensitivity to the electrode pads and possible paresthesia sensations when the affected area is stimulated. Extracranial approaches offer targeted treatment usually over a smaller distribution than intracranial but with the possibility of less severe adverse effects or complications.

Patient Selection

There are many approaches to neuromodulation and each presents its own risks, invasiveness, and potential for complication. Different approaches may vary in selection criteria but there are general criteria that the treating physician or team should consider before determining candidacy for neuromodulation therapy. Apart from a few transcutaneous stimulators, many neuromodulator therapies are performed via implanted electrodes. Implant criteria include: a patient's failure of first-line therapies, the surgical approach can be safely performed, the patient is an appropriate candidate for a surgical procedure, a stimulation trial was successful, the patient understands the risks and benefits of the procedure, the patient has undergone a psychological evaluation and deemed an adequate candidate [8]. Additional considerations that may preclude a patient from implantation of neuromodulatory devices include a need for long-term anticoagulation, MRI compatibility of devices, presence of an implanted pacemaker, comorbidities such as the history of drug abuse, poor medical compliance, current medico-legal issues, and inadequate support system. When considering an intracranial technique, a history of epilepsy and the inability to communicate the nature of their pain adequately should be considered relative contraindications. Although many neuromodulation techniques show promise, they are still under investigation and the hardware, such as leads and generators, are often used off-label. At this time, patients selected for neuromodulation are most likely to be part of an investigation.

Techniques

Deep Brain Stimulation

The use of deep brain stimulation has been primarily studied for the treatment of headache disorders including migraine and trigeminal autonomic cephalgias(TACs) such as cluster headache and SUNCT/SUNA. Targets for stimulation included the ventral tegmental area, subthalamic nucleus, and posterior hypothalamus [9, 10]. Data suggests that deep brain stimulation was effective at reducing the number of episodes but was less effective at decreasing the acute pain or aborting acute attacks [10]. Interestingly, therapeutic onset was not immediate, taking months of stimulation before having a positive effect but this therapeutic effect was also observed to extend beyond the end of stimulation, sometimes years beyond [10].

As an intraparenchymal procedure deep brain stimulation is a higher risk treatment. Serious complications include intracerebral hemorrhage and seizure [10]. Other complications include lead migration, infection, intraventricular hemorrhage, altered appetite and thirst, dizziness, syncope, diplopia, paroxysmal sneezing, and even death [10, 11]. As with other implanted devices requiring leads be tunneled and connected to a generator, lead failure or fracture, infection of lead or generator pocket and generator failure are also possible complications.

High Cervical Spinal Cord Stimulation

Evidence suggests that the high cervical spinal nerve branches communicate with and can modulate the activity of the trigeminal nucleus caudalis via the trigemino-cervical complex [10, 12]. Through this pathway, it is possible to use neuromodulation of the occipital nerves to treat facial pain. See Fig. 15.1 for an illustration of the

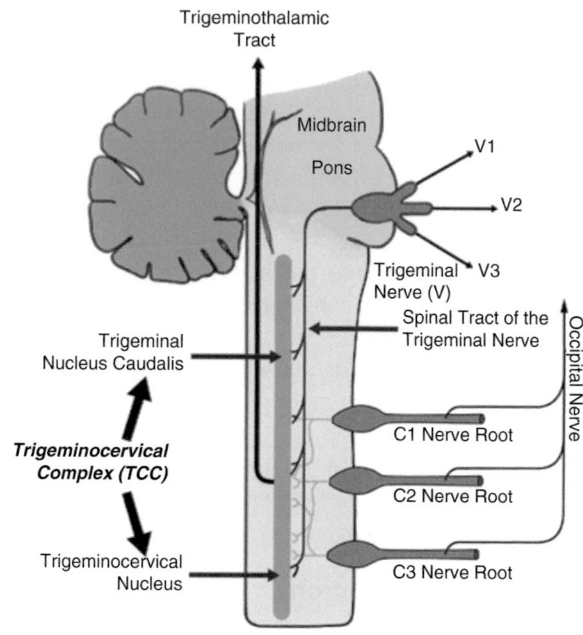

Fig. 15.1 A depiction of the connection between the trigeminal nerve and the cervical spinal nerves. Reprinted with permission from: Antony A, Mazzola A, Dhaliwal G, Hunter C. Neurostimulation for the treatment of chronic head and facial pain: A literature review. Pain Physician 2019; 22:447–477

trigeminocervical complex. Therefore, neuromodulation of the dorsal column in the regions of C1–C3 could theoretically provide therapeutic benefits for trigeminal pathologies.

The majority of available data is pooled from small studies using spinal cord stimulators in the high cervical region to treat migraine, cluster headache, and SUNCT/SUNA. A reduction of pain by more than 50% was reported at a rate of 40–70% of implanted patients with roughly 50% of patients having a reduction in headache days [12–14]. Another small study by Papa et al reported promising results in the treatment of Eagle Syndrome [15]. Little data is currently available as to the efficacy and safety of high cervical spinal cord stimulation for the treatment of other trigeminal nerve pain pathologies. There is theoretical benefit and the positive data from HA and TACs is promising but more research is required.

Technique for placement is similar to the placement of spinal cord stimulators at other levels but may vary based on practitioner and available hardware. A Tuohy needle is advanced to the epidural space, the stim lead is advanced through the needle and guided to the high cervical spinal cord along the dorsal column. Figure 15.2 demonstrates the placement of a spinal cord stimulator lead in the area of the high cervical spine. In one study, a C1 posterior arch laminectomy was performed to place a paddle-style lead. Studies with unilateral lead placement did report incidences of pain location switching to the non-stimulated side. Reported adverse events included lead migration, lead disconnections, and lead infection. Additional adverse effects of spinal cord stimulation can include paresthesia, spinal cord injury, bleeding, paralysis, and even death.

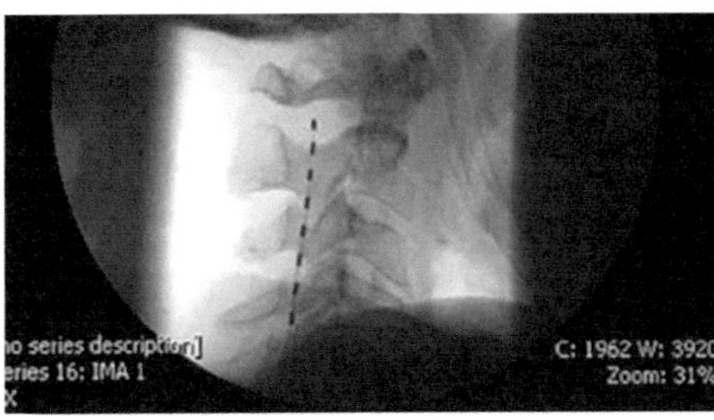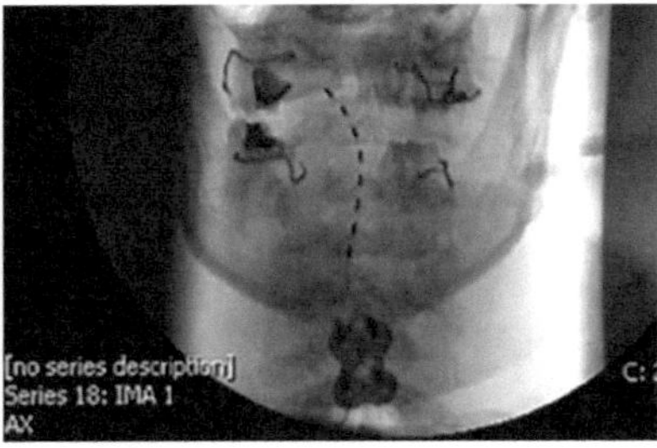

Fig. 15.2 Fluoroscopic image of high spinal cord stimulator. Reprinted with permission from: Antony A, Mazzola A, Dhaliwal G, Hunter C. Neurostimulation for the treatment of chronic head and facial pain: A literature review. Pain Physician 2019; 22:447–477

Gasserian Ganglion Stimulation

The gasserian ganglion, also called semilunar ganglion, has been studied in the treatment of trigeminal neuralgia, trigeminal neuropathic pain such as anesthesia dolorosa and post-herpetic neuralgia, and persistent idiopathic facial pain. The gasserian ganglion offers a unique target for neuromodulation as it contains nerves of all three major trigeminal divisions. Therefore, neuromodulation of this ganglion could theoretically produce therapeutic effects in any desired facial region. Another potential benefit of targeting the gasserian ganglion is the possible reduction of serious post-operative adverse events compared to other intracranial procedures; risks such as intraparenchymal bleeding, epidural bleeding, and seizures.

The ganglion can be stimulated by advancing a stimulator lead through the foramen ovale and into Meckel's cave. This is usually achieved by a Hartel anterior approach, where a long needle is advanced from an insertion point lateral of the oral commissure to the foramen ovale. Intraoperative fluoroscopy and even CT supported guidance can be used to place the needle tip at the target. From there the lead is advanced through the foramen ovale and into Meckel's cave. The lead is then tunneled subcutaneous to an implanted generator. See Fig. 15.3a–c for fluoroscopic images of lead placement for a gasserian ganglion electrode.

A small case series of 10 patients with trigeminal neuropathic pain by Machado et al found that 8/10 of patients responded well to a trial of stimulation. Only 3 out the 5 remaining patients in the study at the 12 months follow-up reported more than 50% relief. Lead migration resulting in loss of efficacy was a primary complication [16]. A large study by Waidhauser and Steude performed trial stimulation for 149 patients with trigeminal neuropathic pain; of the 149 trialed, 81 went on to permanent implantation and the authors report that more than 80% of implanted patients had long-term pain relief [16]. Additional small studies have demonstrated the therapeutic benefit of gasserian ganglion stimulation for patients with persistent idiopathic facial pain and refractory trigeminal neuralgia [17, 18].

Although theorized to be of less risk than motor cortex or deep brain stimulation, no studies are yet available to compare the adverse event rates between these techniques. From the available reports, gasserian ganglion stimulation shares the

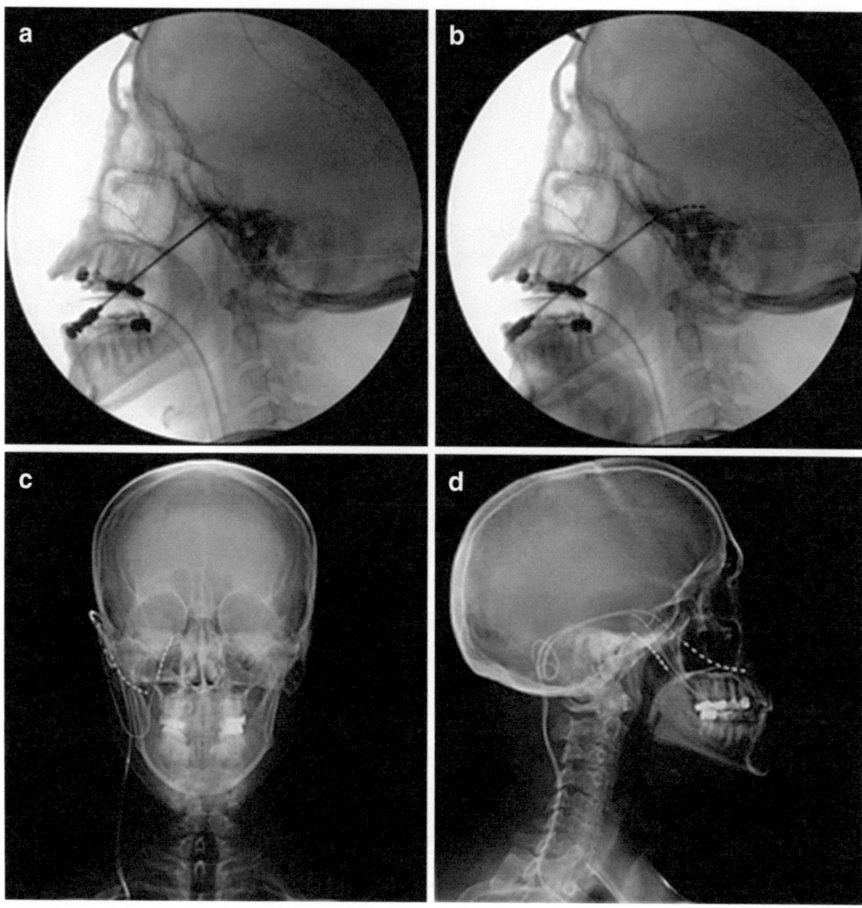

Fig. 15.3 Imaging studies showing percutaneous trigeminal nerve stimulator placement. (**a**) Intraoperative fluoroscopic image of intracranial lead placement. The stylet has been advanced to cannulate the foramen ovale. (**b**) The stylet has been removed, and the lead has been advanced into Meckel's cave. (**c**) Anteroposterior and lateral radiographs demonstrating lead placement for the infraorbital nerve stimulator lead and gasserian ganglion trigeminal nerve. Reprinted with permission from: McMahon T, Torah M, Betley N, et al. Percutaneous trigeminal nerve stimulation for persistent idiopathic facial nerve pain: A case series. World Neurosurgery 2019; 126: e1379–e1386

common adverse events such as lead migration requiring revision, lead perforation, infection along a lead or at the generator site, and generator failure. In addition to these shared adverse events, stimulation of the gasserian ganglion also presents additional risks as the stimulator lead is advanced intracranially and placed in the epidural space. For example, one study reported a patient with a CSF leaking from their incision site that resolved without intervention. The gasserian ganglion may prove to be a powerful target for neuromodulation with reduced risks compared to highly invasive interventions but more study and data is required to determine its safety and efficacy in the treatment of trigeminal nerve pathologies.

Sphenopalatine Ganglion Stimulation

The sphenopalatine ganglion (SPG) sits extracranially within the pterygopalatine fossa and presents a possible target for neuromodulation. SPG stimulation has been studied in small cases series for the treatment of persistent idiopathic facial pain with promising results of a high percentage of implanted patients experiencing relief out to a 24-month follow-up. The largest and highest level of evidence studies investigated the utility of SPG stimulation on cluster headache. The Pathway CH1 trial, an RCT with sham procedure control, also found that SPG stimulation could provide relief for acute attacks and reduced the frequency of attacks. The effect continued throughout the 24-month follow-up period [19]. A follow-up study, the Pathway CH2 trail is a multicenter double-blinded randomized control trial with preliminary results demonstrating SPG stimulation to be superior for the treatment of acute attack when compared to the sham-control [20]. Schytz et al performed a double-blind cross-over trial investigating the utility of stimulation and comparing high frequency, 80–120 Hz, vs. low frequency, 5 Hz. They found that high-frequency stimulation had a positive effect on aborting acute attacks whereas low-frequency stimulation possibly increased the rate of attacks. The observed increase in attacks was believed to be due to the low-frequency 5 Hz stimulation effect on parasympathetic outflow. High-frequency SPG stimulation for refractory cluster headache has been recognized by expert consensus in Europe [12].

An SPG micro-stimulation device has also been approved in Europe for the treatment of cluster and migraine headaches. These devices do not require the implantation of a generator and contain no power source. Instead, they are controlled by a remote held to the cheek and powered from this remote inductively. Figure 15.4 depicts the placement of a sphenopalatine microstimulator. A post-market study of the SPG micro-stimulation device, Pathway R-1, was conducted to assess safety and

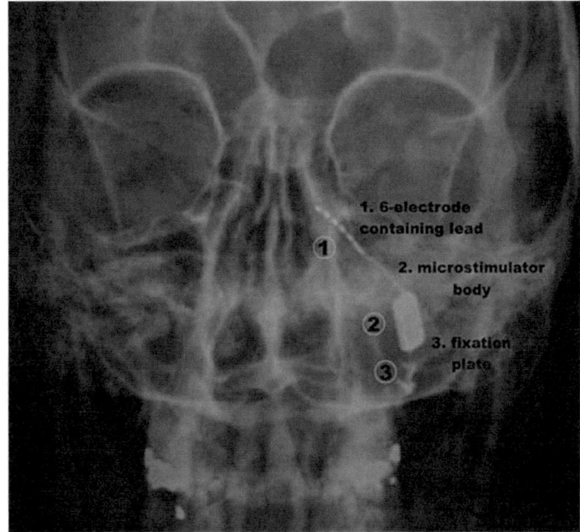

Fig. 15.4 An x-ray demonstrating placement of a Sphenopalatine ganglion microstimulator. Reprinted with permission from: Antony A, Mazzola A, Dhaliwal G, Hunter C. Neurostimulation for the treatment of chronic head and facial pain: A literature review. Pain Physician 2019; 22:447–477

efficacy. Barloese et al reported their observations of 85 treated patients after a 12-month follow-up period. They found that roughly 32% of all patients were able to treat their acute attacks and 55% of the chronic headache patients had a reduction in headache frequency. The study also found that 67% of patients taking abortive medications for acute attacks were able to reduce use by roughly 50%. Seventy percent of patients with chronic headaches were also able to reduce or even stop the use of preventive medications. More than half of all patients in the study also reported improvement in headache impact and quality of life measurements [21].

Trigeminal Nerve Stimulation

The trigeminal nerve can be targeted at branches of its multiple divisions, extracranial ganglion, and intracranial ganglion. Branches such as infraorbital, supraorbital, maxillary, mandibular, and auriculotemporal have all been studied and are promising targets for neuromodulation therapies [12]. Small cases series studies performed throughout the last two decades have demonstrated promising results of targeted trigeminal branch neuromodulation. Most small studies observed how neuromodulation targeted at specific trigeminal nerve branches affected a mix of pathologies. The patients in these trials suffered anesthesia dolorosa, post-herpetic neuralgia, PIFP, atypical facial pain, and refractory trigeminal neuralgia [12, 17]. The sample size for the observational studies ranged from 3 to 30 patients with a mix of trigeminal pathologies within and between the studies. Each study performed a neurostimulation trial, usually lasting approximately 1 week, with a successful trial, defined as >50% reduction in reported pain, occurring for 70–80% patients tested.

While the techniques used for each study varied a small degree, each study used multipolar leads tunneled subcutaneously via coude or Tuohy needle to target the supraorbital and/or infraorbital nerves depending on a patient's identified region of pain. The leads were tunneled into place from temporal incisions anterior to the ear and near the hairline. Positioning was typically monitored and confirmed using intraoperative fluoroscopy. The leads were then tunneled subcutaneously posterior to the ear to generators placed in either the infraclavicular or axillary pocket. Figure 15.3c depicts the placement of a peripheral nerve stim lead at the infraorbital nerve.

Primary end points focused on reduction in reported pain scores. Response rate averaged about 70–80% of permanently implanted patients achieving pain relief of 50% or more for the larger studies while one three patient study reported only one patient responding to therapy. Patient follow-up ranged from a few months to 4 years with continued therapeutic effect for early responders. The investigators did not report an increase in response as stimulation continued over time. The investigators found that many patients were able to decrease their prescribed pain medications and some patients were able to stop all medications.

Reported complications during the trials occurred in roughly 30–40% of permanently implanted patients. The most common complications included: skin erosion, infection at the surgical site requiring extraction of lead and generator, lead migration requiring placement revision, seroma, allodynia over the lead, and lead and battery malfunction [12, 17]. Migration of the stimulation lead was one of the most common complications, despite attempts to anchor the lead at the insertion site. This resulted in the loss of therapeutic effect and required replacement of the lead. These complications are not specific to neuromodulation at the trigeminal branches but can occur with nearly all neuromodulatory implanted devices at our current level of technology. As electrical lead and generator technology continuously advances, complications such as lead failure and migration would be expected to decrease.

Neurostimulation of the trigeminal nerve branches has also been studied for the treatment of other painful pathologies within the trigeminal distribution such as migraine and trigeminal autonomic cephalalgias (TACs). Schoenen et al performed a randomized sham procedure control trial with 59 pts. The trial targeted the supraorbital and supratrochlear nerves. At the 3 months follow-up the treatment group had significantly few migraine days per month compared to the sham procedure control group [12]. A small case study has shown that targeted trigeminal branch neurostimulation could be an effective treatment for trigeminal autonomic cephalalgias.

Occipital Nerve Stimulation

The occipital nerves are branches of the C2 and C3 nerve roots. As previously discussed in the high cervical spine stimulation section, the second and third cervical spinal nerve branches communicate with the trigeminal nucleus caudalis through the trigeminocervical complex. Through this pathway, it is possible to use neuromodulation of the occipital nerves to treat facial pain. Occipital nerve stimulation has primarily been studied for the treatment of headache disorders such as migraine and those falling under the category of trigeminal autonomic cephalalgias.

A number of small studies since the mid-2000s have reported promising data with the treatment of TACs by occipital nerve neuromodulation. The pathology most studied was cluster headache but there are positive results for SUNCT/SUNA, hemicrania continua, and paroxysmal hemicrania as well [10]. In general, about two-thirds of patients with permanently implanted stimulators had a significant reduction in either pain severity or the number of attacks per month [10]. Interestingly, many studies showed that the full therapeutic effect could take months of stimulation to achieve. Another interesting finding was that patients with unilateral stimulators reported the anatomical laterality of their symptoms switched after initiation of therapy. The adverse effects reported are comparable to other implanted devices with the most common being a pain in the area of operation, shock-like sensation contributed to kinked leads, and repeat operation for lead migration or generator failure [10]. See Fig. 15.5 for images of occipital nerve lead placement.

There have been two larger multicenter RCTs investigating the efficacy of occipital nerve stimulation on migraine. The ONSTIM trial, sponsored by Medtronic, was single-blinded and studied adjustable stimulation vs preset stimulation vs

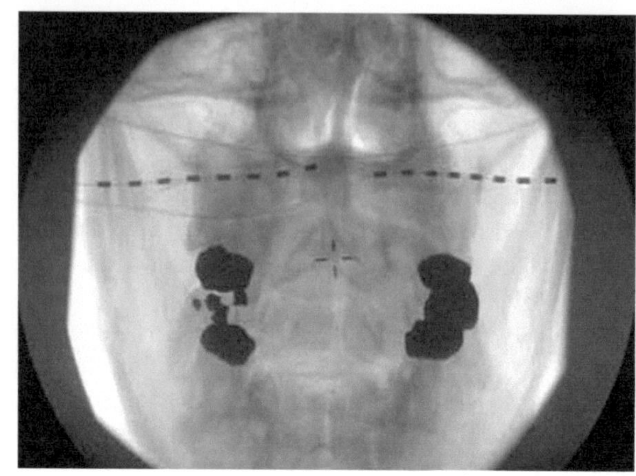

Fig. 15.5 Fluoroscopic image of occipital nerve stimulator. Reprinted with permission from: Antony A, Mazzola A, Dhaliwal G, Hunter C. Neurostimulation for the treatment of chronic head and facial pain: A literature review. Pain Physician 2019; 22:447–477

medical management. At the 3-month follow-up, 39% of patients within the adjustable group had a reduction in the number of headache days or more than 3-pt reduction in their VAS pain score [12]. The study reported that 24% of implant patients suffered lead migration. St. Jude Medical also sponsored a large multicenter, double-blind, RCT for chronic migraine. At the 3 months follow-up only 30% of patients in the treatment group had a reduction in daily VAS pain scores. One-year follow-up however demonstrated a reduction in the number of headache days as well as a reduction in headache disability indices. This trial also reported a high post-operative adverse event rate of 70% with 40% requiring surgical intervention. More research, investigation, and device development are required to reduce the rate of lead migration, one of the most common reported adverse events and a common cause for surgical revision.

Through its high cervical spine communication, the occipital nerve is a possible target for the treatment of trigeminal nerve pathologies. Current data has demonstrated promising results for the treatment of migraine and trigeminal autonomic cephalalgias. With promising results for the treatment of trigeminal nerve-related pathologies and known neural communication, occipital nerve stimulation could be a therapy for other trigeminal nerve pathologies but more investigation is required to determine its utility.

Vagal Nerve Stimulation

Vagal nerve stimulation has been previously studied for the treatment of epilepsy and depression. During the studies for depression, the investigators found that patients with concomitant headache disorders also experienced an improvement in their headaches. Small sample-sized case series and retrospective studies have demonstrated that roughly 50% of patients that have an implanted vagal nerve stimulator have had improvement in their migraine or cluster headache [12].

Non-invasive vagal nerve stimulation (nVNS) is another possible treatment for migraine and TACs. Electrical stimulation is applied transcutaneously. An RCT evaluating its use for migraines initially found no benefit at 2 months but when the trial was extended to 8 months, ~50% of patients had a reduction in headache days [12]. Transcutaneous Vagal Nerve Stimulation, tVNS, has also been studied in the treatment for cluster headache. In addition, small case series show possible benefits in other TACs such as paroxysmal hemicranias and hemicrania continua [9, 10, 12]. The technique significantly reduces risk to the patient but there are still reports of adverse effects such as skin irritation associated with the conducting gel. The PREVA, ACT1, and ACT2 studies were all randomized control trials evaluating the utility of tVNS treatment for cluster headache. The PREVA trial demonstrated that an nVNS protocol performed twice a day reduced cluster headache attack frequency. The ACT1 trial found nVNS to be a beneficial treatment for acute cluster headache attacks, but only for those patients with episodic cluster headache [22]. The ACT2 trial confirmed the results from the ACT1 studied; nVNS was a possible treatment for acute cluster headache attacks for those patients with the episodic disease and not for those patients classified as having chronic cluster headache [23].

Peripheral Nerve Field Stimulation

Peripheral nerve field stimulation (PNFS) is the placement of stimulatory electrical leads within the innervated region of a peripheral nerve. One potential benefit is that lead placement does not need to be in the immediate vicinity of the targeted nerve. The placement of the lead can therefore be targeted into the region of pain as identified by the patient.

Stimulation leads are placed via Tuohy or coude needles inserted through small incisions in the patient's temporal area. Some investigators have attempted to place the leads near anatomical landmarks [24]. Other investigators attempted to maximize a leads contact within a patient identified area of pain [25]. Another possible location included placing the stimulation lead within the hyperalgesia strip, identified by the patient, and outside of the area of allodynia [26]. Those using anatomical landmarks frequently used intraoperative fluoroscopy while other investigators only performed post-operative x-rays. Although techniques differed between the various studies, the reported outcomes were all very similar. Without more data or direct comparison, no technique can be declared superior. Another important aspect of placement may be lead depth. Data from PNFS for low back pain has indicated that the optimal depth for A-beta and A-delta fiber stimulation occurs at roughly 1 cm [27, 28]. The skin thickness of the face is notably thinner than the lower back and depending on the area 1 cm depth may not be achievable. More data to guide optimal lead placement is needed.

Several small studies have investigated PNFS as a treatment for recurrent classical trigeminal neuralgia, classical trigeminal neuralgia, trigeminal neuropathy due to Multiple Sclerosis and radiation, post-herpetic neuralgia, persistent idiopathic facial pain, migraine, and occipital neuralgia. The studies demonstrated that roughly 60–80% of patients with implanted PNFS experienced more than 50% reduction in reported pain [12, 24–26, 29]. Reported complications included lead dislocation and migration, lead infection, and generator failure/dislocation.

Discussion

Multiple neuromodulatory targets have been identified and tested for the treatment of head and facial pain pathologies. While all show promise of therapeutic benefit, there is little overall data of efficacy and safety. The highest level of data currently available comes from randomized control trials studying migraine and cluster headache. There have been no randomized control trials of neuromodulation techniques for other trigeminal nerve pathologies. The best data has come from prospective or retrospective observational studies, case series, or case reports.

There have been no studies directly testing the superiority of one technique or target of neuromodulation to another for the treatment of any trigeminal nerve pathology. There has been no study comparing safety or complication rates of one technique to another. Despite this, there are inherent differences in risks and complications for current neuromodulation techniques. Intracranial surgery for the placement of deep brain stimulators has greater risks compared to a stimulation lead placed in the epidural space, which has a greater risk than a subcutaneous lead which has a greater risk than a transcutaneous stimulator. Advancements in the field of neuromodulation are continuous. Smaller, less invasive electrodes that can utilize more sophisticated programming are continuously being developed. One focus for significant technological development should be on maintaining the lead position after deployment. One of the most common adverse events reported in trials of various targets was lead migration. This typically resulted in a loss of therapeutic effect and required an additional surgical operation to correct, exposing the patient to the risks of another surgery. The understanding of applied electrical current to change neuron activity will continue to advance and as our knowledge base advances so will our technology. Neuromodulation has the promise of a new and evolving therapy for previously difficult to treat and debilitating pain pathologies but as with any new treatment it requires continued study and development.

References

1. Krames E, Peckham PH, Rezai AR. Neuromodulation. Amsterdam: Elsevier/Academic Press; 2009.
2. Nayak R, Banik RK. Current innovations in peripheral nerve stimulation. Pain Res Treat. 2018:1–5. https://doi.org/10.1155/2018/9091216.
3. Maniam R, Kaye AD, Vadivelu N, Urman RD. Facial pain update: advances in neurostimulation for the treatment of facial pain. Curr Pain Headache Rep. 2016;20:24.
4. Kolodziej MA, Hellwig D, Nimsky C, Benes L. Treatment of central deafferentation and trigeminal neuropathic pain by motor cortex stimulation: report of a series of 20 patients. J Neurol Surg A Cent Eur Neurosurg. 2016;77:52–8.

5. Tomycz ND, Deibert CP, Moossy JJ. Cervicomedullary junction spinal cord stimulation for head and facial pain. Headache. 2011;51:418–25.
6. Goadsby PJ, Bartsch T, Dodick DW. Occipital nerve stimulation for headache: mechanisms and efficacy. Headache. 2008;48:313–8.
7. Deer TR, Mekhail N, Petersen E, et al. The appropriate use of neurostimulation: stimulation of the intracranial and extracranial space and head for chronic pain. Neuromodulation. 2014;17:551–70.
8. Atkinson L, Sundaraj SR, O'Callaghan J, Teddy P, Salmon J, Semple T, Majedi PM. Recommendations for patient selection in spinal cord stimulation. J Clin Neurosci. 2011;18:1295–302.
9. Burish MJ, Rozen TD. Trigeminal autonomic cephalalgias. Neurol Clin. 2019;37:847–69.
10. Wei DY, Jensen RH. Therapeutic approaches for the management of trigeminal autonomic cephalalgias. Neurotherapeutics. 2018;15:346–60.
11. Leone M, Cecchini AP. Deep brain stimulation in headache. Cephalalgia. 2016;36:1143–8.
12. Antony AB, Mazzola AJ, Dhaliwal GS, Hunter CW. Neurostimulation for the treatment of chronic head and facial pain: a literature review. Pain Physician. 2019;22:447–77.
13. Lambru G, Trimboli M, Palmisani S, Smith T, Al-Kaisy A. Safety and efficacy of cervical 10 kHz spinal cord stimulation in chronic refractory primary headaches: a retrospective case series. J Headache Pain. 2016;17:66.
14. Arcioni R, Palmisani S, Mercieri M, et al. Cervical 10 kHz spinal cord stimulation in the management of chronic, medically refractory migraine: a prospective, open-label, exploratory study. Eur J Pain. 2016;20:70–8.
15. Papa A, Ferrara M, Buonanno P, Santoro V, Servodio C, Servillo G. A novel approach with spinal cord stimulation for the treatment of chronic pain in Eagle's syndrome: a case report. Chronic Pain Manag CPMT-112; 2018. https://doi.org/10.29011/2576-957X/100012
16. Machado A, Ogrin M, Rosenow J, Henderson J. A 12-month prospective study of gasserian ganglion stimulation for trigeminal neuropathic pain. Stereotact Funct Neurosurg. 2007;85:216–24.
17. Mcmahon JT, Tora MS, Bentley JN, Texakalidis P, Campbell MA, Keifer OP, Boulis NM. Percutaneous trigeminal nerve stimulation for persistent idiopathic facial pain: a case series. World Neurosurg. 2019;126:1379–86.
18. Kustermans L, Van Buyten JP, Smet I, Coucke W, Politis C. Stimulation of the gasserian ganglion in the treatment of refractory trigeminal neuropathy. J Cranio-Maxillofac Surg. 2017;45:39–46.
19. Schoenen J, Jensen RH, Lantéri-Minet M, et al. Stimulation of the sphenopalatine ganglion (SPG) for cluster headache treatment. Pathway CH-1: a randomized, sham-controlled study. Cephalalgia. 2013;33:816–30.
20. Goadsby PJ, Sahai-Srivastava S, Kezirian EJ, et al. Safety and efficacy of sphenopalatine ganglion stimulation for chronic cluster headache: a double-blind, randomised controlled trial. Lancet Neurol. 2019;18:1081–90.
21. Barloese M, Petersen A, Stude P, Jürgens T, Jensen RH, May A. Sphenopalatine ganglion stimulation for cluster headache, results from a large, open-label European registry. J Headache Pain. 2018; https://doi.org/10.1186/s10194-017-0828-9.
22. Silberstein SD, Mechtler LL, Kudrow DB, Calhoun AH, Mcclure C, Saper JR, Liebler EJ, Engel ER, Tepper SJ. Non-invasive vagus nerve stimulation for the acute treatment of cluster headache: findings from the randomized, double-blind, sham-controlled ACT1 study. Headache. 2016;56:1317–32.
23. Goadsby PJ, Coo IFD, Silver N, et al. Non-invasive vagus nerve stimulation for the acute treatment of episodic and chronic cluster headache: a randomized, double-blind, sham-controlled ACT2 study. Cephalalgia. 2017;38:959–69.
24. Lenchig S, Cohen J, Patin D. A minimally invasive surgical technique for the treatment of posttraumatic trigeminal neuropathic pain with peripheral nerve stimulation. Pain Physician. 2012;15:725–32.

25. Klein J, Sandi-Gahun S, Schackert G, Juratli TA. Peripheral nerve field stimulation for trigeminal neuralgia, trigeminal neuropathic pain, and persistent idiopathic facial pain. Cephalalgia. 2015;36:445–53.
26. Feletti A, Santi GZ, Sammartino F, Bevilacqua M, Cisotto P, Longatti P. Peripheral trigeminal nerve field stimulation. Neurosurg Focus. 2013; https://doi.org/10.3171/2013.7.focus13228.
27. Mørch CD, Nguyen GP, Wacnik PW, et al. Mathematical model of nerve fiber activation during low back peripheral nerve field stimulation: analysis of electrode implant depth. Neuromodulation. 2014;17:218–25.
28. Abejón D, Deer T, Verrills P. Subcutaneous stimulation: how to assess optimal implantation depth. Neuromodulation. 2011;14:343–8.
29. Ellis JA, Munne Mejia JC, Winfree CJ. Trigeminal branch stimulation for the treatment of intractable craniofacial pain. J Neurosurg. 2015;123:283–8.

Infusion Therapy

16

Nathan J. Rudin

Introduction

Infusion therapies have been successfully employed to treat chronic pain refractory to other treatment. Conditions treated by infusion include complex regional pain syndrome [1], chronic refractory headache [2], painful peripheral neuropathies [3], cancer-related neuropathic pain [4, 5], postherpetic neuralgia [6], and fibromyalgia [7, 8]. As a severe and often challenging neuropathic pain condition, trigeminal neuralgia (TN) is a logical target for infusion therapies.

The literature on infusion for TN is small, primarily consisting of case reports, small studies, and literature reviews. Much research remains to be done before the clinician can readily identify the best infusion candidates, use the most effective medications and doses, and have a solid expectation of outcome. Of the drugs discussed, only lidocaine has sufficient evidence to warrant the inclusion of specific therapeutic recommendations in this chapter. Other candidate medications are more briefly discussed.

Intravenous (IV) or Subcutaneous (SQ) Lidocaine

Lidocaine, a blocker of sodium channels in the neuronal cell membrane [9], blocks depolarization of afferent neurons, causing temporary regional anesthesia with a half-life of 120 min. Interestingly, lidocaine also exerts antinociceptive effects when given intravenously (IV), and the duration of analgesia may last for days or weeks [10], making intermittent infusions an effective treatment for some

N. J. Rudin (✉)
Department of Orthopedics and Rehabilitation, University of Wisconsin School of Medicine and Public Health, Madison, WI, USA
e-mail: rudin@rehab.wisc.edu

A. Abd-Elsayed (ed.), *Trigeminal Nerve Pain*,
https://doi.org/10.1007/978-3-030-60687-9_16

individuals. Werdehausen et al. demonstrated that lidocaine's metabolites enhance the synaptic concentration of glycine, a major inhibitory neurotransmitter, by inhibiting glycine transporter 1, which removes glycine from the synapse. This mechanism could produce the longer-term analgesia seen after systemic lidocaine administration [11].

Evidence Lidocaine is the most evaluated and safest available infusion therapy for neuropathic pain. A Cochrane review of controlled clinical trials concluded that systemic lidocaine (and its oral analogs mexiletine, tocainide, and flecainide) are safe, better than placebo, and as effective as other analgesics [12], though there is room for substantial further investigation.

Lidocaine infusion has been employed to treat refractory TN, though few reports have been published. Chaudhry and Friedman [13] report a single case of complete relief of TN symptoms with continuous IV lidocaine infusion, 60–120 mg/h, for 72 h. Stavropoulou and colleagues [14] conducted a randomized double-blind placebo-controlled trial of IV lidocaine in 20 patients with TN, with (active) lidocaine 5 mg/kg is given in 5% dextrose, versus (control) 5% dextrose alone, over 1 h. Each patient received 4 infusions, 2 active and 2 control in random order, spaced 2 days apart. The active group reported significant decreases in pain, allodynia, and hyperalgesia that lasted at least 24 h after infusion.

Indications TN refractory to other treatments, including acute exacerbations of TN pain. Lidocaine may be employed where oral agents have been insufficiently helpful or as an adjunct to oral therapies. If effective, it may be used as maintenance therapy, or as a temporizing measure while awaiting decompression or other definitive treatment.

Contraindications Table 16.1 contains contraindications assembled by the University of Wisconsin Hospital and Clinics for consideration prior to initiating systemic lidocaine therapy. Available evidence was of low quality, so recommendations are conservative.

Screening

- Baseline lab work. Values should be normal within 1 week of the initial infusion.
  - Potassium, magnesium, serum creatinine, ALT/SGPT
- Twelve-lead electrocardiogram. Should be done within 1 month of the initial infusion.

IV Dose

- Trial dose: 5 mg/kg (maximum: 500 mg) over 60 min. If suboptimally effective, consider retrial at higher dose (max 7.5 mg/kg) or weekly infusions × 3.
- Maintenance dose: 3–7.5 mg/kg (maximum 750 mg) over 60 min.

Table 16.1 Contraindications to IV lidocaine therapy

Absolute contraindications
• Conduction block with the following findings
– Stokes-Adams syndrome
– Wolff-Parkinson-White syndrome
– Severe degrees of SA, AV, or intraventricular heart block (e.g., 2nd degree), except in patients with a functioning artificial pacemaker
• Allergy to lidocaine or other amide local anesthetics
• Pregnancy
• Age less than 6 months (secondary to increased risk of toxicity related to immature hepatic function and increased free lidocaine levels).
Relative contraindications
• Chronic alcoholism or substance abuse (due to risk for additive CNS adverse events, evaluate on an individual basis if the benefit is greater than the risk).
• ECG Findings
– PR interval >200 ms
– QRS complex >120 ms
– Bifascicular block regardless of QRS complex duration
• Age 6 months–1 year (secondary to increased risk of toxicity related to immature hepatic function and increased free lidocaine levels)
• Patients who are unable to self-report adverse events
• Seizure history or at risk for seizure
• Advanced age/poor functional status
• Renal dysfunction
• Hepatic dysfunction
• Drug–drug interactions
– Medications that induce CYP1A2 (the primary enzyme responsible for metabolism) or CYP3A4 (a minor enzyme involved in metabolism) decrease lidocaine concentrations, but therefore increase active metabolites which are renally eliminated.
– Medications that inhibit CYP1A2 and CYP3A4 (will increase lidocaine concentrations).
– Antiarrhythmic agents (concern for additive cardiac toxicity-concomitant use should be evaluated by a cardiologist prior to initiating IV lidocaine for pain).

SQ Dose Continuous SQ infusion can be employed for maintenance dosing with systemic lidocaine and is an effective modality for those whose analgesic response to lidocaine is of short duration (days or less), making intermittent infusion impractical. The test dose is the same as for IV lidocaine. The usual maintenance dose is 0.5–3 mg/kg/h, using ideal body weight for the calculation. SQ lidocaine tends to be less acceptable than intermittent infusion due to the discomfort of the SQ infusion catheter, technical issues, and limited coverage by health insurers.

Risks Lidocaine toxicity is directly related to the serum drug level. Intravenous lidocaine is well tolerated at the doses used above; calibrating the dose to body weight improves tolerability. In 69 patients with neuropathic pain, flat-rate infusions at 500 mg/30 min (16.7 mg/min) were safe and effective but produced adverse effects (mainly lightheadedness) in 88% of patients, necessitating a reduction of the infusion rate and/or total dose [16]. In children and adolescents with chronic pain, doses up to 21.6 mg/kg, given over 6 h, were safe, effective, and well tolerated [17]. Routine cardiac monitoring is not required but may be appropriate in individuals with higher arrhythmia risk. Severe toxicity can be prevented by monitoring vital signs, level of consciousness, and pain ratings throughout the infusion.

- *Mild toxicity* includes numbness and tingling in fingers, toes, around the mouth; blurred vision; tinnitus; a metallic taste; lightheadedness, drowsiness.
  - Treatment: Slow the infusion rate; if symptoms are more severe, pause the infusion until they resolve, then resume infusion at a slower rate.
- *Moderate toxicity* can include more pronounced drowsiness (patient can still be aroused), severe dizziness, tremor, nausea, vomiting, altered blood pressure, and pulse.
  - Treatment: Discontinue the infusion. Patients are monitored until adverse effects resolve. Alert a physician.
- *Severe toxicity* can include loss of consciousness or severe drowsiness, confusion, myoclonus, seizure, cardiac conduction abnormalities.
  - Treatment: Discontinue the infusion. Seizure may be controlled using lorazepam. Treat hypotension with IV hydration. For very severe symptoms, use lipid infusion to reduce toxicity.

Other Agents

Ketamine

Ketamine is a noncompetitive antagonist of the N-methyl-D-aspartate (NMDA) glutamate receptor and profoundly affects ascending nociceptive transmission. It has been used as an anesthetic for decades and is well known to inhibit acute nociceptive pain in subanesthetic concentrations [18]. Like lidocaine, it alleviates some forms of neuropathic pain, with relief outlasting the anticipated half-life of the drug; this suggests effects beyond NMDA-receptor antagonism alone [19].

Evidence Three of seven female patients with post-traumatic trigeminal pain (not classic TN) experienced transient pain relief (1–3 days) with subanesthetic doses of ketamine (0.4–1.8 mg/kg). There have been no formal studies of ketamine as a treatment for TN itself.

Side Effects Ketamine has a narrow therapeutic window and side effects may be seen even at relatively low doses. These may include hallucinations, panic attacks, agitation, somnolence, nausea, vomiting, cardiovascular hyperactivity, and hepatoxicity.

Clinical Guidelines Little guidance is available regarding candidate selection, protocols, or indications for intravenous ketamine infusion to treat neuropathic pain. A 2018 guideline from three pain societies [20] provides recommendations, but these are consensus-based and therefore subjective. A more focused meta-analysis suggests that IV ketamine does provide "significant short-term analgesic benefit in patients with refractory chronic pain [19]." Neither the guideline nor the meta-analysis specifically addresses TN. At this time insufficient evidence exists to support IV ketamine as a TN therapy.

Phenytoin and Fosphenytoin

The anticonvulsant phenytoin produces voltage-dependent blockade of voltage-gated sodium channels, blocking high-frequency, sustained repetitive sodium action potentials (as classically seen in epileptic seizures). Phenytoin has been used to treat neuropathic pain conditions and fibromyalgia, though evidence for such use remains weak [21].

Evidence Phenytoin and its IV-administered prodrug, fosphenytoin have been reported to be effective for the treatment of otherwise intractable TN, but only two single-case reports and a three-case series have been published [22–24]. Doses of 11–18 mg/kg were used, some as a single infusion over 20–30 min, others as incremental doses every 10 min. Relief of 2–20 days was reported. Further study is required before recommending the use of these drugs as infusions for TN treatment.

Side Effects Phenytoin and fosphenytoin have significant potential side effects including altered mentation, gum hyperplasia, excessive hair growth, rash, marrow suppression, and hepatic dysfunction.

Magnesium

Magnesium is a cofactor in hundreds of reactions throughout the body and is necessary for the active transport of calcium and potassium across cell membranes. Magnesium naturally blocks NMDA receptors and therefore may exert analgesic effects in neuropathic pain states [25]. Magnesium is typically given intravenously as the sulfate ($MgSO_4$) and orally as the oxide or citrate. Higher oral doses are often used as laxatives. IV magnesium is an effective treatment for acute migraine [26] and reduces migraine symptoms when given as part of an oral supplement [27].

Evidence Weak evidence is available for $MgSO_4$'s efficacy in acute TN pain. A single case report showed 80% relief of TN pain for 4 h after 30 mg/kg $MgSO_4$ given IV over 30 min. Arai and colleagues [28] produced pain relief in 9 patients with TN by infusing 1.2 g $MgSO_4$ plus 100 mg lidocaine weekly over 1 h for 3 weeks.

Side Effects Magnesium's most common side effects are gastrointestinal, including diarrhea, nausea, and vomiting. Hypermagnesemia may be seen with overuse of magnesium laxatives or with overdose of IV $MgSO_4$. It is a dangerous electrolyte imbalance that can cause hypotension, respiratory depression, cardiac arrythmia, and death.

Chlormethiazole

Zurak and colleagues [29] reported successful pain reduction using IV 0.8% chlormethiazole (3–10 days, 5–6 h/infusion) every other day in an uncontrolled study of 16 patients with TN. Follow-up period was short and no firm conclusions could be drawn. Evidence quality is weak. Chlormethiazole is a barbiturate-type sedative-hypnotic with high toxicity and addiction potential and is not recommended for TN treatment, though these results might inspire better-designed studies employing related, less toxic agents.

In conclusion, a growing body of evidence exists to support the use of IV lidocaine as a safe and well-tolerated treatment for neuropathic pain. For TN itself, the literature is sparser, but the evidence is promising. Providers and institutions with expertise and comfort in the use of lidocaine for chronic pain may find it an effective addition to the treatment arsenal for TN. Other candidate drugs have very weak evidence, high potential toxicity, or both. Considerable further study is required before infusion therapies become a regular part of TN management.

References

1. Xu J, Yang J, Lin P, Rosenquist E, Cheng J. Intravenous therapies for complex regional pain syndrome: a systematic review. Anesth Analg. 2016;122:843–56.
2. Pomeroy JL, Marmura MJ, Nahas SJ, Viscusi ER. Ketamine infusions for treatment refractory headache. Headache. 2017;57:276–82.
3. Kvarnstrom A, Karlsten R, Quiding H, Emanuelsson BM, Gordh T. The effectiveness of intravenous ketamine and lidocaine on peripheral neuropathic pain. Acta Anaesthesiol Scand. 2003;47:868–77.
4. Buchanan DD, JM F. A role for intravenous lidocaine in severe cancer-related neuropathic pain at the end-of-life. Support Care Cancer. 2010;18:899–901.
5. Papapetrou P, Kumar AJ, Muppuri R, Chakrabortty S. Intravenous lidocaine infusion to treat chemotherapy-induced peripheral neuropathy. A A Case Rep. 2015;5:154–5.
6. Rowbotham MC, Reisner-Keller LA, Fields HL. Both intravenous lidocaine and morphine reduce the pain of postherpetic neuralgia. Neurology. 1991;41:1024–8.
7. Albertoni Giraldes AL, Salomao R, Leal PD, Brunialti MK, Sakata RK. Effect of intravenous lidocaine combined with amitriptyline on pain intensity, clinical manifestations and the concentrations of IL-1, IL-6 and IL-8 in patients with fibromyalgia: a randomized double-blind study. Int J Rheum Dis. 2016;19:946–53.
8. Marks DM, Newhouse A. Durability of benefit from repeated intravenous lidocaine infusions in fibromyalgia patients: a case series and literature review. Prim Care Companion CNS Disord. 2015;17(5):10.
9. Kosharskyy B, Almonte W, Shaparin N, Pappagallo M, Smith H. Intravenous infusions in chronic pain management. Pain Physician. 2013;16:231–49.

10. Backonja M, Gombar KA. Response of central pain syndromes to intravenous lidocaine. J Pain Symptom Manag. 1992;7:172–8.
11. Werdehausen R, Kremer D, Brandenburger T, Schlosser L, Jadasz J, Kury P, Bauer I, Aragon C, Eulenburg V, Hermanns H. Lidocaine metabolites inhibit glycine transporter 1: a novel mechanism for the analgesic action of systemic lidocaine? Anesthesiology. 2012;116:147–58.
12. Challapalli V, Tremont-Lukats IW, McNicol ED, Lau J, Carr DB. Systemic administration of local anesthetic agents to relieve neuropathic pain. Cochrane Database Syst Rev. 2019;2019 https://doi.org/10.1002/14651858.CD003345.pub2.
13. Chaudhry P, Friedman DI. Intravenous lidocaine treatment in classical trigeminal neuralgia with concomitant persistent facial pain. Headache. 2014;54:1376–9.
14. Stavropoulou E, Argyra E, Zis P, Vadalouca A, Siafaka I. The effect of intravenous lidocaine on trigeminal neuralgia: a randomized double blind placebo controlled trial. ISRN Pain. 2014;2014:853826.
15. Buck K, Christensen H, Bazinski M. Systemic lidocaine for the treatment of pain—adult/pediatric—inpatient/ambulatory/emergency department clinical practice guideline. Madison, WI: UW Health Center for Clinical Knowledge Management; 2019.
16. Hutson P, Backonja M, Knurr H. Intravenous lidocaine for neuropathic pain: a retrospective analysis of tolerability and efficacy. Pain Med. 2015;16:531–6.
17. Mooney JJ, Pagel PS, Kundu A. Safety, tolerability, and short-term efficacy of intravenous lidocaine infusions for the treatment of chronic pain in adolescents and young adults: a preliminary report. Pain Med. 2014;15:820–5.
18. Mathisen LC, Skjelbred P, Skoglund LA, Oye I. Effect of ketamine, an NMDA receptor inhibitor, in acute and chronic orofacial pain. Pain. 1995;61:215–20.
19. Orhurhu V, Orhurhu MS, Bhatia A, Cohen SP. Ketamine infusions for chronic pain: a systematic review and meta-analysis of randomized controlled trials. Anesth Analg. 2019;129:241–54.
20. Cohen SP, Bhatia A, Buvanendran A, Schwenk ES, Wasan AD, Hurley RW, Viscusi ER, Narouze S, Davis FN, Ritchie EC, Lubenow TR, Hooten WM. Consensus guidelines on the use of intravenous ketamine infusions for chronic pain from the American Society of Regional Anesthesia and Pain Medicine, the American Academy of Pain Medicine, and the American Society of Anesthesiologists. Reg Anesth Pain Med. 2018;43:521–46.
21. Birse F, Derry S, Moore RA. Phenytoin for neuropathic pain and fibromyalgia in adults. Cochrane Database Syst Rev. 2012;2012(5):CD009485.
22. Cheshire WP. Fosphenytoin: an intravenous option for the management of acute trigeminal neuralgia crisis. J Pain Symptom Manag. 2001;21:506–10.
23. Tate R, Rubin LM, Krajewski KC. Treatment of refractory trigeminal neuralgia with intravenous phenytoin. Am J Health Syst Pharm. 2011;68:2059–61.
24. Vargas A, Thomas K. Intravenous fosphenytoin for acute exacerbation of trigeminal neuralgia: case report and literature review. Ther Adv Neurol Disord. 2015;8:187–8.
25. Gröber U, Schmidt J, Kisters K. Magnesium in prevention and therapy. Nutrients. 2015;7:8199–226.
26. Bigal ME, Bordini CA, Tepper SJ, Speciali JG. Intravenous magnesium sulphate in the acute treatment of migraine without aura and migraine with aura. A randomized, double-blind, placebo-controlled study. Cephalalgia. 2002;22:345–53.
27. Gaul C, Diener HC, Danesch U, Migravent® SG. Improvement of migraine symptoms with a proprietary supplement containing riboflavin, magnesium and Q10: a randomized, placebo-controlled, double-blind, multicenter trial. J Headache Pain. 2015;16:516.
28. Arai YC, Hatakeyama N, Nishihara M, Ikeuchi M, Kurisuno M, Ikemoto T. Intravenous lidocaine and magnesium for management of intractable trigeminal neuralgia: a case series of nine patients. J Anesth. 2013;27:960–2.
29. Zurak N, Randic B, Poljaković Z, Vöglein S. Intravenous chlormethiazole in the management of primary trigeminal neuralgia resistant to conventional therapy. J Int Med Res. 1989;17:87–92.

Balloon Compression of the Trigeminal Nerve

Priodarshi Roychoudhury, Vitaliano Di Grazia, Vwaire Orhurhu, and Alaa Abd-Elsayed

Introduction

Trigeminal neuralgia (TN), or tic douloureux, is a chronic pain syndrome characterized by recurrent attacks of lancinating facial pain occurring in the distribution of one or more divisions of the trigeminal nerve [1].

The International Headache Society (IHS) divides TN into two distinct categories: "classical" and "symptomatic."

The "Classical" form of the disorder (Type 1, or TN1) causes intermittent severe burning pain, with each attack lasting for up to 2 min [2].

The "atypical" form TN (Type 2, or TN2) in contrast is described as constant, burning, and stabbing, pain though of lesser severity than TN1. Diagnosis of TN relies on the identification of a paroxysmal occurrence of each episode with the definite demarcation between onset and termination [3].

Patients may have identifiable vascular compression of the trigeminal nerve, caused by tumor, multiple sclerosis, or an arteriovenous malformation. Pain onset

P. Roychoudhury (✉)
Department of Anesthesia and Pain Management, Toronto General Hospital, University of Toronto, Toronto, ON, Canada

V. Di Grazia
Department of Pain Management, Toronto Western Hospital, University of Toronto, Toronto, ON, Canada

V. Orhurhu
Department of Anesthesia, Critical Care and Pain Medicine, Massachusetts General Hospital, Harvard Medical School, Boston, MA, USA

A. Abd-Elsayed
Department of Anesthesiology, University of Wisconsin School of Medicine and Public Health, Madison, WI, USA

A. Abd-Elsayed (ed.), *Trigeminal Nerve Pain*, https://doi.org/10.1007/978-3-030-60687-9_17

can be triggered even by minimal stimulation such as talking, chewing, or light touch of the overlying skin, most often unilateral.

The diagnosis of TN is primarily clinical and based on the exclusion of other diseases. TN spontaneously resolves in 63% of patients with a total absence of symptoms for years. The condition is not fatal; however, even fear of an impending attack can be debilitating for patients [4].

History of the Procedure

When TN becomes refractory to medical management, surgery becomes imminent. Glycerol rhizolysis, thermocoagulation, and balloon compression are well established in the treatment of TN.

In 1983, Mullan [5] first described balloon compression consecutively to the operative data reported by Shelden [6] in 1955, that established preference of decompression with a blunt dissector over simple decompression of the fifth nerve.

In 1995, Brown demonstrated that large myelinated axons, involved in the sensory trigger, were mostly injured while small myelinated fibers were relatively preserved during this mechanical compression [7].

The ideal goal of the procedure was analgesia without side effects.

The technique still remains as one of the most popular surgical procedures practiced today.

The trigeminal nerve also provides touch and pain sensation to the nasal sinuses, inner aspect of the nose, mouth, and anterior two-thirds of the tongue.

The mechanism of action of this technique is not yet perfectly understood. Interesting hypothesis is that the balloon compression on the nerve fibers causes anatomic injury different from the one caused by thermal or chemical energy as in the radiofrequency rhizotomy or in the glycerol injection techniques.

Nerve compression using a Fogarty catheter evokes a depression of response of nerve fibers but preserves the response of the ganglion cells, so that balloon compression specifically relieves trigeminal pain affecting the large myelinated fibers, which are involved in the sensory triggers.

Indications

1. Patients who have failed medical therapy for classic TN.
2. TN in association with multiple sclerosis. However, symptom recurrence is seen to be higher and requires multiple procedures, as compared to non-multiple sclerosis patients.
3. Young patients are willing to accept the associated mild numbness which might occur after surgery.

Contraindications

In addition to contraindications such as uncorrected coagulopathy, sepsis, or infection at the site of the procedure, hemodynamic instability, and lack of consent, it is contraindicated in atypical facial pain or post-herpetic pain and contralateral masseter weakness. It is important to have a thoughtful risk/benefit analysis and use clinicians' judgment in the decision-making process.

Pre-procedural Preparation

Informed consent is obtained after the risks, benefits, and alternatives are clearly outlined. An intravenous line is placed in a pre-procedure room. The site of the procedure is labeled, and the patient is transported to the procedure room, where the patient is positioned on a radiolucent procedure table in a supine position. Fluoroscope is used to guide needle placement. Standard American Society of Anesthesiologists (ASA) monitors are used for monitoring. A pre-procedural time out is performed to confirm the patient's identity, allergies, procedure site, body position, and necessary equipment. The majority of patients require general anesthesia with intratracheal intubation.

Techniques

Device and positioning:
   The procedure requires a Fluoroscope and the following materials:

- A hollow metallic introducer (HI) 14 gauge with a sharp tip, with a silicone catheter (SC) allowing the blood or the cerebrospinal fluid (CSF) to escape in case of vessel injury or dural tear.
- A number 4 Fogarty catheter to inflate the balloon, and.
- A contrast medium.

   The patient lies in the supine position, with the neck and thorax slightly flexed with the nose at the top. Thus, strict sagittal X-rays can be obtained during the following surgical steps.

Surgical Procedure

Involved the following two steps.

Foramen Ovale Cannulation

Three skin landmarks are marked on the cheek.
   Using the classical *Hartel's route* [8] (Fig. 17.1):

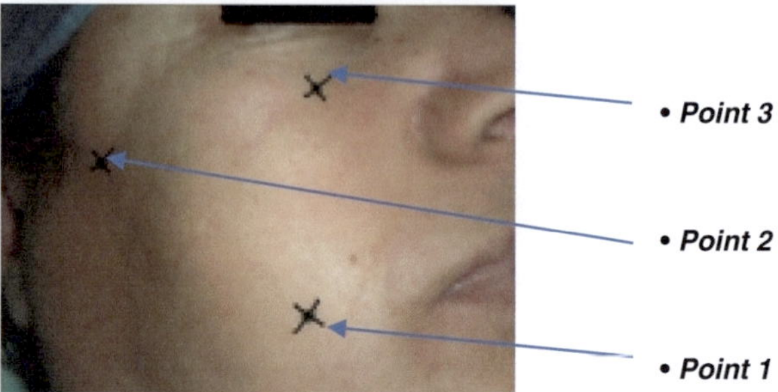

Fig. 17.1 Landmarks of the Hartel's route. The first corresponds to the location of the skin puncture:2.5 cm lateral to the angle lip. The second is on the inferior edge of the zygomatic arch, 3 cm anterior to the external auditory canal. The third is on the line joining the first point to the pupil on the inferior edge of the orbit. Reprinted with permission from Abdennebi B, Guenane L. Technical considerations and outcome assessment in retrogasserian balloon compression for treatment of trigeminal neuralgia. Series of 901 patients. Surg Neurol Int 2014; 5:118 [8]

1. The first corresponds to the location of the skin puncture: 2.5 cm lateral to the angle lip.
2. The second is on the inferior edge of the zygomatic arch, 3 cm anterior to the external auditory canal.
3. The third is on the line joining the first point to the pupil on the inferior edge of the orbit.

After surgical cleaning of the affected hemi face, the HI is inserted in the first landmark (Fig. 17.3). While advancing it forward, we must remember, that the direction of the foramen oval (FO) cannulation is corresponding to the intersection of two planes, one lateral between points 1 and 2, and the other sagittal between points 1 and 3. Three anatomical structures are successively traversed: the cheek, then the pterygomaxillary fossa, and finally the FO.

The neurosurgeon's index finger is kept in close contact with the inner side of the cheek (Fig. 17.2). It helps to guide the introducer without penetrating into the oral cavity. However, Bleeding might occur in the pterygomaxillary fossa through the HI or within the cheek, due to the injury of branches of the internal maxillary artery or of the veins of the pterygoid venous plexus. In that case, the procedure needs to be abandoned, and hemostasis is obtained by external compression of the cheek. The surgery can be attempted at a later date.

Multiple endeavors are required at times to penetrate the FO. Bony landmarks, depicted on biplane fluoroscopy, help to guide HI steering. The first is in close contact with the introducer with the projection of the posterior extremity of the horizontal plate of the palatine bone observed on the X-rays sagittal view (Fig. 17.3).

The second is the direction of the HI, which should be the bisector of the angle composed by the superior edge of the petrous bone and the clivus (Fig. 17.3).

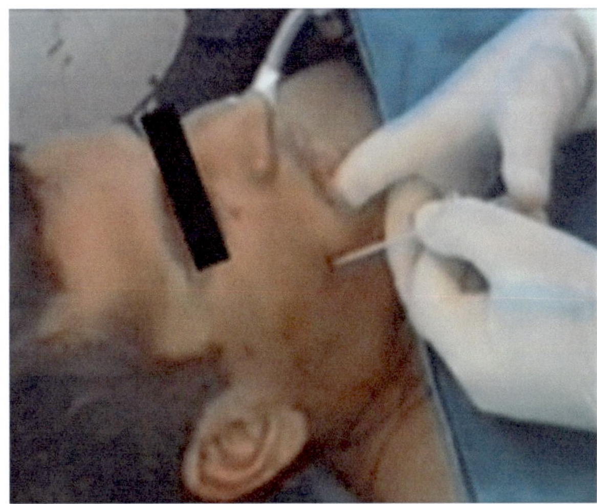

Fig. 17.2 Skin puncture for balloon compression in a patient under general anesthesia. Reprinted with permission from Abdennebi B, Guenane L. Technical considerations and outcome assessment in retrogasserian balloon compression for treatment of trigeminal neuralgia. Series of 901 patients. Surg Neurol Int 2014;5:118 [9]

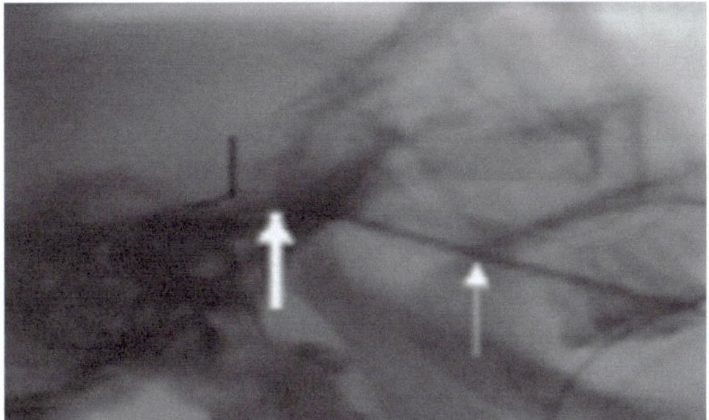

Fig. 17.3 Sagittal X-ray showing the metallic hollow introducer, in close contact with the posterior extremity of the horizontal plate of the palatine bone, thin white arrow, at the level of the foramen ovale, thick white arrow. In black lines: the clivus and the superior edge of the petrous bone. Reprinted with permission from Abdennebi B, Guenane L. Technical considerations and outcome assessment in retrogasserian balloon compression for treatment of trigeminal neuralgia. Series of 901 patients. Surg Neurol Int 2014;5:118 [9]

The crucial step is the engagement of the FO, recognized on seeing and feeling the masseter muscles shrinking. The advancement of the HI is interrupted from that moment, in order to avoid its penetration inside the skull.

Balloon Inflation

The HI is withdrawn while the plastic catheter is gently advanced upwards 3–4 mm towards the gasserian ganglion. CSF drops, coming from the trigeminal cistern, may exit through the stylet at the skin orifice. The Fogarty Catheter's balloon is filled with Contrast Medium in order to check its patency and to realize the air evacuation.

Next, the Fogarty catheter is inserted into the hub of the Silicon Catheter so that the extremity corresponding to the deflated balloon is located *ahead*. Once the optimal location of the balloon is ensured under fluoroscopy with a first small inflation with 0.3 cc of contrast medium, the definitive inflation of the balloon is finally achieved with 0.7 cc for 6 min.

Bradycardia might occur, with a diminution of the blood pressure at this stage. The last sagittal X-ray shows the thin SC and the balloon in a pear shape on both sides of the clivus: The body and the stalk of this image correspond, respectively, to the Gasserian ganglion and to the triangular plexus. When the duration mentioned earlier is completed, the balloon is deflated and all the other stuff is removed [8].

Risks and Complications

Numbness is a goal of the procedure, although the majority of the patients indicate that their numbness is mild and tolerable. The small percentage of patients with severe numbness. Associated with the numbness are several other elements which are a consequence of the motor innervation of the trigeminal nerve. Patients may complain of otalgia, related to weakness of the tensor tympani muscle. The jaw might deviate in some to the contralateral side due to pterygoid weakness. Rarely, patients have developed hemotympanum from blood entering the eustachian tube.

Dysesthesias are rare and rarely bothersome. There may be a sense of intermittent "crawling" perception. Often, numbness is localized in the perioral area of V2 and V3 if the balloon is positioned properly radiographically. Further medial placement of the catheter at the porous trigeminus by using a more lateral entrance point if V1 numbness is desired.

Arrhythmias from the bradycardia and cardiac pacing are rare. Complications of the brief hypertensive response have never been seen. The needle used is larger than a radiofrequency needle, hence can be more painful at the puncture site. An ice pack is placed on the cheek afterward for several hours to reduce pain and swelling.

A randomized controlled study from the University of Sao Paolo, Brazil in 2010 on 55 patients showed that the use of local anesthetics during the trigeminal balloon compression for TN can have a preventive role for the risk of cardiovascular events [9].

Cold sores may emerge several days after the procedure as is the case with other trigeminal manipulations, but prophylactic treatment with acyclovir has not been routinely done unless there is a known propensity. One death has been reported associated with intraoperative bleeding, but the needle, in that case, was incorrectly placed far too deep beyond the foramen ovale.

Temporary sixth nerve palsy can also occur, presumably from balloon overinflation and cavernous sinus compression. According to a study from Functional Neurosurgery Unit, Department of Neurosurgery, Medical School of Patras, Patras, Greece on 79 patients in 2009 this resulted from irregular balloon shape and inflation of the balloon towards the sellar floor [10].

Lasting corneal anesthesia is rare, although a brief reduction in the reflex has been seen. Keratitis or anesthesia is unlikely because of selective compressive injury to large myelinated fibers only.

Post-procedural Care

The patient should be monitored in the recovery room for at least an hour after the procedure. The patient's pain level is recorded before and after the procedure to assess response to the anesthetic with a numeric rating scale. Vital signs and neurological functions are assessed and documented before discharge. Fall prevention protocols are followed to minimize the risks of injury. Written discharge instructions include limiting activities the day of the procedure; and contacting the physician if there is any weakness, fever, chills, or erythema or induration at the site of the procedure.

Clinical Pearls and Trouble Shooting

1. If *the balloon is inflated too far* into the porous trigeminus, it can slip farther into the pre-pontine cistern.
2. If a *pear shape is not seen*, the balloon may not have been advanced far enough to have entered the porous trigeminus. The lateral view on fluoroscopy will show whether the balloon has reached the clival line.
3. If advancement of the catheter still does not lead to a pear shape, or if inflation pressure is near the 550-mm Hg, the catheter might have penetrated the dura.
4. The best chance of success is to remove the needle and catheter and reposition them using a stylet, thereby preventing the catheter to slide through the same path, repeatedly penetrating the dura in the same site.
5. Incase venous bleeding occurs, the needle is repositioned at the foramen, by advancing slightly until firmly engaged under lateral fluoroscopic screening, preventing excessive advancement into the middle fossa.
6. If there are concerns for subarachnoid bleeding a CT scan should be done.
7. Drowsiness is not expected, and if it occurs, should lead to further investigation.
8. Subarachnoid bleeding might simulate aseptic meningitis, with fever, headache, and confusion lasting for 24–48 h. Such patients complain of the headache immediately upon awakening and need symptomatic treatment.
9. If pain is not relieved the procedure may be repeated, but one should wait for at least a week since the secondary injury to the nerve may cause progressive injury and pain relief may occur in the next several days.
10. If *numbness* is bothersome, the patient should that the assured that numbness will decrease notably during the first several days after surgery.
11. Severe numbness might not resolve but improve.
12. Jaw weakness might last for several weeks.
13. In case of pain resistant to compression, despite numbness in the appropriate divisions, the possibility of trigeminal neuralgia must be re-examined.

Outcome and Recurrence

Long-term pain recurrence varies between 20 and 43%, and immediate pain relief is higher than 90%. Recurrence rates are lower with microvascular decompression: 4–30%.

Late regeneration of damaged nerves might be a factor leading to higher recurrence rates.

The effectiveness of percutaneous balloon compression in the treatment of patients with TN recurrence after other surgical techniques has been a matter of debate.

Factors Affecting Outcome

1. Shape of the Balloon: A retrospective study from the Department of Neurosurgery, Umeå University Hospital, Umeå; and Karolinska University Hospital, Stockholm, Sweden in 2010 on 87 PBC's demonstrated longer pain relief, using a pear-shaped balloon than non-pear-shaped balloons [11].
2. Balloon opening pressure: Procedural pressure patterns of the balloon opening pressure and the initial compression pressure are important.

    A study from *Department of Neurosurgery Chang Gung University & Chang Gung Memorial Hospital, Taoyuan, Taiwan* in 2003 on 75 patients, showed how a computerized pressure monitoring system has proven to be accurate, reliable, and extremely useful for monitoring the PBC procedure [12].
3. Balloon Compression time: affect the results as well. The aforesaid group in a study *on* 80 patients with intractable third-branch trigeminal (V3) neuralgia, showed that the shorter duration of PBC had lesser side effects. At 1-year follow-up, the incidence of recurrence rate was slightly higher in the patients who received 60-s compression compared to 180-s compression, but there was no significant statistical difference [13].
4. Whether patients with first or second branch TN require longer compression duration needs further study.

    Brown et al. in a study in 56 patients reported PBC for a duration of 1–1.5 min with an intraluminal balloon pressure of 1140–1215 mm Hg reduces the occurrence of masseter muscle weakness, dysesthesias, and severe numbness without reducing the degree of pain relief achieved in patients with classic TN [14].
5. Pain relief is usually present after the patient is fully awake from anesthesia but has, on occasion, been delayed for several days.

Review of Literature

Comparison with other techniques: The Department of Neurosurgery, Wessex Neurological Centre, Southampton, UK in a study involving 393 procedures performed for 210 patients over 19 years reported longer pain relief with PBC than glycerol and thermocoagulation. PBC led to numbness and a few minor and transitory complications. Moreover, PBC following previous percutaneous procedures was found to be highly effective [15].

Recurrence following other procedures: Nicola Montano et al. reviewed the outcome of PBC on 22 patients with recurrence of TN after previous procedures. The group observed an excellent outcome in 16 out of 22 (72.72%) patients and a good outcome in the remaining six. No patients had uncontrolled pain. The lack of history of MS ($p = 0.0174$), the pear-like shape of the balloon at the operation ($p = 0.0234$), and a compression time <5 min ($p\backslash0.05$) were associated with pain-free survival. Considering these results, they concluded that PBC is a useful technique for patients whose pain recurs after other procedures [16].

In Multiple sclerosis(MS): The Department of Neurosurgery, Institute of Neurological Science, Glasgow, UK, found PBC to be effective in the treatment of trigeminal neuralgia in patients with MS in 80 patients (17 with MS and 63 non-MS) from January 2000 to January 2010 but, however, symptom recurrence was higher compared to non-MS patients [17].

References

1. Montano N, Conforti G, Di Bonaventura R, Meglio M, Fernandez E, Papacci F. Advances in diagnosis and treatment of trigeminal neuralgia. Ther Clin Risk Manag. 2015;11:289–99.
2. Krafft RM. Trigeminal neuralgia. Am Fam Physician. 2008;77:1291–6.
3. McMillan R. Trigeminal neuralgia—a debilitating facial pain. Rev pain. 2011;5:26–34.
4. Cruccu G, Finnerup NB, Jensen TS, Scholz J, Sindou M, Svensson P, et al. Trigeminal neuralgia: new classification and diagnostic grading for practice and research. Neurology. 2016;87:220–8. Describing a new classification system for TN
5. Mullan S, Lichtor T. Percutaneous microcompression of the trigeminal ganglion for trigeminal neuralgia. J Neurosurg. 1983;59(6):1007–12.
6. Shelden CH, Pudenz RH, Freshwater DB, Crue BL. Compression rather decompression for trigeminal neuralgia. J Neurosurg. 1955;12:123–6.
7. Brown JA, Hoeflinger B, Long PB, Gunning WT, Rhoades R, Bennet-Clarke CA, et al. Axon and ganglion cell injury in rabbits after percutaneous trigeminal balloon compression. Neurosurgery. 1996;38:993–1004.
8. Abdennebi B, Guenane L. Technical considerations and outcome assessment in retrogasserian balloon compression for treatment of trigeminal neuralgia. Series of 901 patients. Surg Neurol Int. 2014;5:118.
9. Tibano AT, de Siqueira SRDT, da Nóbrega JCM, et al. Cardiovascular response during trigeminal ganglion compression for trigeminal neuralgia according to the use of local anesthetics. Acta Neurochir. 2010;152:1347–51.
10. Kefalopoulou Z, Markaki E, Constantoyannis C. Avoiding abducens nerve palsy during the percutaneous balloon compression procedure. Stereotact Funct Neurosurg. 2009;87(2):101–4.
11. AsPlund P, Linderoth B, Bergenhei AT. The predictive power of balloon shape and change of sensory functions on outcome of percutaneous balloon compression for trigeminal neuralgia. J Neurosurg. 2010;113:498–507.
12. Lee S-T, Chen J-F. Percutaneous trigeminal ganglion balloon compression for treatment of trigeminal neuralgia—part I: pressure recordings. Surg Neurol. 2003;59:63–7.
13. Lee ST, Chen JF. Percutaneous trigeminal ganglion balloon compression for treatment of trigeminal neuralgia—part II: results related to compression duration. Surg Neurol. 2003;60:149–54.

14. Brown JA, Pilitsis JG. Percutaneous balloon compression for the treatment of trigeminal neuralgia: results in 56 patients based on balloon compression pressure monitoring. Neurosurg Focus. 2005;18:E10.
15. Noorani I, Lodge A, Vajramani G, Sparrow O. Comparing percutaneous treatments of trigeminal neuralgia: 19 years of experience in a single centre. Stereotact Funct Neurosurg. 2016;94(2):75–85. https://doi.org/10.1159/000445077.
16. Montano N, Papacci F, Cioni B, et al. The role of percutaneous balloon compression in the treatment of trigeminal neuralgia recurring after other surgical procedures. Acta Neurol Belg. 2014;114:59–64. https://doi.org/10.1007/s13760-013-0263-x.
17. Martin S, Teo M, Suttner N. The effectiveness of percutaneous balloon compression in the treatment of trigeminal neuralgia in patients with multiple sclerosis. J Neurosurg. 2015;123(6):1507–11. https://doi.org/10.3171/2014.11.jns14736.

Wendell Lake

Introduction

Trigeminal neuralgia is a common cause of neuropathic face pain. The prevalence of the disease is between 0.03 and 0.3%. Women are three times as likely to be affected as men. The mean age of patients with trigeminal neuralgia is over 60 years [1]. Some studies estimate that 50% of patients with trigeminal neuralgia will not be adequately managed with medical therapy [2]. This presents a challenge for clinicians since many trigeminal neuralgia patients will fail medical management and several older patients will have significant co-morbidities precluding invasive procedures. Because of this many have proposed radiosurgery as a reasonable treatment alternative that may improve symptom control but does not require general anesthesia or an invasive procedure.

Historically, trigeminal neuralgia was one of the first diseases treated with radiosurgery with the first treatment beginning in 1953. Since that time several studies have demonstrated the safety and long-term efficacy of radiosurgery for the treatment of trigeminal neuralgia. Various dosages and targeting techniques have been reported in the radiosurgical treatment of trigeminal neuralgia [3]. Like many more invasive treatment methods, several side effects have been reported with radiosurgery for trigeminal neuralgia. The most common side effect of radiosurgery for trigeminal neuralgia is facial sensory changes. A significant minority of patients have long-term pain recurrence following radiosurgical treatment for trigeminal neuralgia, but this is a problem familiar for all other treatments of this difficult illness [4].

Given its efficacy and favorable side effect profile, stereotactic radiosurgery will continue to be an important part of the management armamentarium for Trigeminal Neuralgia.

W. Lake (✉)
University of Wisconsin-Madison, Madison, WI, USA
e-mail: lake@neurosurgery.wisc.edu

© The Author(s), under exclusive license to Springer Nature
Switzerland AG 2021
A. Abd-Elsayed (ed.), *Trigeminal Nerve Pain*,
https://doi.org/10.1007/978-3-030-60687-9_18

Historical Advent

Trigeminal neuralgia was one of the first illnesses effectively treated with radiosurgery. Difficult surgical access to the trigeminal ganglion and the severely debilitating nature of the illness were drivers in the early application of radiosurgery to this illness. Relatively safe, durable outcomes were reported in early radiosurgical treatment series. The advent of MRI scanning and image merger techniques further improved the accuracy and safety of the procedure [5]. Since its advent, thousands of trigeminal neuralgia patients have been treated with radiosurgery by various methods.

Radiosurgical Modalities for Treatment of Trigeminal Neuralgia

Various methods have been described for the radiosurgical treatment of trigeminal neuralgia. The radiation delivery method, radiation dose, and radiation target vary by center. Here we discuss these three parameters.

The radiation delivery method for radiosurgery can be Gamma Knife (GK), linear accelerator (LINAC), or cyberknife (CK). All three of these methods aim beams of radiation from multiple angles at a specific target, in this case, the trigeminal nerve. These beams converge at a specific point. At the convergent point, the radiation dose is very high. As one moves away from the point where the beams converge the dose falls off rapidly. This allows an ablative radiation dose to be delivered to the trigeminal nerve at or near its origin from the brain stem without exposing other critical areas of the brain and surrounding structures to a damaging level of radiation, see Fig. 18.1.

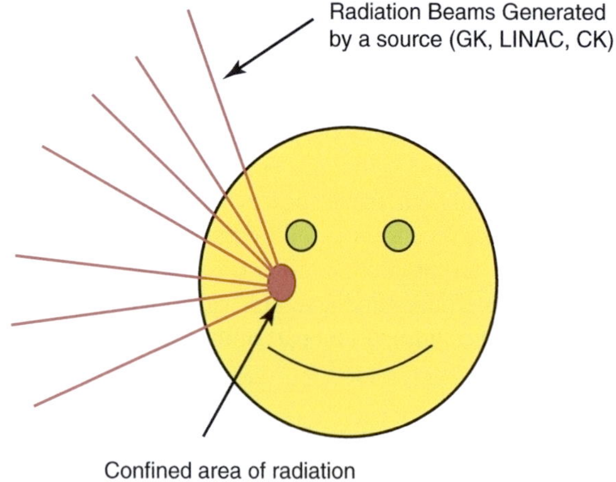

Fig. 18.1 Radiation beams from multiple angles converge at a given target resulting in a confined area of damage at the radiosurgical target. Radiation beams from different angles may be generated by a source that moves relative to the patient, in the case of LINAC and CK, or by using multiple different radiation emitting sources placed at specific positions relative to the patient GK

Linear Accelerator (LINAC), Gamma knife (GK), and Cyberknife (CK) all deliver ionizing electromagnetic radiation. For GK the patient's head is placed inside a helmet-like device, then various stationary radioactive Cobalt-60 gamma-emitting sources are uncovered to produce radiation beams intercepting the target from various angles. In the case of LINAC and CK. In the case of LINAC and CK, a microwave field inside of a waveguide accelerates electrons that collide with heavy metals creating high energy X-rays. These X-rays are then focused on the radiosurgical target from multiple different directions as the machine moves relative to the patient's head. This results in a radiosurgical lesion. LINAC is differentiated from CK in that the LINAC radiation emitters only move around the patient's head in different rotational arcs whereas CK is affixed to a robotic arm and can make non-rotational movements. GK, LINAC, and CK are all accepted methods for radio-surgical treatment of trigeminal neuralgia. Developments in image science, such as MRI CT merging, and computerized radiosurgical planning have substantially improved the accessibility and safety of radiosurgery over the past two decades [6]. The largest series of patients have been treated with GK but substantial numbers of patients have been treated with all three modalities resulting in similar outcomes [3].

Radiosurgical Technique in the Treatment of Trigeminal Neuralgia

Parameters that can be varied in the radiosurgical treatment of trigeminal neuralgia are many but three major variables are frequently reported: dose, stereotactic target-ing system, and anatomical target.

Dose

In a systematic review that evaluated over 5600 patients treated with GK the mean maximal doses ranged from 71 to 90 Gy. The same study compiled results from approximately 511 patients treated with LINAC and 263 patients treated with CK and the mean maximal dose ranges in these studies were 70–90 Gy and 65–81 Gy respectively. For GK the dose was reported at the 100% isodose line whereas the dose for LINAC and CK were reported at the 80 or 90% isodose line.

Head Fixation

In the case of GK, the patient is immobilized in a rigid stereotactic frame that allows the patient to be rigidly fixed to the table. This frame-based system facilitates pre-cise targeting but requires pins to be placed into the skin abutting the skull. Frames may subject patients to some discomfort and some infection risk but are generally tolerated by most with the addition of local anesthesia and anxiolytic and or pain medication [3]. LINAC radiosurgical treatment generally uses frame immobilization but some centers have switched to thermoformed face masks. CK uses thermoformed face masks. If the stereotactic system, either CK or LINAC, employs a thermoplastic face mask then image guidance or real-time image assisted targeting is required with either X-rays or infrared imaging [4, 7].

If a stereotactic frame is used in the radiosurgical treatment procedure then appropriate placement is critical. The projection of the trigeminal ganglion on the lateral portion of the patient's face is at a point approximately 1.5 cm anterior and superior to the external auditory meatus. The bottom of the frame must be below this point and the angle of the frame should be parallel to the line drawn from the orbit to the external auditory meatus. This angle ensures that the frame parallels the course of the nerve from the pons to Meckel's cave, where the preganglionic segment connects to the ganglion [8].

Targeting

The anatomical position of the target in radiosurgery for trigeminal neuralgia varies between centers, and ranges from posterior targeting up to targeting the\anterior portion of the nerve in the cistern. Generally, the total distance ranges from 0 mm, which is at the nerve's junction with the pons, up to 8 mm anterior which is the point where the nerve joins with the ganglion in Meckel's cave. In the case of posterior targeting, some portion of the pons is within the 20 or 30% isodose line and receives a significant dose of radiation. This more posterior target may be associated with a higher rate of long-term pain improvement but some studies have also reported a higher rate of facial numbness [3, 9]. A more anterior target, at the trigeminal ganglion itself, was used early in the history of radiosurgical treatment. This target may be associated with a lower rate of facial hypesthesia but may also be associated with a lower rate of durable treatment effect in some studies. This however is controversial and others have found that the anterior target has similar pain relief with lower complications [10]. Currently, there is level 2 evidence to suggest the use of an anterior target [3].

Some initial work suggested that the durability of pain relief may be proportional to the length of the cisternal nerve segment exposed to radiation. Given this finding, authors began to suggest the use of more than one isocenter during radiation treatment planning to permit a greater length of the trigeminal nerve to be exposed to radiation. A double-blinded randomized controlled trial compared treatment with one versus two isocenters. In this study they found no difference in pain relief with a 36 month follow-up period, but treatment with two isocenters did result in a higher proportion of patients with bothersome facial numbness [11]. In general, most centers now tend towards the use of a single 4 mm isocenter [7]. Figure 18.2 provides a schematic summary of targeting methods superimposed on thin-cut T2 sequence MRI imaging of the cisternal segment of the trigeminal nerve [3].

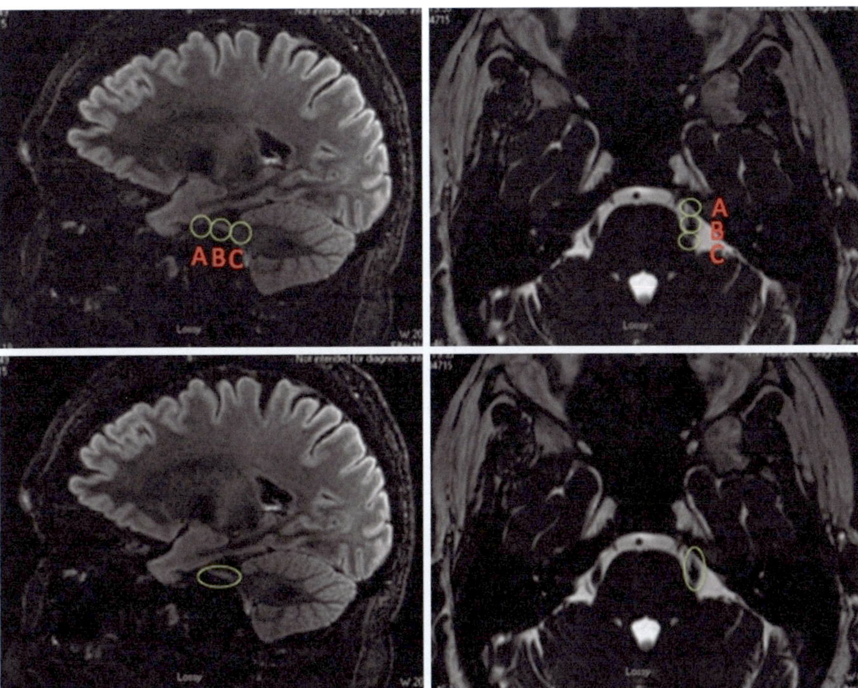

Fig. 18.2 Upper two panes represent a schematic of radiosurgical 4 mm isocenters in the anterior, mid-cisternal, and posterior positions. Usually only one is employed in a given treatment. Lower two panes provide a schematic for a treatment plan with two non-concentric isocenters. Scales are approximate

Outcomes of Radiosurgery for Trigeminal Neuralgia

Thousands of patients have been treated with radiosurgery for trigeminal neuralgia. The results of many treatments have been published in case series format and often long-term follow-up is available. GK has the most extensive case series publication but LINAC and CK also have a significant number of published case series. To discuss the outcomes of radiosurgical treatment of trigeminal neuralgia an introduction to the grading of facial pain is necessary. In the discussion of outcomes other relevant factors that should be addressed include time to response, long-term freedom from pain, rate of patients undergoing additional procedures aimed at treatment of trigeminal neuralgia and radiosurgery related complications.

Measurement Scales in Radiosurgical Studies

A variety of grading scales may be used in various studies of radiosurgery for the treatment of trigeminal neuralgia, but the Barrow Neurological Institute (BNI) Pain Intensity score is used in many studies. For this scale the patient's pain is graded on a Roman numeral scale I–V, see Table 18.1 [12].

Table 18.1 Barrow neurological institute pain intensity score

Grade	Pain description
I	No pain, no medications
II	No medications required, occasional pain
III	Some pain, adequately controlled with medications
IV	Some pain, not adequately controlled with medications
V	Severe pain or no pain relief

Like most types of neuropathic pain, Trigeminal neuralgia is a multifaceted problem. Therefore, other authors have characterized the outcomes by examining the quality of life and functionality post-treatment. As expected in patients with pain relief there was a significant improvement in the quality of life and functionality [13, 14].

Time to Pain Relief

Unlike invasive surgical procedures, radiosurgical treatment of trigeminal neuralgia usually requires a time period prior to realization of pain relief. Reported time to pain relief varies between case series and modalities. When case series are aggregated the mean time to pain relief was on average 15–78 days for GK and 28–81 days for LINAC. Usually, pain relief is thought to have reached its maximum level by 180 days [3].

Freedom from Pain

Like all treatment methods for trigeminal neuralgia, radiosurgery fails in a significant minority of patients. The failure of the therapy to control pain generally increases with increasing time. Comparison patients treated with GK, CK, and LINAC showed no statistically significant difference in mean or median rates of freedom from pain (BNI Pain intensity score of I–III). All three methods demonstrated freedom from the pain of approximately 85% once a response had occurred. Freedom from pain without medication (BNI Pain intensity score of I) was usually around 50% and not statistically different between treatment methods of GK, CK, or LINAC. As previously mentioned time to pain response was usually on the order of 1 month or more and maximal pain relief response was thought to occur around 180 days [3].

Recurrence

Reported pain recurrence rates for GK range from 0 to 52%, for LINAC 19–63%, and for CK 16–33%. The recurrence rate on average is 25% for GK and 32% for LINAC. This was statistically significant for BNI pain intensity score grades of III and IV. Meaning that the rates were the same between the two modalities for patients that realized no pain improvement.

On average time to pain recurrence was 6–48 months for GK, 8–20 months for LINAC, and 1–43 months for CK. There was not enough data on the recurrence time frame to draw meaningful conclusions as to rather one radiosurgical method was superior to others. However, it can be concluded that a significant number of patients do experience a recurrence of pain following these treatments [3].

Sustained pain relief with long-term follow-up is rarely studied. Limited data showed that at 7 years pain relief was maintained in 22–60% of patients with GK treatment and at 10 years maintained pain relief with GK treatment ranged from 30 to 45% but fewer studies were available [4, 15]. Long-term maintenance of pain control has even more limited data in the LINAC literature. At 3 years 60% were still reported to have pain relief in one study [16].

Complications

Radiosurgery for treatment of trigeminal neuralgia has a very favorable safety profile and is sometimes chosen as a first-line treatment for patients that suffer from significant co-morbidities or are of advanced age. Patients undergoing radiosurgery generally do not face the risk of cerebrospinal fluid leak and wound infection that microvascular decompression patients face. Serious life-threatening complications such as vasculopathy or aneurysm formation and rupture are very rare [17].

The most common serious complication is keratitis or corneal damage due to loss of sensation in the area of the cornea. In GK studies keratitis is reported in up to 7% of treated patients while in LINAC studies keratitis is reported in up to 3.6%. Some case series in GK, CK, and LINAC report no patient developing keratitis. The complication of keratitis has been reported to correspond with the amount of brainstem receiving a significant dose of radiation in some studies [18].

Facial hypesthesia (numbness) and dysesthesia are the most common complications associated with radiosurgery for trigeminal neuralgia. In GK up to 52% of patients in some series endorse some form of altered facial sensation. Some studies have actually shown a positive association with facial numbness and sustained pain relief. In some cases the sensation may be severely altered to the point that it is painful for the patient but the rate of this complication is generally under 5%. Eye dryness is a common complaint, ~20% in some case series, following radiosurgery for trigeminal neuralgia and is generally associated with numbness in the ophthalmic distribution of the trigeminal nerve [15, 18]. Overall, patients treated with radiosurgery for trigeminal neuralgia must be followed closely for the development of any ophthalmological complications.

Table 18.2 provides a summary of complications, outcomes, and mean time to recurrence for various radiosurgical treatment methods. Good pain control is described as BNI Pain Intensity score I–III in the table meaning no pain without medications, occasional pain without medications, or adequate control of pain with mediations.

Table 18.2 Outcomes and complications in radiosurgery for trigeminal neuralgia with various modalities

Modality	BNI pain intensity score I–III (%)	Mean time to pain relief onset (days)	Mean recurrence rate (%)	Mean time to recurrence (months)	Complication
GK	85	15–78	25	6–48	Hypesthesia 22% Keratitis 0–7% Dry eye 0–22%
LINAC	88	28–81	32	7–20	Hypesthesia 28% Keratitis 0–3.6% Dry Eye 0–20%
CK	79	–	26	9	Hypesthesia 29% Other complications not reported in CK

Columns 1 and 2 do not represent statistically significant differences
Mean time to pain relief was not reported in a sufficient number of CK studies
BNI Barrow Neurological Institute, *GK* Gamma Knife, *LINAC* Linear Accelerator, *CK* Cyberknife

Attempts have been made to categorize trigeminal neuralgia patient-specific factors such that outcomes of radiosurgery can be predicted. Factors evaluated include: presence of atypical symptoms, presence of multiple sclerosis, age, prior surgical procedures, post-treatment numbness, neurovascular conflict on MRI, and post-treatment nerve enhancement.

In general, older patients, age >70 years, are found to fare better with radiosurgery as are patients with typical pain. Here typical pain is defined as intermittent lancinating pain with little inter-episode pain or dysesthesias [3, 19]. Patients with post-treatment numbness are also more likely to have a durable treatment response in some studies but others refute this finding [15]. Interestingly, patients with neurovascular conflicts identified on preprocedural MRI do not have a lower rate of pain relief with radiosurgical treatment of trigeminal neuralgia. This likely relates to the fact that most cases of typical trigeminal neuralgia are thought to be associated with neurovascular conflict. Therefore, the presence of neurovascular conflict may be a surrogate for typical face pain [20]. Post-treatment MRI has shown gadolinium enhancement of the trigeminal nerve in some studies. Some of the case series found that this effect was in the majority of patients while in other series it was the minority of patients. This enhancement was found to have no obvious effect on either pain relief or durability of the procedure [21, 22].

Prior surgery and atypical pain character have both been found to be associated with lower rates of pain freedom and durability of pain relief in trigeminal neuralgia patients treated with radiosurgery. However, radiosurgery is not contraindicated in patients that have undergone prior surgical decompression or ablation. In many cases, practitioners employ radiosurgery as a salvage treatment after surgery and it has shown significant pain relief. In one study 91% of patients reported initial pain relief following radiosurgery as a salvage therapy, although only 50% of patients reported continued pain improvement at the 5-year mark [3, 23]. Both diabetes mellitus and multiple sclerosis have been found to negatively correlate with pain improvement in trigeminal neuralgia following radiosurgery [3, 4]. This raises suspicion that these illnesses either alter the mechanism of the neuralgia or the response of the nerve to treatment.

In conclusion, Radiosurgery is a safe and effective, albeit imperfect, treatment for trigeminal neuralgia. A large amount of data in the form of extensive case series and one randomized controlled trial support the use of this treatment. Severe complications are rare and the most common complications include facial numbness and dry eye on the treatment side. The use of this treatment technique is warranted both as a primary treatment strategy and also as a salvage treatment therapy for patients that have undergone prior treatment with invasive procedures such as open surgery or rhizotomy. Technological advancement has allowed greater access to radiosurgery over the past two decades improving both ease of use and safety. Future efforts in following patients treated with radiosurgery over longer time intervals are warranted and may allow improved patient selection based on individualized patient factors.

References

1. De Toledo IP, et al. Prevalence of trigeminal neuralgia: a systematic review. J Am Dent Assoc. 2016;147:570–576.e2.
2. Jones MR, et al. A comprehensive review of trigeminal neuralgia. Curr Pain Headache Rep. 2019;23:74.
3. Tuleasca C, et al. Stereotactic radiosurgery for trigeminal neuralgia: a systematic review. J Neurosurg. 2018;130:733–57.
4. Régis J, et al. The very long-term outcome of radiosurgery for classical trigeminal neuralgia. Stereotact Funct Neurosurg. 2016;94:24–32.
5. Kondziolka D, Perez B, Flickinger JC, Lunsford LD. Gamma knife radiosurgery for trigeminal neuralgia. Prog Neurol Surg. 1998;14:212–21. https://doi.org/10.1159/000062032.
6. Deinsberger R, Tidstrand J. Linac radiosurgery as a tool in neurosurgery. Neurosurg Rev. 2005;28:79–88; discussion 89–90.
7. Richards GM, et al. Linear accelerator radiosurgery for trigeminal neuralgia. Neurosurgery. 2005;57:1193–200; discussion 1193–200.
8. Gurney SP, Ramalingam S, Thomas A, Sinclair AJ, Mollan SP. Exploring the current management idiopathic intracranial hypertension, and understanding the role of dural venous sinus stenting. Eye Brain. 2020;12:1–13.
9. Goss BW, et al. Linear accelerator radiosurgery using 90 gray for essential trigeminal neuralgia: results and dose volume histogram analysis. Neurosurgery. 2003;53:823–8; discussion 828–30.
10. Park S-H, et al. The retrogasserian zone versus dorsal root entry zone: comparison of two targeting techniques of gamma knife radiosurgery for trigeminal neuralgia. Acta Neurochir. 2010;152:1165–70.
11. Flickinger JC, et al. Does increased nerve length within the treatment volume improve trigeminal neuralgia radiosurgery? A prospective double-blind, randomized study. Int J Radiat Oncol Biol Phys. 2001;51:449–54.
12. Chen HI, Lee JYK. The measurement of pain in patients with trigeminal neuralgia. Clin Neurosurg. 2010;57:129–33.

13. Herman JM, et al. Repeat gamma knife radiosurgery for refractory or recurrent trigeminal neuralgia: treatment outcomes and quality-of-life assessment. Int J Radiat Oncol Biol Phys. 2004;59:112–6.
14. Petit JH, Herman JM, Nagda S, DiBiase SJ, Chin LS. Radiosurgical treatment of trigeminal neuralgia: evaluating quality of life and treatment outcomes. Int J Radiat Oncol Biol Phys. 2003;56:1147–53.
15. Kondziolka D, et al. Gamma Knife stereotactic radiosurgery for idiopathic trigeminal neuralgia. J Neurosurg. 2010;112:758–65.
16. Smith ZA, et al. Dedicated linear accelerator radiosurgery for trigeminal neuralgia: a single-center experience in 179 patients with varied dose prescriptions and treatment plans. Int J Radiat Oncol Biol Phys. 2011;81:225–31.
17. Dominguez L, et al. Ruptured distal superior cerebellar artery aneurysm after gamma knife radiosurgery for trigeminal neuralgia: a case report and review of the literature. World Neurosurg. 2020;135:2–6.
18. Matsuda S, Serizawa T, Sato M, Ono J. Gamma knife radiosurgery for trigeminal neuralgia: the dry-eye complication. J Neurosurg. 2002;97:525–8.
19. Han JH, et al. Long-term outcome of gamma knife radiosurgery for treatment of typical trigeminal neuralgia. Int J Radiat Oncol Biol Phys. 2009;75:822–7.
20. Erbay SH, et al. Association between neurovascular contact on MRI and response to gamma knife radiosurgery in trigeminal neuralgia. Neuroradiology. 2006;48:26–30.
21. Massager N, Abeloos L, Devriendt D, Op de Beeck M, Levivier M. Clinical evaluation of targeting accuracy of gamma knife radiosurgery in trigeminal neuralgia. Int J Radiat Oncol Biol Phys. 2007;69:1514–20.
22. Alberico RA, Fenstermaker RA, Lobel J. Focal enhancement of cranial nerve V after radiosurgery with the Leksell gamma knife: experience in 15 patients with medically refractory trigeminal neuralgia. AJNR Am J Neuroradiol. 2001;22:1944–8.
23. Little AS, Shetter AG, Shetter ME, Kakarla UK, Rogers CL. Salvage gamma knife stereotactic radiosurgery for surgically refractory trigeminal neuralgia. Int J Radiat Oncol Biol Phys. 2009;74:522–7.

Wendell Lake

Introduction

Over the past several decades microvascular decompression (MVD) has become increasingly popular as a primary treatment for patients with trigeminal neuralgia who have failed medical management. Trigeminal neuralgia was one of the first diseases treated by neurosurgical intervention due to its severity. Surgical treatment strategies have evolved significantly over the past century. At this point, there is a large collection of case series supporting the durable and effective nature of MVD. Certain patient factors may provide prognostic information and assist in patient selection for this procedure. Although MVD is one of the most effective known treatments for trigeminal neuralgia there are a significant minority of patients that will have a recurrence of pain following the treatment. As a surgical procedure microvascular decompression has a risk of complications including cerebrospinal fluid leak, facial numbness, hearing loss, wound infection, and stroke. In the coming years, MVD will likely continue to evolve with new techniques and instruments aimed at improving safety and efficacy [1, 2].

Historical Advent and Surgical Views on the Etiology of Pain

Surgical treatment of trigeminal neuralgia is closely linked to the history of neurosurgery. Surgical treatment of this illness was described as early as the eighteenth century. Early in the twentieth-century surgical treatment of trigeminal neuralgia was associated with significant potential for morbidity and even death. Nonetheless, due to the severe and often progressive nature of this illness many patients were still

W. Lake (✉)
University of Wisconsin-Madison, Madison, WI, USA
e-mail: lake@neurosurgery.wisc.edu

© The Author(s), under exclusive license to Springer Nature
Switzerland AG 2021
A. Abd-Elsayed (ed.), *Trigeminal Nerve Pain*,
https://doi.org/10.1007/978-3-030-60687-9_19

willing to undergo surgical treatment. Early established treatments for trigeminal neuralgia involved a temporal craniotomy and sectioning of a significant portion of the trigeminal nerve. Many patients undergoing treatment by this Spiller-Frazier procedure were subject to risk of profound facial numbness and weakness. Walter Dandy further refined trigeminal nerve sectioning by performing a posterior fossa craniotomy to reach the nerve as opposed to the previously recommended temporal craniotomy. This posterior fossa approach improved visualization of the nerve and Dandy discovered that many patients suffering from classic trigeminal neuralgia had an artery abutting and displacing the nerve.

Recalling the observations of Dandy, and having the new tool of the operating microscope at his disposal, Peter Janetta performed operative exploration of the posterior fossa on patients suffering from trigeminal neuralgia. Finding vascular compression of the fifth nerve, he implemented the use of microsurgical techniques and placed teflon cushions to displace the compressing blood vessels. At this point, the procedure was termed microvascular decompression, also known as MVD. Janetta also carried out research to examine the Obersteiner-Redlich zone of the trigeminal nerve where the myelination of the nerve transitions from peripheral schwann cell-mediated myelination to central oligodendrocyte mediated myelination. It was theorized that classic trigeminal neuralgia may be related to neurovascular compression mediating demyelination and resulting ephaptic transmission of nerve impulses [3]. Since that time there has been some evolution regarding the understanding pain mechanisms in trigeminal neuralgia and factors other than demyelination and vascular compression may be involved in some patients [4]. Additionally, the microsurgical and operative techniques have evolved in MVD allowing greater safety and efficacy for this operation [5]. In recent years, the use of MVD as a surgical treatment has increased as the use of percutaneous ablative surgical treatments has declined [6].

Patient Selection

Patient selection is a key factor in determining MVD success. Virtually all patients undergoing MVD will have had some form of medication trial and surgical treatment is reserved for patients who have failed to have adequate pain control with medication. An individual patient's likelihood of success from treatment with MVD cannot be predicted precisely. However, there are several patient factors described in the literature, which have been associated with either an increased or a decreased likelihood of pain relief following the MVD procedure. Important factors include the character of the pain, disease duration, divisions of the nerve involved, and patient age [6].

Pain Character

When examining a patient to determine if they are suitable for MVD it is imperative to make the diagnosis of trigeminal neuralgia. Specific criteria for the diagnosis are reviewed in depth in Chap. 4. This is critical because some types of headache, atypical facial pain, and other types of neuropathic pain can masquerade as trigeminal neuralgia and in general these illnesses do not respond durably to treatment with MVD. Briefly, to make the diagnosis of trigeminal neuralgia the patient should have unilateral lancinating facial pain seconds to 2 min in duration. The patient should be predominantly pain free between attacks. Frequent triggers of the pain include talking, eating, touching the face, or brushing the teeth. The majority of patients evaluated for surgery will initially respond to carbamazepine or oxcarbazepine, but with time the dose will escalate until the patient has side effects or the medication is no longer effective. Many patients will have spontaneous remissions of pain and episodic recurrences. The mandibular (V3) or maxillary (V2) branches are most commonly affected with patients frequently complaining of jaw pain or upper lip pain.

Patients with constant pain or long-lived episodes of pain (i.e., attacks lasting hours) should be considered for alternative diagnoses, such as atypical facial pain or a headache disorder. If a patient has a neurological deficit this should be explored until a diagnosis is made. Generally, patients with trigeminal pain resulting from demyelinating disorders, tumors, or inflammatory diseases do not respond to MVD well and most centers do not recommend the MVD in these cases [1].

Once the diagnosis of idiopathic trigeminal neuralgia is made the pain can be further characterized as either Burchiel type 1 or Burchiel Type 2 pain. Burchiel Type 1 trigeminal neuralgia is characterized by patients classifying >50% of their pain as episodic and Burchiel Type 2 trigeminal neuralgia is classified by patients having >50% of their pain classified as constant [7]. This classification is important in setting patient expectations regarding MVD surgery because data has accumulated demonstrating that patients with Burchiel Type 1 trigeminal neuralgia are more likely to be pain free following MVD surgery when compared with patients classified as having Burchiel Type 2 trigeminal neuralgia [6].

Preoperative Imaging

Patient history and examination are important in making the diagnosis of idiopathic trigeminal neuralgia and may have prognostic value regarding the possible outcomes of MVD. Additional workup with MRI imaging of the brain is routine in patients evaluated for MVD. MRI of the brain allows exclusion of tumors, inflammation, and demyelination and this further supports a diagnosis of idiopathic trigeminal neuralgia. Many centers specifically employ thin cut MRI imaging in the region of the trigeminal nerve root entry zone to look for vascular compression. In many cases, the vascular compression is due to a loop of the superior cerebellar artery abutting and even displacing the nerve [8, 9]. Figure 19.1 demonstrates a patient with typical findings of trigeminal nerve compression by a loop of the superior cerebellar artery.

The degree of vascular compression and the source of vascular compression may predict which patients respond well to MVD. Some studies demonstrate that patients with arterial as opposed to venous neurovascular compression are more likely to have good results with MVD. Patients with compression from the superior cerebellar artery as opposed to other arterial structures, such as a dolichoectatic basilar

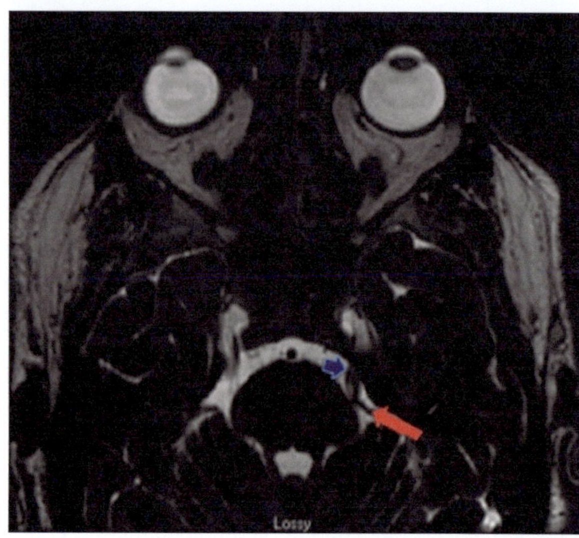

Fig. 19.1 Thin cut axial T2 weighted fast imaging employing steady state MRI at the level of the trigeminal nerve root entry zone. The blue arrow denotes the cisternal segment of the trigeminal nerve and the red arrow denotes the superior cerebellar artery in contact with the trigeminal nerve. This patient underwent left MVD and was pain free without medication at follow-up

artery may be more likely to have a good response with MVD [6]. Some authors have quantified the degree of trigeminal nerve displacement in a case series of patients. They found that patients with obvious nerve deformity or displacement due to the arterial compression may respond better to MVD than those with contact alone and better than those with no obvious signs of vascular contact [10]. High-quality MRI imaging of the symptomatic trigeminal nerve can also assist in surgical planning by informing the surgeon of the location of the offending vessel. This improves operative efficiency and makes it less likely that a significant compressing vessel will be missed [8, 9].

Some centers do continue to advocate for surgical posterior fossa exploration in patients without vascular compression on MRI despite the sensitivity of MRI in detecting blood vessels. In some studies up to 30% of patients presenting with trigeminal neuralgia Burchiel Type 1 have no evidence of neurovascular compression on imaging. On average these patients are more likely to be younger and female. For these patients posterior fossa exploration, followed by internal neurolysis of the trigeminal nerve if no compression is found, may represent an option with some efficacy in pain relief. Internal neurolysis consists of separating fascicles of the trigeminal nerve using small instruments and microsurgical techniques [4, 11].

In summary high-quality MRI imaging of the brain, usually with thin cuts through the trigeminal nerve root entry zone, is a routine part of the preoperative workup for trigeminal neuralgia at most centers. The imaging rules out diseases that mimic idiopathic trigeminal neuralgia and do not respond to MVD. It also allows the surgeon to localize the likely offending vessel. Despite the sensitivity and specificity of this imaging, some centers proceed with operative exploration of the posterior fossa in patients with typical symptoms of trigeminal neuralgia even if no vascular compression is seen on MRI. Additional imaging with CT scan of the maxillofacial region should be considered for patients with atypical symptoms, a history of facial trauma, dental concerns, or concerns for sinus disease [8, 9].

Procedure

A wealth of resources are available describing the surgical nuances of MVD and several excellent operative videos are also available [12–15]. Here some of the key steps of MVD are described.

The first step of the surgery is preoperative evaluation. This consists of disease diagnosis and preoperative imaging as previously described. The patient must undergo preoperative pulmonary and cardiac clearance as well. Medical clearance and evaluation of comorbid conditions are crucial in this population since many of these patients are advanced in age, average age is >55 years. Some have suggested that older patients should be more strongly considered for less invasive interventions such as radiosurgery or percutaneous ablation procedures. However, these procedures are generally less durable than MVD and have a higher associated rate of facial numbness. Others have advocated for MVD even in elderly patients if they do not have significant comorbidities. In one meta-analysis, 36 elderly patients (mean age 73 years) were compared to 53 non-elderly patients (mean age 53 years). In this series pain outcomes were the same for both groups. Also, the complication was low and equivalent in both the elderly and non-elderly [16]. Other studies have shown similar findings [17, 18]. In general, patients should be strongly considered for MVD if they have typical Burchiel Type 1, evidence of vascular compression, and an acceptable level of operative risk regardless of whether they are elderly or not.

MVD is performed under general anesthesia. Total IV anesthesia with an agent such as Propofol is generally used so the patient can undergo brain stem auditory evoked response (BAER) monitoring during the surgery. Some centers also choose to perform facial nerve monitoring during the surgery. When BAERs are monitored the operative and nonoperative sides are both monitored and compared to detect any degradation in response from the operative side. Data in the form of case series is available to recommend BAER monitoring. The use of BAER monitoring during surgery may reduce the risk of hearing loss. Particularly, it prompts the surgeon as to when they should relax retraction on the cerebellum, which if prolonged may result in stretch of the cochlear nerve and postoperative deafness [19–21].

After induction of anesthesia and initiation of BAER monitoring. The patient is positioned usually by turning the head such that the operative side is up and the junction of the transverse sinus and sigmoid sinus is at the highest point in the operative field. A curvilinear incision is created on the operative side behind the ear to create exposure of the retrosigmoid area and the transverse sigmoid junction. A retrosigmoid craniotomy or craniectomy is created with a drill and care is taken to occlude any mastoid air cells encountered. Occlusion of these air cells is important because it reduces the risk of CSF leak. Once the craniotomy is created, the dura is opened and tacked up. The operating microscope or endoscope is brought into the field. Some CSF is drained to provide brain relaxation and microsurgical dissection is carried out to identify the trigeminal nerve and vessels compressing it in the area of the nerve root entry zone. Either teflon or ivalon sponges are placed to separate the vessels from the nerve. Then the scope is removed and the dural is closed. The craniotomy defect is closed either with the patient's own bone, cement, or a combination of the two. The deep layers and skin are closed [15].

During the microsurgical dissection, it is crucial that the surgeon pay close attention to the amount of retraction placed on the cerebellum. Excessive retraction may damage the cerebellar tissue or lead to excessive traction on the cochlear nerve resulting in hearing loss. Changes in BAERs beyond a given threshold warn of excessive traction on the cochlear nerve. Appropriate craniotomy size, brain relaxation by cerebrospinal fluid drainage, and mannitol administration are established techniques to minimize retraction [15, 19].

Another important point regarding complication avoidance during the microsurgical dissection relates to the superior petrosal vein. This vein, which can be singular or in the form of a venous complex, is often encountered in the operative corridor while approaching the trigeminal nerve root entry zone. Excessive brain relaxation or retraction can result in tearing the vein and cause uncontrolled bleeding that complicates the operation. When this vein is obstructing the operative approach to the trigeminal nerve the surgeon is faced with a dilemma. If it is torn inadvertently the resulting bleeding is difficult to control and can lead to complications. Unfortunately, if it is taken prophylactically this can also result in complications. Case series have reported 1–30% complication rates when sacrificing the superior petrosal vein. Because of the unknown repercussions, preservation of the vein should be considered [22].

Another factor to consider during surgery is the method of separating compressing blood vessels from the trigeminal nerve. Original reports focused on the use of teflon sponges to separate the vessels from the nerve (Fig. 19.2) [5, 12]. The use of ivalon sponges has also been described and is associated with a similar success and

Fig. 19.2 Surgical separation between the vessel and the trigeminal nerve

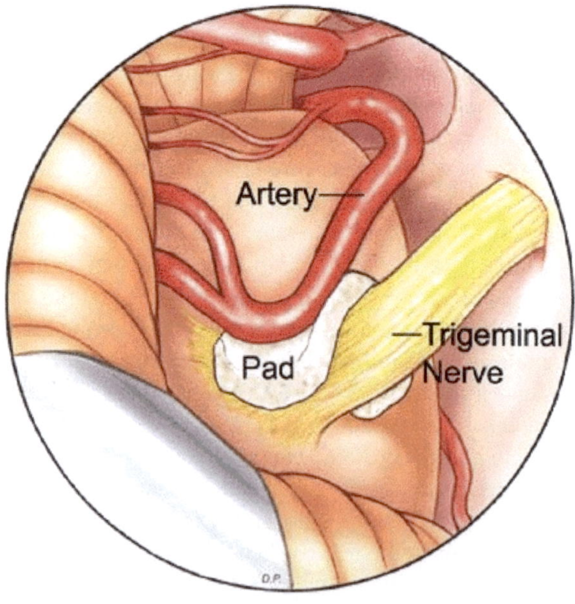

complication rate [23]. Other authors have advocated creating a sling with sutures or glue and autologous tissues to separate the nerve and blood vessels [24, 25].

Outcomes

There are various operative nuances in patient selection and performance of the MVD procedure. This variation makes review of the operative outcomes complex given the heterogeneous nature of the patients and procedures performed. Comparing outcomes for MVD and other treatments such as radiosurgery are made even more difficult by the fact that there is no standardized outcome reporting measure for trigeminal neuralgia in these studies. Many authors choose the Barrow Neurological Institute Pain Intensity Scale (see Table 16.1), but other scales are also used and some authors rank outcomes qualitatively only [2]. Still, some groups have compiled results and compared patient outcomes with discussion of prognostic factors [6, 16, 26, 27].

The initial pain freedom results following MVD are very favorable with systematic reviews of case series reporting ~90% or greater initial freedom from pain [26, 27]. Given the non-randomized nature of these studies, and the inherent lack of controls available in surgical studies, this evidence is level 3 at best. Any intervention is, of course, subject to the placebo effect as well and this must be considered for this intervention as well. Therefore, a better measure of MVD success is generated when patients are followed for longer periods of time, as placebo effects are generally short lived. Even at longer term follow-up, a substantial proportion of patients who underwent MVD are pain free. A recent meta-analysis including 3897 patients showed 76% pain free at a follow-up of 1.7 ± 1.3 years [6]. Another meta-analysis that compared radiosurgery and MVD found that long-term pain free rates ranged from 69 to 92% compared to 10–80% for gamma knife radiosurgery. Long-term follow for MVD patients in this study ranged from 1 to 8 years. In this meta-analysis, initial pain relief from radiosurgery was low compared to MVD, which is to be expected because the effects of radiosurgery are delayed. MVD also had a lower recurrence rate compared to radiosurgery, 15 versus 19%, but this was not statistically significant [26].

Patient outcomes for MVD vary. Several patient factors are thought to influence the patient's prognosis with regards to pain improvement after MVD. Among these factors are duration of disease, pain type (either Type 1 or Type 2 trigeminal neuralgia), and type of vascular compression. In general, a shorter duration of disease (< or = 5 years) seems to portend a better outcome with surgical decompression of the nerve. It is theorized that a long disease duration may lead to permanent nerve damage or sensitization that mitigates improvement due to operative intervention [6]. Classification of trigeminal neuralgia either Type 1 or Type 2 was proposed by Burchiel [7]. Following MVD patients with a more substantial episodic pain component, Type 1 trigeminal neuralgia, had higher rates of pain freedom, compared to those with more constant pain, Type 2 trigeminal neuralgia. When comparing Type 1 and Type 2 trigeminal neuralgia patients undergoing MVD the rate of pain

Table 19.1 Factors associated with and not associated with a higher likelihood of sustained pain freedom following MVD as compiled from a meta-analysis of pain outcomes [6]

Patient characteristics	Associated improved outcomes following MVD
Type 1 Trigeminal neuralgia	Yes
Type 2 Trigeminal neuralgia	No
Arterial neurovascular compression	Yes
Venous neurovascular compression	No
Obvious arterial compression on MRI	No
Sex of patient	No
Laterality of disease (right vs. left)	No
Number of trigeminal nerve divisions affected	No
Disease duration </= 5 years	Yes

freedom at long-term follow-up was 74 and 60%. Arterial compression as opposed to venous compression was associated with better rates of pain freedom following MVD. The superior cerebellar artery as the compressing agent was also associated with better long-term postoperative pain freedom. Patient factors that did not seem to provide prognostic information about outcome following MVD were as follows: patient sex, number of trigeminal nerve divisions involved, and side of the disease [6]. Table 19.1 provides a summary of patient factors associated with higher likelihood of pain freedom following MVD.

Complications

MVD is a safe and effective treatment for appropriately selected patients that suffer from trigeminal neuralgia. Nonetheless, as an invasive surgical procedure complications are possible. Many of the complications are those associated with any cranial surgery. Here we review rates of some significant complications and provide special attention to those that have a stronger association with MVD.

First, mortality is rarely associated with this surgery. Rates reported in case series range from 0 to 0.4%. Cerebrospinal fluid leak is one of the more common major complications reported around 3% of the time. Usually, this can be managed with lumbar drain, CSF shunt, and/or wound revision. Infection is rare and similar in rate compared to other craniotomy procedures. In several case series, it is reported 1–2% of the time and is treated by antibiotics and/or wound washout. Hematoma, either intraparenchymal or extra-axial is similarly rare, 0.2–1% [1, 6].

Cranial nerve-related complications bear special consideration in the case of MVD. Numbness and dysesthesias in the trigeminal nerve occur in a significant minority of patients, 5–10%. However, these rates are actually low in comparison with ablative procedures. For comparison, approximately half of patients undergoing radiosurgery report significant alteration in trigeminal sensation. Because of the proximity of the surgical corridor to the edge of the tentorium, and hence the trochlear nerve, diplopia, and trochlear nerve palsy are occasionally reported, <1% [1, 6].

As the surgeon approaches the trigeminal nerve for decompression the facial nerve and cochlear nerve are in close proximity. Therefore, there is special risk for damage to these nerves. The rate of hearing loss is reported in approximately 1% of cases and rates of facial nerve injury are similar. In general, most centers that routinely perform this surgery monitor brain stem auditory evoked responses in an effort to modulate cerebellar retraction and reduce the risk of hearing loss. The use of brain stem auditory evoked responses to reduce hearing loss have been extensively described in the literature [19–21].

With regard to stratifying patient risk, even elderly patients with good functional status and lack of significant comorbidities can be considered for MVD. In studies comparing patients with an average age in the 50s to another patient group with an average age in the 70s it was found that the groups had similar outcomes in pain improvement and a similar low complication rate. Even the number of days hospitalized showed no statistically significant difference [16–18].

In conclusion, since its advent in the 1960s MVD has increasingly become the standard of care for treating patients with medically intractable classic idiopathic trigeminal neuralgia. While complications are possible, rare life-altering or life-ending events are rare in appropriately selected patients. Outcomes are excellent compared to other treatment methods with approximately 76% of patients reporting significant pain relief at long-term follow-up. Large case series have been compiled allowing review of patient factors that may be associated with better surgical outcomes including, shorter duration of disease, type 1 trigeminal neuralgia, and presence of arterial compression. Rates of MVD utilization will likely continue to rise in the future as surgical technique continues to improve and excellent outcomes in the treatment of trigeminal neuralgia are increasingly reported.

References

1. Zakrzewska JM, Coakham HB. Microvascular decompression for trigeminal neuralgia: update. Curr Opin Neurol. 2012;25:296–301.
2. Nova CV, Zakrzewska JM, Baker SR, Riordain RN. Treatment outcomes in trigeminal neuralgia—a systematic review of domains, dimensions and measures. World Neurosurg X. 2020;6:100070.
3. Patel SK, Liu JK. Overview and history of trigeminal neuralgia. Neurosurg Clin N Am. 2016;27:265–76.
4. Magown P, Ko AL, Burchiel KJ. The spectrum of trigeminal neuralgia without neurovascular compression. Neurosurgery. 2019;85:E553–9.
5. Kaufmann AM, Price AV. A history of the Jannetta procedure. J Neurosurg. 2019;132:639–46.
6. Holste K, Chan AY, Rolston JD, Englot DJ. Pain outcomes following microvascular decompression for drug-resistant trigeminal neuralgia: a systematic review and meta-analysis. Neurosurgery. 2020;86:182–90.
7. Burchiel KJ. A new classification for facial pain. Neurosurgery. 2003;53:1164–6; discussion 1166–7.
8. Seeburg DP, Northcutt B, Aygun N, Blitz AM. The role of imaging for trigeminal neuralgia: a segmental approach to high-resolution MRI. Neurosurg Clin N Am. 2016;27:315–26.
9. Hughes MA, Frederickson AM, Branstetter BF, Zhu X, Sekula RF Jr. MRI of the trigeminal nerve in patients with trigeminal neuralgia secondary to vascular compression. AJR Am J Roentgenol. 2016;206:595–600.

10. Leal PRL, et al. Preoperative demonstration of the neurovascular compression characteristics with special emphasis on the degree of compression, using high-resolution magnetic resonance imaging: a prospective study, with comparison to surgical findings, in 100 consecutive patients who underwent microvascular decompression for trigeminal neuralgia. Acta Neurochir. 2010;152:817–25.
11. Ko AL, et al. Long-term efficacy and safety of internal neurolysis for trigeminal neuralgia without neurovascular compression. J Neurosurg. 2015;122:1048–57.
12. Jannetta PJ, McLaughlin MR, Casey KF. Technique of microvascular decompression. Technical note. Neurosurg Focus. 2005;18:E5.
13. Tomasello F, et al. Microvascular decompression for trigeminal neuralgia: technical refinement for complication avoidance. World Neurosurg. 2016;94:26–31.
14. Cohen-Gadol AA. Microvascular decompression surgery for trigeminal neuralgia and hemifacial spasm: naunces of the technique based on experiences with 100 patients and review of the literature. Clin Neurol Neurosurg. 2011;113:844–53.
15. Forbes J, Cooper C, Jermakowicz W, Neimat J, Konrad P. Microvascular decompression: salient surgical principles and technical nuances. J Vis Exp. 2011;5(53):e2590.
16. Sekula RF Jr, et al. Microvascular decompression for elderly patients with trigeminal neuralgia: a prospective study and systematic review with meta-analysis. J Neurosurg. 2011;114:172–9.
17. Javadpour M, Eldridge PR, Varma TRK, Miles JB, Nurmikko TJ. Microvascular decompression for trigeminal neuralgia in patients over 70 years of age. Neurology. 2003;60:520.
18. Pollock BE, Stien KJ. Posterior fossa exploration for trigeminal neuralgia patients older than 70 years of age. Neurosurgery. 2011;69:1255–9; discussion 1259–60.
19. Sindou M, Fobé JL, Ciriano D, Fischer C. Hearing prognosis and intraoperative guidance of brainstem auditory evoked potential in microvascular decompression. Laryngoscope. 1992;102:678–82.
20. Friedman WA, Kaplan BJ, Gravenstein D, Rhoton AL Jr. Intraoperative brain-stem auditory evoked potentials during posterior fossa microvascular decompression. J Neurosurg. 1985;62:552–7.
21. Radtke RA, Erwin CW, Wilkins RH. Intraoperative brainstem auditory evoked potentials: significant decrease in postoperative morbidity. Neurology. 1989;39:187–91.
22. Narayan V, et al. Safety profile of superior petrosal vein (the vein of Dandy) sacrifice in neurosurgical procedures: a systematic review. Neurosurg Focus. 2018;45:E3.
23. Pressman E, et al. Teflon™ or Ivalon®: a scoping review of implants used in microvascular decompression for trigeminal neuralgia. Neurosurg Rev. 2020;43:79–86.
24. Liu J, et al. Biomedical glue sling technique in microvascular decompression for trigeminal neuralgia caused by atherosclerotic vertebrobasilar artery: a description of operative technique and clinical outcomes. World Neurosurg. 2019;128:e74–80.
25. Steinberg JA, et al. Tentorial sling for microvascular decompression in patients with trigeminal neuralgia: a description of operative technique and clinical outcomes. J Neurosurg. April 1;2018:1–6. https://doi.org/10.3171/2017.10.JNS17971.
26. Mendelson ZS, et al. Pain-free outcomes and durability of surgical intervention for trigeminal neuralgia: a comparison of gamma knife and microvascular decompression. World Neurosurg. 2018;112:e732–46.
27. Sharma R, et al. Microvascular decompression versus stereotactic radiosurgery as primary treatment modality for trigeminal neuralgia: a systematic review and meta-analysis of prospective comparative trials. Neurol India. 2018;66:688–94.

Peripheral Neurectomy for Treatment of Trigeminal Neuralgia

Priodarshi Roychoudhury, Andrés Rocha Romero, Ahmed Raslan, and Alaa Abd-Elsayed

Introduction

Trigeminal Neuralgia is a chronic pain disorder that can be difficult to diagnose and treat. According to the third edition of the International Classification of Headache Disorders, TN is a disorder characterized by recurrent unilateral brief electric shock-like pain, triggered by innocuous stimuli, abrupt in onset and termination, limited to the distribution of one or more divisions of the trigeminal nerve [1]. For the vast majority of TN patients, pain affects one side of the face, and in the rare occasions of bilateral TN, it independently affects each side of the face. TN in its chronic state is characterized by longer-lasting, medically refractory pain, and neuroanatomical morphological changes [2]. TN has unpredictable periods of complete remission due to a reduction in excitability and partial remyelination.

Since it was described as early as the first century AD in the writings of Aretaeus, treatment has evolved from bloodletting, application of arsenic bandages, cobra venom, nutritious diet, hydrotherapy, electrotherapy to high-end surgical interventions.

P. Roychoudhury (✉)
Department of Anesthesia and Pain Management, Toronto General Hospital, University of Toronto, Toronto, ON, Canada

A. R. Romero
Hospital de Trauma, Centro Nacional de rehabilitacion, San Jose, Costa Rica

A. Raslan
Department of Neurological Surgery, Oregon Health and Science University, Portland, OR, USA

A. Abd-Elsayed
Department of Anesthesiology, University of Wisconsin School of Medicine and Public Health, Madison, WI, USA

A. Abd-Elsayed (ed.), *Trigeminal Nerve Pain*, https://doi.org/10.1007/978-3-030-60687-9_20

The available surgeries for TN can be classified as destructive (trigeminal nerve sensory function intentionally destroyed), or non-destructive (trigeminal nerve decompressed, with sensory function usually preserved) [3].

Peripheral neurectomy is a minimally invasive surgical method of destruction of the peripheral branches of the trigeminal nerve that can be carried out as an outpatient procedure, and is indicated for patients who have failed medical therapy, ganglionlysis, or have severe cardiopulmonary disease and are unable to tolerate a suboccipital craniectomy for microvascular decompression.

History

Peripheral neurectomy was practiced for the first time in the eighteenth century with limited success. Successful neurectomy of the inferior maxillary nerve was reported by Joseph Pancoast in 1840. In 1851, J. M. Carnochan described successful resection of the maxillary nerve and removal of Meckel's ganglion from the foramen rotundum to the infraorbital foramen. It has been also done for the supraorbital, supratrochlear, infratrochlear, lacrimal nerves, infraorbital nerve, and inferior alveolar, lingual, and mental nerves since then.

Pathogenesis of Hyperexcitability of the Peripheral Branches of the Trigeminal Nerve

Classical TN is caused by demyelination of the trigeminal nerve at the junction of central and peripheral myelin which leads to a series of physiologic changes that leads to neuronal hyperexcitability and increased firing which leads to the behavioral effect (Pain), this is well described under the so-called "ignition theory" [4]. Demyelination may reach a level that allows ions to move in and out of axon, resulting in the inability to immediately re-establish resting potential. Axons tend toward a state of depolarization, making them hyperexcitable and hyperactivity of primary afferents may induce central sensitization of wide-dynamic-range neurons in the spinal trigeminal nucleus. Pain might become unbearable and refractory to medical management. Demyelination is caused by vascular compression in about 70% of patients, typically by an artery at the cerebellopontine cistern. Other causes of TN include multiple sclerosis plaques in pons or trigeminal root entry zone, tumors (such as epidermoid tumor, meningioma, neurinoma), arteriovenous malformation, aneurysm, skull base bone deformity, connective tissue disease and dural arteriovenous fistula are causes of secondary TN [2, 5].

Peripheral neurectomy is a minimally invasive surgical method of destruction of the peripheral branches of the trigeminal nerve. It can be done for the supraorbital, supratrochlear, infratrochlear, lacrimal nerves, infraorbital nerve, inferior alveolar, lingual, and mental nerves.

Neurectomies remove the sensory receptors of the peripheral nerves, producing dense numbness along the distribution of the eradicated nerve and degenerative changes in the ganglion.

Indications

1. TN is refractory to medication or needs dosages that will result in significant side effects.
2. Elderly patients or severely debilitated patients in whom MVD or percutaneous ablative procedures are contraindicated.
3. Patients with recurrence of pain following a percutaneous radiofrequency thermocoagulation.
4. Patients unwilling to accept the anesthesia that would result from a root or ganglion destruction.

Contraindications

1. Uncorrected coagulopathy
2. Sepsis or infection at the site of the procedure
3. Hemodynamic instability
4. Lack of consent
5. Contraindication to Local Anesthesia or General Anesthesia

It is important to have a thoughtful risk/benefit analysis and use clinicians' judgment in the decision-making process.

Anatomic Considerations

The nerve is named "trigeminal," because of its three major branches: the ophthalmic (V1), maxillary (V2), and mandibular (V3). The trigeminal nerve exits the brainstem from the ventrolateral pons, entering a small fossa just posterior and inferolateral to the cavernous sinus called Meckel's cave. The trigeminal ganglion, also known as the Gasserian ganglion, lies in Meckel's cave and is the sensory ganglion of the trigeminal nerve.

The ophthalmic division (V1) travels through the inferior part of the cavernous sinus to exit through the superior orbital fissure. The maxillary division (V2) exits via the foramen rotundum and the mandibular division (V3) via the foramen ovale.

The trigeminal nerve also provides touch and pain sensation to the nasal sinuses, inner aspect of the nose, mouth, and anterior two-thirds of the tongue.

In also provides pain sensation for the supratentorial dura mater, while the dura of the posterior fossa is innervated by CN X and upper cervical roots.

Pre-procedural Preparation

The procedure can be performed on an outpatient basis usually with light sedation. Informed consent is obtained after the risks, benefits, and alternatives are clearly outlined. An intravenous line is placed in a pre-procedure room. The site of the procedure is labeled, and the patient is transported to the procedure room, where the patient is positioned on the procedure table. Sometimes it is done under general anesthesia with endotracheal intubation. This can be also performed using an endoscope. Patients are monitored with standard ASA monitors that include three-lead electrocardiography, pulse oximetry, and noninvasive blood pressure measurement at least every 5 min. A pre-procedure time out is performed to confirm the patient's identity, allergies, procedure site, body position, and necessary equipment.

Technique

Supraorbital Neurectomy (Branch of the Ophthalmic Division)

It is approached extraorally through the upper eyebrow incision; the nerve is identified and avulsed by reeling on a hemostat [6]. The remnants of the nerve are cauterized. Double layered closure is recommended (Fig. 20.1).

Infraorbital Neurectomy (Branch of the Maxillary Division)

The Infraorbital nerve is accessed via the maxillary vestibular approach. The infraorbital foramen is visualized, and the infraorbital nerve and its peripheral branches are identified. Avulsion of the nerve is then performed from the soft tissues and from the infraorbital canal by reeling on a hemostat. The remnants of the nerve are cauterized deep in the foramen (Fig. 20.2).

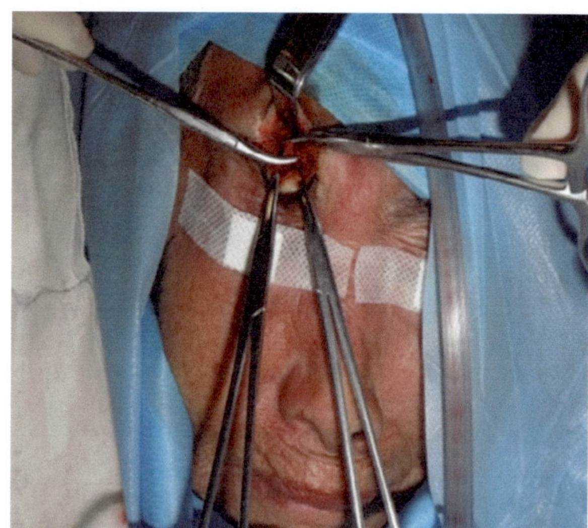

Fig. 20.1 Supraorbital neurectomy through an upper eyebrow incision. (Reprinted with permission from Lamichhane NS, Du X, Li S, Poudel DC. Effectiveness of peripheral neurectomy in refractory cases of trigeminal neuralgia. J Orofac Sci 2016;8:86–91.)

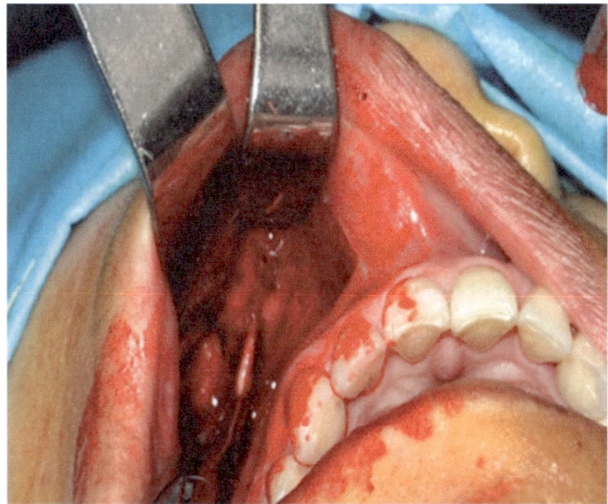

Fig. 20.2 Infraorbital Neurectomy via Maxillary vestibular approach. (Reprinted with permission from Lamichhane NS, Du X, Li S, Poudel DC. Effectiveness of peripheral neurectomy in refractory cases of trigeminal neuralgia. J Orofac Sci 2016;8:86–91.)

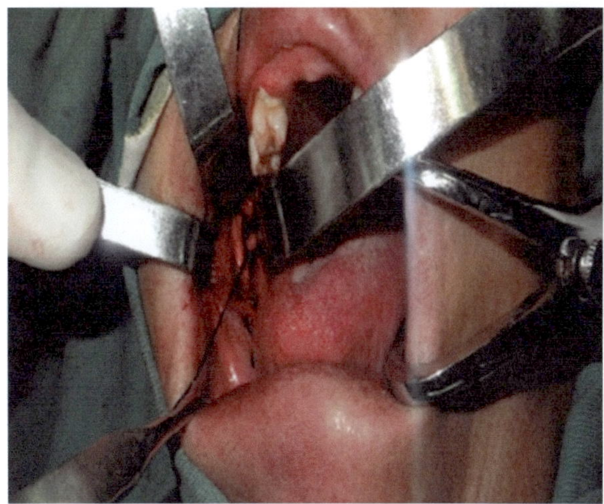

Fig. 20.3 Inferior alveolar neurectomy. (Reprinted with permission from Lamichhane NS, Du X, Li S, Poudel DC. Effectiveness of peripheral neurectomy in refractory cases of trigeminal neuralgia. J Orofac Sci 2016;8:86–91.)

Inferior Alveolar Neurectomy (Branch of the Mandibular Division)

An incision is taken extending lingually and buccally along the anterior border of the ascending ramus, followed by deepening of its medial aspect by means of blunt dissection. The temporalis and medial pterygoid muscles are split, and the nerve is located. Two heavy black linen threads are looped around the nerve using a nerve hook and divided between the two threads. The remnants of the nerve are cauterized deep in the foramen (Fig. 20.3).

Post-procedural Care

The patient should be monitored in the recovery room for at least a few hours after the procedure. The patient's pain level is recorded before and after the procedure to assess response with a numeric rating scale. Vital signs and neurological functions are assessed and documented before discharge. Written discharge instructions include limiting activities the day of the procedure; routine antibiotics and contacting the physician if there is any sign of infection like fever, chills, or erythema or induration at the site of the procedure.

Complications

Loss of facial sensation in the appropriate division is inevitable. Facial edema and bruising are common. No major complications are reported [6].

When comparing to percutaneous or central procedures, complications are always minor (Table 20.1).

Table 20.1 Complications following surgical management of trigeminal neuralgia

Approaches	Complications reported	Consolidated rate of complications (%)
Peripheral	Hypoesthesia, dysesthesia, paresthesia High requirement of analgesics Persisting paroxysms several days after neurectomy	39.46
Percutaneous	Diminished corneal reflex Anesthesia dolorosa Masseter weakness and paralysis Permanent palsy of the abducent nerve CSF leakage Aseptic meningitis Carotid cavernous fistula	65.42
Central	Deaths (0.2%) Brain stem infarction (0.1%) Ipsilateral hearing loss (1%) Hypoesthesia, disappearance of corneal reflection, masticatory atonia, paraesthesia, trachyphonia, hearing loss, vertigo or tinnitus CSF leakage, hearing loss and persistent diplopia Facial numbness (36%) Persistent paresthesia (15.8%) Hypoesthesia, disappearance of corneal reflection, masticatory atonia, paraesthesia, trachyphonia, hearing loss, vertigo or tinnitus CSF leakage, hearing loss and persistent diplopia Facial numbness (36%) Persistent paresthesia (15.8%)	10.41

Reprinted with permission from V. Yuvaraj, B. Krishnan et al.: Efficacy of Neurectomy of Peripheral Branches of the Trigeminal Nerve in Trigeminal Neuralgia: A Critical Review of the Literature J. Maxillofac. Oral Surg, 2018

Recurrence of pain following neurectomy might involve other branches of the same division of the trigeminal nerve, the intact collateral branches, or the main ascending trunk remaining after the neurectomy, associated with neuroma formation in the excised nerve, and demyelination and central sensitization [6].

Recurrence

It is economical, less morbid, and can be performed in patients with extremes of age, debility, or significant systemic diseases with limited life expectancy and refractory cases. One of the problems that may arise following peripheral neurectomy is spontaneous peripheral nerve regeneration and recurrence of pain.

Recurrence following the first infraorbital neurectomy is reported between 12 and 15 months, after the second is reported between 9 and 12 months. Recurrence following first surgery on the mandibular nerve is reported between 15 and 18 months, after the second procedure was 12.3 months on an average. The calculated prediction of the average time of remission was in agreement with the actual duration of painlessness [6]. According to a critical review [6] recurrence is still higher compare to central procedures (Table 20.2).

Attempts have been made to prevent peripheral nerve regeneration by obliterating the canal or foramen where nerves were avulsed, using materials like gold foil, silver plugs, bone, fat, bone wax, steel screws, and amalgam [7]. This has helped in prolonging remission by up to 10 years [8–10].

In conclusion, while peripheral neurectomies cannot be recommended for routine purposes due to the inferior outcome compared to standard neurosurgical procedures, nevertheless, they present a safe and effective procedure for a certain subset of patients where neurosurgical interventions are either not possible or not desired. Undiagnosed central pathologies may partly explain the unsatisfactory results associated with peripheral neurectomies.

Table 20.2 Pain recurrence rates following surgical intervention in trigeminal neuralgia

Approach	Pain relief (in %)	Duration of pain relief (years)	Rate of recurrence (in %)
Peripheral	53.13	2	15.34
Percutaneous procedures	62.38	2.4	18.33
Central procedures	76.062	10	7.81

Reprinted with permission from V. Yuvaraj, B. Krishnan et al.: Efficacy of Neurectomy of Peripheral Branches of the Trigeminal Nerve in Trigeminal Neuralgia: A Critical Review of the Literature J. Maxillofac. Oral Surg, 2018

References

1. Headache Classification Committee of the International Headache Society (IHS) The International Classification of Headache Disorders, 3rd edition. Cephalalgia 2018;38(1):1–211.
2. Maarbjerg S, Di Stefano G, Bendtsen L, Cruccu G. Trigeminal neuralgia—diagnosis and treatment. Cephalalgia. 2017;37(7):648–57.
3. Parmar M, Sharma N, Modgill V, Naidu P. Comparative evaluation of surgical procedures for trigeminal neuralgia. J Maxillofac Oral Surg. 2013;12(4):400–9.
4. Devor M, Amir R, Rappaport H. Pathophysiology of trigeminal neuralgia: the ignition hypothesis. Clin J Pain. 2002;18(1):4–13.
5. Foley PL, Vesterinen HM, Laird BJ, et al. Prevalence and natural history of pain in adults with multiple sclerosis: systematic review and meta-analysis. Pain. 2013;154(5):632–42. https://doi.org/10.1016/j.pain.2012.12.002.
6. Zhu S, Rong Q, Chen S, Li X. Pterygopalatine fossa segment neurectomy of maxillary nerve through maxillary sinus route in treating trigeminal neuralgia. J Cranio-Maxillofac Surg. 2013;41(7):652–6.
7. Kumar P, Maleedi S, Goud SS. Peripheral neurectomy: a surgical option for trigeminal neuralgia involving inferior alveolar nerve. J Headache Pain Manag [Internet] 2017;02(02). Available from http://headache.imedpub.com/peripheral-neurectomy-a-surgical-option-for-trigeminal-neuralgia-involving-inferior-alveolar-nerve.php?aid=19844
8. Ali FM, Prasant MC, Aher VA, Safiya T, Pai D, Kar S. Peripheral neurectomies: a treatment option for trigeminal neuralgia in rural practice. J Neurosci Rural Pract. 2012;03(02):152–7.
9. Lamichhane NS, Du X, Li S, Poudel DC. Effectiveness of peripheral neurectomy in refractory cases of trigeminal neuralgia. J Orofac Sci. 2016;8:86–91.
10. Yuvaraj V, Krishnan B, et al. Efficacy of neurectomy of peripheral branches of the trigeminal nerve in trigeminal neuralgia: a critical review of the literature. J Maxillofac Oral Surg. 2018;18(1):15–22.

Ketty Thertus

Pain Psychology

It is well established that chronic pain is associated with distress and adverse psychological outcomes. The relationship between pain and psychiatric disorders is bidirectional: an adverse emotional environment can function as both the cause and effect of persistent pain. In working with patients with pain disorders, the biological reductionist model can tend to be short-sighted, exacerbate poor outcomes, and alienate patients from aspects of care that will enable their restoration to function [1, 2]. Newer theoretical explanations for pain and the positive outcomes seen with interdisciplinary pain clinics provide a basis and support for interventions beyond those that focus solely on biological factors [3, 4]. This chapter will review psychological factors related to chronic pain and trigeminal neuralgia, and the available intervention and management strategies.

To understand approaches to the psychological challenges that arise when treating a patient with trigeminal neuralgia, the clinician must first understand the complexity of emotional, behavioral, and cognitive responses to acute and chronic pain. Gatchel described stages of pain to explain the potential struggles in the transition from acute to chronic pain. Stage one is marked by typical emotional reactions such as fear, anxiety, and worry in the acute pain state. In stage two, helplessness, anger, and distress arise with pain that persists beyond what is expected for acute pain [5]. The transition from acute to chronic pain results in alterations in neural networks involved in memory, attention, mood, motivation, perception, and learning, and these changes have ramifications on pain perception and global functioning. Physical and emotional symptoms are processed among overlapping pathways that

K. Thertus (✉)
University of Wisconsin School of Medicine and Public Health, Madison, WI, USA
e-mail: thertus@wisc.edu

© The Author(s), under exclusive license to Springer Nature
Switzerland AG 2021
A. Abd-Elsayed (ed.), *Trigeminal Nerve Pain*,
https://doi.org/10.1007/978-3-030-60687-9_21

influence each other [6]. The diathesis–stress model describes the process by which emotional responses develop in individuals. These emotional responses to pain are informed both by the person's preexisting psychological traits, and any stressors related to their socioeconomic conditions [7].

A biopsychosocial approach to pain management is essential for improved functional outcomes because the experience of pain is a subjective state affected by psychosocial factors [8]. As described by Engel, the biopsychosocial approach highlights that care for medical conditions requires attention to the psychological, social, and behavioral aspects of illness beyond the biological explanation of the disease state [9]. This comprehensive approach is beneficial for pain states because psychosocial inputs can inform how pain is reported and modulated and can disrupt the course of medication treatment [2, 8]. Additionally, pain functions as a chronic stressor that leads to changes in thought processes and behaviors that can perpetuate the negative experience and intensity of pain. A biomedical approach would not adequately address the psychosocial sequelae of chronic pain, such as interpersonal relationship strain, occupational impairment, disruptions to identity, and loss of engagement in pleasurable activities [6, 8]. Psychological vulnerabilities such as anger, neuroticism, psychological distress, the quality of the relationship with a spouse, job dissatisfaction, positive or negative perceptions before treatment, a history of trauma, and maladaptive beliefs are related to poor treatment outcomes. Functional decline is associated with catastrophizing, a lower sense of self-efficacy, pessimism, lower educational level, a personality disorder, or a history of maladjustment. A strong therapeutic alliance between the physician and the patient promotes a positive, successful treatment course [2, 8]. A clinician who utilizes a biopsychosocial approach can conceptualize pain not just as a symptom but also as an experience encompassing biological, psychological, and social variables [10]. This approach equips the clinician to identify factors that will delay or prevent pain relief or restoration of functioning, even as medication or surgical treatments are trialed.

The subjectivity of the experience of pain is a complex process involving various neural pathways between the cortical and limbic systems involved in emotional regulation and cognition. An individual's interpretations and responses to pain have been attributed to an interplay among the structures, as described in Melzack's "body-self neuromatrix" theory of pain. This theory describes the experience of pain stemming from the neural network involving the thalamocortical, limbic, and somatosensory systems functioning to drive, process, and mediate pain-related emotional, cognitive, and interoceptive information [3]. The areas described in the "neuromatrix" such as the prefrontal cortex, the insula, and the limbic system, are regions also found to be dysfunctional in major depressive disorder [3, 11]. Additionally, major depressive disorder could be associated with diminished ability to modulate pain due to changes to the frontal-limbic neurocircuitry [12]. There has been evidence for both structural and functional deficits in areas involved in emotional processing in trigeminal neuralgia patients. Pain relief led to a resolution in pathways between the frontal cortex and amygdala regions [13]. The evidence for neurochemical alterations highlights the plasticity and sensitivity of the brain in response to pain, which explains why there is a risk for the development of psychological disturbance. It may also inform therapeutic intervention strategies [6, 14].

Psychiatric and Psychological Comorbidities

There is limited evidence examining psychological experiences and quality of life for patients with trigeminal neuralgia but, a few studies have shown that the condition is associated with an increased risk for depressive, anxiety, and insomnia disorders [15–17]. The characteristics of trigeminal neuralgia pain and the associated triggers are distressing and detrimental to a person's quality of life given the severity, the unpredictable recurrences, and the relatively benign triggers associated with essential activities of daily living such as brushing one's teeth, talking, drinking, and eating [18]. Trigeminal neuralgia is described as one of the most severe clinical pain states [19]. It is an overwhelming sensory experience characterized as severe and rapid, with intermittent repetitive bursts. The periodic quality of the pain may lead to a state of hypervigilance, anticipatory fear, and avoidance of activities [18, 20, 21]. Severe pain can be triggered by non-noxious stimuli such as light touch to the face that could serve to interfere with human connection and lead to social isolation. The quality of interpersonal and occupational life diminishes with time given the high recurrence rates of trigeminal neuralgia [22]. In studies, 31% of patients with orofacial pain have been found to have an anxiety disorder, and 28% were found to meet the criteria for depression [20]. Patients with trigeminal neuralgia and chronic facial pain have higher levels of pain intensity than those with atypical facial pain and reported higher levels of depression, anxiety, and disability [23].

A 2015 qualitative review conducted by Allsop et al. that utilized focus groups to elucidate the subjective experience of people with trigeminal neuralgia identified themes that patients struggled with: (1) diagnosis and support, (2) living in fear of pain, (3) isolation and social withdrawal, and (4) medication burden and cure seeking. Choice quotes from patients provided by the study highlight the distress from the pain, isolation, and the burden of medication effects:

> It's as if somebody has just hit you in the face for no reason whatsoever, and you just want to hit back.
>
> I couldn't even have my tea in front of my children or my husband because I felt I looked like a freak. …you're in pain and feel like you're contorted.
>
> I gave up doing gas work; I couldn't guarantee that I could concentrate on it enough to do it… I chopped [off] the ends of three fingers, I wasn't concentrating … I was thinking about the pain instead of what I was doing…
>
> I couldn't calculate, I lost my mental arithmetic, it disappeared I just could not think…So yeah, it did affect me…. [21]

Anxiety in chronic pain disorders is associated with increased sensitivity to pain due to decreased pain threshold and tolerance. Depression and anxiety are linked to exacerbated physical symptoms via somatic amplification, misinterpretation, and autonomic hyperactivity. Anger is a common response in those with pain conditions and is correlated with higher levels of pain, depression, and disability [5, 8, 24]. Anxiety or anger may build in initial stages of pain because of frequent delays in diagnosis for trigeminal neuralgia or during treatment stages in relation to the side effect burden of medications [21].

The relationship between sleep and pain has been described as bidirectional and reciprocal in pain literature [25, 26]. Disturbed sleep may indirectly increase pain by potentiating negative affect, which in turn perpetuates insomnia. Direct effects of sleep deficits on pain include hyperalgesia via disruptions to endogenous opioid production or via alternate pain pathway changes. Pain intensity and depressed mood are frequent predictors of low sleep quality, and sleep disruptions consistently predict chronic pain relapses [26–28]. Historically, trigeminal neuralgia was not initially thought to awaken patients from sleep. However, there is now more evidence that pain may disrupt sleep due to nighttime awakening [19]. Fifty-five to eighty percent of patients with chronic nonmalignant pain report sleep disturbance. In a sample of patients with neuropathic pain, 68% were found to have "strongly or mostly disturbed sleep." Almost two-thirds of patients with trigeminal neuralgia experience awakenings triggered by innocuous sensations [29]. A survey study of orofacial pain patients revealed that 22.6% of those with trigeminal neuralgia self-reported pain-related awakenings [30]. Another survey of patients with trigeminal neuralgia, with additional input from their partners, found that 31% of patients experience awakenings due to pain [19].

The suicide rate in chronic pain patients has been reported as two to three times higher than the general population; therefore, a review of suicide risk factors is necessary for the care of patients with chronic pain [31]. General suicide risk factors include any psychiatric diagnosis, a family history of suicide, male gender, unmarried relational status, low social support, medical illness, unemployment, a disruptive change in social or economic status, substance abuse, personality disorder, access to a firearm, recent hospital discharge, living alone, older age, white race and prior suicide attempts [31, 32]. Insomnia and a longer duration of pain may increase the risk of suicidal ideation in pain patients [33]. Chronic pain patients have higher prevalence rates of suicidal ideation and a history of suicide attempts compared to the general population. Sensitive times include when the patient perceives or faces lower recovery chances or a failed surgical intervention [31]. The risk remains independently elevated even when depression, anxiety, and substance abuse are controlled for [34]. Catastrophizing and avoidance may increase the risk of suicidality. Catastrophizing and depression are the two most constant predictors of the occurrence and magnitude of suicidal ideation. In one study, a suicide plan, a risk factor for suicide, was found in chronic pain patients five times more than in healthy controls. In patients with chronic pain, a history of prior suicide attempts is 1.6–3.25 times higher than healthy controls. The presence of worker's compensation and litigation are other risk factors for suicidality seen in chronic pain patients in a rehabilitation program [35].

Trigeminal neuralgia has historically been referred to as the "suicide disease"; however, there has not been conclusive data documenting the rates of death by suicide [36]. The suicide risk for trigeminal neuralgia can be considered in relation to data generated from the study of other painful headache syndromes: migraine and cluster headache. A prospective study found that in patients with cluster headaches, there was a significant increase in passive and active suicidal ideation, suicidal planning, and suicide attempt during attacks. Suicidal ideation prior to attacks predicted suicidal ideation during attacks. More headache-related functional impact and longer disease duration were also associated with suicidal ideation [37]. Primary headaches consist of 1% of the all-cause suicide rate with cluster and migraine headaches as a cause for 70–80% of the headache-associated suicide deaths. Cluster headaches appear to have more risk than migraine headaches, and in one case series, 2% of cluster headache patients attempted suicide [38, 39]. In the Trejo-Gabriel-Galan retrospective study, which interviewed neurologists regarding their cases, trigeminal neuralgia was not the leading cause of headache-related suicide in any country, but it did account for 25% of headache-related suicide attempts. The author noted that cluster headache is associated with restlessness and increased psychomotor behavior, contrasted with the decreased motor behavior seen in trigeminal neuralgia, which may decrease the risk of a suicide attempt [38]. The review by Allsop et al. discussed above obtained two quotes from patients highlighting suicidal ideation: *"If I couldn't get the pills I would commit suicide"* and *"I would probably have put a bullet through my brains because the pain was so intense"* [21].

Universal precautions guidelines were proposed for clinicians to use to assess, manage, and stratify risk factors in patients with chronic pain [40]. Utilizing universal precautions has been shown to detect, deter, and reduce suicidality in a retrospective review of chronic, non-cancer pain patients. Precautions enable screening for depression, which can improve health outcomes, mainly if it facilitates access to interventions [41]. There are limitations to screening as many patients who commit suicide deny suicidality when seeing their clinician in the month before death. It is unclear if screening reduces rates. While not all patients are comfortable with questioning, most patients appreciate the inquiry as the thoughts often represent distress they experience as they are seeking care, and inquiry helps to decrease their sense of isolation. Nonjudgmental, open inquiry about thoughts can provide relief for patients who are struggling. The clinician should ask about intent, access to means, destabilizing symptoms such as acute worsening of pain or insomnia, and precipitating stressors or losses with despair. Protective factors such as a sense of responsibility to relationships, pets or work, religious beliefs, and social supports are included in the assessment. People with imminent intent or plans, who cannot control their urges should be referred for emergent evaluation by mental health clinicians [32].

The anticonvulsant medications that are recommended as part of trigeminal neuralgia treatment are associated with adverse cognitive or psychiatric side effects that the clinician should remain attentive to and evaluate for in management. Certain antiepileptics such as carbamazepine, valproate, lamotrigine, and oxcarbazepine have mood-stabilizing effects [42]. Yet, there is a statistically significant increase in suicidality in patients taking antiepileptic medications. The rates and magnitude of suicidal behavior are low, and a protective effect from the medications have been found in other studies, potentially due to achieving relief for the indicated condition [42, 43]. Gabapentin and lamotrigine may be associated with aggression in children and adults with learning disabilities or mental handicaps. Insomnia may occur with lamotrigine, phenytoin, and carbamazepine. There are cases of phenytoin-induced encephalopathy, and phenytoin at toxic levels can induce psychotic symptoms. Topiramate has been associated with causing depressive symptoms [44]. Case reports have linked baclofen to behavioral disinhibition and drug-induced mania [45]. Delirium and psychosis may occur with baclofen withdrawal [46]. Deficits in memory, concentration, attention, mental processing, and motor speed have been described with the anticonvulsant medications, exacerbated by combination treatment [47]. The side effects of medications for trigeminal neuralgia are potential contributors to psychological distress and social and occupational dysfunction. The Allsop et al. review included narratives of people struggling with the cognitive side effects of treatment. The patients described performance decreases, quitting work due to an accident, or accusations of drug addiction [21].

Mental Status Screening

When following patients with pain through time, it is helpful to assess mental functioning by completing a focused mental status exam. Attention to mood, affect, thought content, thought process, and perception enables the clinician to identify aspects of care that may influence treatment, that may need further assessment and intervention, or that maybe the direct result of certain prescribed medications. The mental status exam elements are subjective (symptoms that the patient reports) and objective (signs observed by the clinician). During an encounter, the clinician should be able to observe patients for objective elements of the mental status exam such as affect and thought process, while also incorporating specific inquiry for those aspects that cannot be determined by observation alone such as mood, suicidal ideation, or reported worries about treatment. Documentation of the mental status exam provides a helpful chronology of the trajectory of specific symptoms for the clinician to follow during visits [2].

Referral to Care

Deciding when to refer a patient for a psychological assessment is dictated by several factors. The decision is influenced by the level of patient interest and motivation. The availability of an appropriate clinician, the patient's locale, or insurance coverage are other limitations to care. Too often, patients with chronic pain are referred to when they have already developed maladaptive cognitions and behaviors or have experienced frustration in their medical care leading to mistrust or anger. Psychological assessment is generally indicated in patients suffering from chronic pain. However, specific indications include:

(a) When psychological dysfunction is observed or suspected
(b) Inadequate recovery such as duration of symptoms beyond typical time course, failure to benefit from treatment, or pain complaints that cannot be explained by physical findings
(c) Substance abuse or aberrant use of prescription medication
(d) Premorbid history of major psychiatric symptoms
(e) Lack of adherence to medical treatment
(f) Suspected cognitive impairment
(g) When a patient has a catastrophic medical condition
(h) Before major surgical or invasive procedures or before the initiation of chronic opioid treatment [2]

The stages of care for the patient in pain have been conceptualized as three stages: primary, secondary, and tertiary care. Acute pain problems are managed during the primary stage, and the focus is on the control of pain symptoms. Psychological interventions involve management of the acute pain stressor but become more pertinent in the secondary and tertiary stages of care if pain persists or recurs. The secondary stage's goal is to prevent physical decline and avoid the progression of psycho-socioeconomic barriers. The tertiary stage of care is for the patient who is suffering from the sequelae of disability, and it is aimed at preventing or relieving permanent disability [4].

In the referral process, the clinician should explore patient expectations of treatment, provide a patient-centered rationale for treatment, and review the patient's understanding of the recommended intervention. This process requires the clinician to achieve comfort with his or her presentation of the information, mainly due to the risk of stigma regarding seeking out psychological care and to the patient's potential perception that the pain is being minimized and seen as not "real" by the clinician. Essential points to relay to the patient are some of the goals of psychotherapy. These include an exploration of one's thoughts, beliefs, and schemas that shape coping abilities in order to enable and empower the individual to decrease negative thought patterns and appraisals that exacerbate pain, decrease pain intensity, and enhance behaviors and skills that lead to an improvement in functioning, esteem, and well-being [48]. Additionally, in any patient with headache, irrespective of any other psychiatric history, stress may be the most salient psychological force in an individual's life. The stress of a persistent headache may overwhelm existing coping mechanisms, rendering them inadequate, and new coping mechanisms may need to be learned [49]. Furthermore, the psychotherapist functions to support the patient in improving interpersonal effectiveness, such as with family members or significant others, and helps the individual to identify methods of creating realistic personal goals and pacing activities [4]. Building positive emotional states, developing a sense of confidence and self-efficacy, and gaining the ability to engage in distraction or relaxation serves to reduce pain sensitivity [20].

The clinician stands to improve the patient's "buy-in" to psychological care by highlighting reductions in disability, discomfort, and distress as the goals of psychotherapy. However, motivational interviewing to assess the patient's readiness for a change to more proactive modalities may be required, including a mutual discussion of the treatment plan, and identifying small goals [50].

Psychological Treatment Modalities

Pharmacotherapy and surgical management remain the primary modalities for the treatment of trigeminal neuralgia. People with intractable pain, limited pain coping, psychiatric comorbidities, or functional decline may require additional treatment strategies. The evidence for the influence of psychological factors on coping with pain and their role in the neurophysiological experience of pain supports the use of psychological interventions [51, 52]. Limitations to psychological treatments occur when clinicians do not readily consider these modalities, when managed care health insurance payers refuse to reimburse interdisciplinary treatments, or due to the patient's beliefs about psychotherapy that prevent engagement [52, 53]. There is a wide breadth of treatment available, including behavior therapy, cognitive therapy, biofeedback, cognitive-behavioral therapy (CBT), acceptance and commitment therapy (ACT), and mindfulness-based therapies. Behavioral therapy focuses on the balance between maladaptive pain behaviors and well behaviors that may influence the person's environment and, thus, either perpetuate or relieve pain [52]. Acceptance and commitment therapy is designed to improve self-compassion, psychological adaptation, and responsiveness to accepting and managing stressors [54]. Mindfulness-based stress reduction aims to enable the patient to develop a detachment from distressing sensations and to improve presence in daily activities. These interventions have evidence for decreasing healthcare utilization, for improvements in pain, distress, and disability, and for improved outcomes in comorbid psychiatric conditions. Some patients may not benefit or may even relapse after some initial stability. Assessing patient interest through motivational interviewing may enhance treatment adherence and response [52]. The choice in treatment modalities may be influenced by patient preference or availability [48].

There are limitations in the evidence for CBT and other psychological interventions for neuropathic pain conditions. Cognitive-behavioral therapy is the predominant psychological intervention for chronic musculoskeletal pain disorders; however, there is a limited amount of randomized controlled trials evaluating this therapy in neuropathic pain and no studies thus far for trigeminal neuralgia [55]. A Cochrane review of CBT for neuropathic pain utilizing two small studies, one for burning mouth syndrome and the other for spinal cord injury, revealed insufficient evidence for the benefit of CBT. The authors noted that each individual study's size was too small to perform statistical analysis, and many other trials did not meet the inclusion criteria for the review. This review highlighted the need for randomized controlled trials for neuropathic pain [55]. While there may be limitations in research methodologies and the strength of evidence for specific conditions, cognitive-behavioral therapy for chronic pain has shown improvements in various elements of the pain experience. In a meta-analysis of studies that compared CBT for chronic pain, excluding headache disorders, to waitlist controls, CBT led to improvements in the experience of pain, cognitive coping and appraisals, pain behaviors, mood, and social functioning [17, 56]. There has been extensive evidence for the use of cognitive-behavioral strategies for headache disorders, and two small studies that indicate ACT may be a helpful modality for headache as well [52]. The avoidant behaviors that develop in orofacial pain patients such as avoidance of mouth opening, facial touch, or social activities are potential targets for psychological interventions [17]. Psychotherapy would provide further benefit for the psychiatric comorbidities of depressive, anxiety, or insomnia disorders that either pre-date or develop as a result of trigeminal neuralgia. These clinical conditions are responsive to cognitive-behavioral interventions [57–60]. For cognitive-behavioral therapy for insomnia (CBT-I) in chronic pain disorders, there have been a few studies evaluating the role in musculoskeletal conditions (osteoarthritis, neck, and back pain) and fibromyalgia. A consistent finding in these small studies revealed improvements in various aspects of sleep, such as sleep latency and total wake time. There were no significant changes found in pain intensity; however, the authors of one review study examining outcomes in CBT vs. non-CBT groups suggested that in their study, effect size differences favored a reduction in pain intensity from CBT [61]. Patients with chronic migraines who completed CBT-I experienced reductions in headache frequency, improved sleep parameters, and further improvement after treatment ended [62]. Patients with neuropathic pain and sleep disturbance may require a combination of pharmacotherapy to target pain and behavioral treatments for the best outcomes [29].

Alternative Modes of Support

Access to specialists due to the insufficient amount of trained clinicians, geographical access, time commitment, and parity in insurance coverage for psychological treatments are some of the limitations that clinicians face in referring their patients to specialty care [52, 63]. Web-based interventions may help ameliorate access challenges. Internet-delivered CBT-I applications such as Sleep Healthy Using the Internet (SHUTi) may help patients with pain interference to manage insomnia [64]. Prescription Digital Therapeutics (PDT) such as SHUTi (now trademarked as Somryst) and web-based delivery of psychoeducation and cognitive-behavioral interventions via sites such as curablehealth.com may be complementary to in-person management or serve as additional support in cases when there is no access to in-person care. Pain-focused programs have been designed to provide information about pain, track symptoms, and educate about self-management strategies. There are no clear clinical guidelines to recommend the design of these programs. The range of content is variable among various applications and websites. A systematic review evaluated various pain-self management programs. These programs do not replace in-person care, and there is still much to be determined about the efficacy for patients in pain and specific pain types. Limitations include the lack of culturally specific interventions, and most programs do not have a comprehensive guide of core self-management skills. In addition to payments required for most programs, technological access and abilities may widen socioeconomic access disparities that patients with chronic pain conditions face more frequently. Depending on individual patient needs, the clinician may recommend web-based applications as part of a patient-centered management plan [65]. Trigeminal neuralgia support groups are another alternative resource for patients and are provided through organizations such as the non-profit Facial Pain Association [66].

In conclusion, trigeminal neuralgia remains a challenging condition for people to endure for many reasons, including the life-altering qualities of the pain, the pain's anatomical location, the nature of the pain leading to delayed diagnosis, the potential burden and limitations of medical interventions, and the degree of functional decline. While there are limitations in the amount and type of evidence for various treatments and interventions for trigeminal neuralgia or the potential psychological sequelae, there is still much to investigate. Brain regions involved in pain and emotion processing have shown neuroplastic improvements in response to various interventions like music, mindfulness exercises, CBT, physical activity, and prayer [14]. It is imperative to consider multiple modes of management and interdisciplinary support to reduce suffering and improve the quality of life for the afflicted.

References

1. Gatchel RJ, McGeary DD, McGeary CA, Lippe B. Interdisciplinary chronic pain management: past, present and future. Am Psychol. 2014;69(2):119–30.
2. Bruns D, Disorbio JM. The psychological assessment of patients with chronic pain. In: Deer T, Leong M, editors. Comprehensive treatment of chronic pain by medical, interventional, and integrative approaches; the American academy of pain medicine textbook on patient management. New York: Springer; 2013. p. 805–27.
3. Melzack R. From the gate to the neuromatrix. Pain Suppl. 1999;82(1):S121–6.
4. Gatchel RJ, Turk DC. Psychosocial factors in pain: critical perspectives. New York: Guilford Press; 1999.
5. Dersh J, Polatin P, Gatchel RJ. Chronic pain and psychopathology: research findings and theoretical considerations. Psychosom Med. 2002;64(5):773–86.
6. Simons L, Elman I, Borsook D. Psychological processing in chronic pain: a neural systems approach. Neurosci Biobehav Rev. 2014;39:61–78.
7. Turk DC, Gatchel RJ. Psychological approaches to pain management, second edition: a practitioner's handbook. New York: Guilford; 2002. p. 39–47.
8. Gatchel RJ, Peng YB, Peters ML, Fuchs PN, Turk DC. The biopsychosocial approach to chronic pain: scientific advances and future directions. Psychol Bull. 2007;133(4):581–624.
9. Engel GL. The need for a new medical model: a challenge for biomedicine. Science. 1977;196(4286):129–36.
10. Leo RJ. Clinical manual of pain management in psychiatry. Arlington: American Psychiatric; 2007.
11. Silz D, Hayley S. Major depressive disorder and alterations in insular cortical activity: a review of current functional magnetic imaging research. Front Hum Neurosci. 2012;6(323):1–14.
12. Terry EL, DelVentura JL, Bartley E, Vincent AL, Rhudy JL. Emotional modulation of pain and spinal nociception in persons with major depressive disorder. Pain. 2013;154(12):2759–68.
13. Zhang Y, Mao Z, Lan L, Ling Z, Liu X, Zhang J, et al. Dysregulation of pain- and emotion-related networks in trigeminal neuralgia. Front Hum Neurosci. 2018;12(107):1–10.

14. Ong WY, Stohler CS, Herr DR. Role of the prefrontal cortex in pain processing. Mol Neurobiol. 2019;56:1137–66.
15. Wu TH, Hu LY, Lu T, Chen PM, Chen HJ, Shen CC. Risk of psychiatric disorders following trigeminal neuralgia: a nationwide population-based retrospective cohort study. J Headache Pain. 2015;16(64):1–8.
16. Jiang C. Risk of probable posttraumatic stress disorder in patients with trigeminal neuralgia. Psychol Health Med. 2019;24(4):493–504.
17. Feinmann C, Newton-John T. Psychiatric and psychological management considerations associated with nerve damage and neuropathic trigeminal pain. J Orofac Pain. 2004;18(4):360–5.
18. McAllister MJ. Trigeminal neuralgia [Internet] [Cited 4 Apr 2020]. Available from https://www.instituteforchronicpain.org/common-conditions/neuralgia/trigeminal
19. Devor M, Wood I, Sharav Y, Zakrzewska JM. Trigeminal neuralgia during sleep. Pain Pract. 2008;8(4):263–8.
20. Carlson CR. Psychological factors associated with orofacial pains. Dent Clin N Am. 2007;51(1):145–60.
21. Allsop MJ, Twiddy M, Grant H, Czoski-Murray C, Mon-Williams M, Mushtaq F, et al. Diagnosis, medication, and surgical management for patients with trigeminal neuralgia: a qualitative study. Acta Neurochir. 2015;157(11):1925–33.
22. Siqueira SRDT, Teixeira MJ, De Siqueira JTT. Severe psychosocial compromise in idiopathic trigeminal neuralgia: case report. Pain Med. 2010;11(3):453–5.
23. Mačianskytė D, Janužis G, Kubilius R, Adomaitienė V, Ščiupokas A. Associations between chronic pain and depressive symptoms in patients with trigeminal neuralgia. Medicina. 2011;47(7):386–92.
24. Greenwood K, Thurston R, Rumble M, Waters SJ, Keefe FJ. Anger and persistent pain: current status and future directions. Pain. 2003;103(1–2):1–5.
25. Almoznino G, Benoliel R, Sharav Y, Haviv Y. Sleep disorders and chronic craniofacial pain: characteristics and management possibilities. Sleep Med Rev. 2017;33:39–50.
26. Finan P, Goodin BR, Smith MT. The association of sleep and pain: an update and a path forward. J Pain. 2013;14(12):1539–52.
27. Fishbain DA, Cole B, Lewis JE, Gao J. What is the evidence for chronic pain being etiologically associated with the DSM-IV category of sleep disorder due to a general medical condition? A structured, evidence-based review. Pain Med. 2010;11(2):158–79.
28. Sayar K, Arikan M, Yontem T. Sleep quality in chronic pain patients. Can J Psychiatry. 2002;47(9):844–8.
29. Ferini-Strambi L. Neuropathic pain and sleep: a review. Pain Ther. 2017;6:19–23.
30. Benoliel R, Eliav E, Sharav Y. Self-reports of pain-related awakenings in persistent orofacial pain patients. J Orofac Pain. 2009;23(4):330–8.
31. Fishbain DA, Goldberg M, Rosomoff RS, Rosomoff H. Completed suicide in chronic pain. Clin J Pain. 1991;7(1):29–36.
32. Stern TH, Fricchione GL, Cassem NH, Jellinek M, Rosenbaum JF, editors. Massachusetts general hospital handbook of general hospital psychiatry. 6th ed. Philadelphia: Elsevier.
33. Tang KY, Crane C. Suicidality in chronic pain: a review of the prevalence, risk factors and psychological links. Psychol Med. 2006;36:575–86.
34. Ilgen MA, Zivin K, McCammon RJ, Valenstein M. Pain and suicidal thoughts, plans and attempts in the United States. Gen Hosp Psychiatry. 2008;30(6):521–7.
35. Fishbain DA, Bruns D, Disorbio JM, Lewis JE. Risk for five forms of suicidality in acute pain patients and chronic pain patients vs pain-free community controls. Pain Med. 2009;10(6):1095–105.
36. Nieto RB, Guasch M, Izquierdo A, Caballero M, Juanola E, Fernanadez A. Suicide risk in refractory chronic migraine, refractory chronic cluster headache, and refractory trigeminal neuralgia. Which is the "suicide disease"? Paper presented at International Headache Congress 2019. 2019 Sept 5–8; Dublin, Ireland. IHC-PO-018.
37. Ji Lee M, Cho S-J, Wook Park J, Kyung Chu M, Moon H-S, Chung P-W, et al. Increased suicidality in patients with cluster headache. Cephalalgia. 2019;39(10):1249–56.

38. Trejo-Gabriel-Galan JA, Aicua-Rapún I, Cubo-Delgado E, Velasco-Bernal C. Suicide in primary headaches in 48 countries: a physician-survey based study. Cephalgia. 2018;38(4):798–803.
39. Rozen TD, Fishman RS. Cluster headache in the United States of America: Demographics, clinical characteristics, triggers, suicidality, and personal burden. Headache. 2012;52:99–113.
40. Gourlay DL, Heit HA. Universal precautions revisited: managing the inherited pain patient. Pain Med. 2009;10(2):S115–23.
41. Gilbert JW, Wheeler GR, Storey BB, Mick G, Richardson G, Westerfield G, et al. Suicidality in chronic noncancer pain patients. Int J Neurosci. 2009;119(10):1968–79.
42. Raju Sagiraju HK, Wang CP, Amuan ME, Van Cott AC, Altalib HH, Pugh MJV. Antiepileptic drugs and suicide-related behavior: is it the drug or comorbidity? Neurol Clin Pract. 2018;8(4):331–9.
43. Britton JW, Shih JJ. Antiepileptic drugs and suicidality. Drug Healthcare Patient Saf. 2010;2:181–9.
44. Schmitz B. Effects of antiepileptic drugs on mood and behavior. Epilepsia. 2006;47(2):28–33.
45. Geoffroy PA, Auffret M, Deheul A, Bordet R, Cottencin O, Rolland B. Baclofen-induced manic symptoms: case report and systematic review. Psychosomatics. 2014;55(4):326–32.
46. Malhotra T, Rosenzweig I. Baclofen withdrawal causes psychosis in otherwise unclouded consciousness. Letter to the editor. J Neuropsychiatr Clin Neurosci. 2009;21(4):476.
47. Reynolds EH, Trimble MR. Adverse neuropsychiatric effects of anticonvulsant drugs. Drugs. 1985;29:570–81.
48. Thorn BE. Cognitive therapy for chronic pain: a step-by-step guide. 2nd ed. New York: The Guilford Press; 2017.
49. Jacobson SA, Folstein MF. Psychiatric perspectives on headache and facial pain. Otolaryngol Clin N Am. 2003;36(6):1187–200.
50. Lipchik GL, Nash JM. Cognitive-behavioral issues in the treatment and management of chronic daily headache. Curr Pain Headache Rep. 2002;6:473–9.
51. Haythornthwaite JA, Benrud-Larson LM. Psychological aspects of neuropathic pain. Clin J Pain. 2000;16(S101–S105):124–9.
52. Turk DC, Gatchel RJ. Psychological approaches to pain management: a practitioner's handbook. New York: Guilford Press; 2018.
53. Schatman ME. The role of the health insurance industry in perpetuating suboptimal pain management. Pain Med. 2011;12(3):415–26.
54. Hayes S, Smith S. Get out of your mind and into your life: the new acceptance and commitment therapy. Oakland: New Harbinger; 2005.
55. Eccleston C, Hearn L, Williams AC. Psychological therapies for the management of chronic neuropathic pain in adults. Cochrane Database Syst Rev. 2015;10:1–30.
56. Morley S, Eccleston C, Williams A. Systematic review and meta-analysis of randomized controlled trials of cognitive behaviour therapy and behaviour therapy for chronic pain in adults, excluding headache. Pain. 1999;80:1–13.
57. Chand SP, Ravi C, Chakkamparambil B, Prasad A, Vora A. CBT for depression: what the evidence says. Curr Psychiatr. 2018;17(9):14–16, 20–23.
58. Hofmann SG, Asnaani A, Vonk IJ, Sawyer AT, Fang A. The efficacy of cognitive behavioral therapy: a review of meta-analyses. Cogn Ther Res. 2012;36(5):427–40.
59. Butler AC, Chapman JE, Forman EM, Beck AT. The empirical status of cognitive-behavioral therapy: a review of meta-analyses. Clin Psychol Rev. 2006;26(1):17–31.
60. Trauer JM, Qian MY, Doyle JS, Rajaratnam SMW, Cunnington D. Cognitive behavioral therapy for chronic insomnia: a systematic review and meta-analysis. Ann Intern Med. 2015;163(3):191–204.
61. Jungquist CR, O'Brien C, Matteson-Rusby S, Smith MT, Pigeon WR, Xia Y, et al. The efficacy of cognitive-behavioral therapy for insomnia in patients with chronic pain. Sleep Med. 2010;11(3):302–9.
62. Smitherman TA, Walters A, Davis RE, Ambrose CE, Roland M, Houle TT, et al. Randomized controlled pilot trial of behavioral insomnia treatment for chronic migraine with comorbid insomnia. Headache. 2016;56(2):276–91.

63. Thomas A, Grandner M, Nowakowski S, Nesom G, Corbitt C, Perlis ML. Where are the behavioral sleep medicine providers and where are they needed? A geographic assessment. Behav Sleep Med. 2016;14(6):687–98.
64. Shaffer KM, Camacho F, Lord HR, Chow PI, Palermo T, Law E, et al. Do treatment effects of a web-based cognitive behavioral therapy for insomnia intervention differ for users with and without pain interference? A secondary data analysis. J Behav Med. 2019;43:503–10.
65. Devan H, Farmery D, Peebles L, Grainger R. Evaluation of self-management support functions in apps for people with persistent pain: systematic review. JMIR Mhealth Uhealth. 2019;7(2) [Internet]. Available from https://www.ncbi.nlm.nih.gov/pmc/articles/PMC6390192/. Accessed 3 May 2020.
66. The Facial Pain Association [Internet]. Available from https://fpa-support.org/. Accessed 3 May 2020.

Algorithms for Management Recommendations

Miles Day, Alaa Abd-Elsayed, and Ben Ashworth

Trigeminal Neuralgia

The trigeminal neuralgia (TN) algorithm seems daunting at first, but it is relatively straightforward once the practitioner has a working knowledge of trigeminal disorders (Table 22.1) [1–8]. For idiopathic TN whether neurovascular compression is present or absent, treatment begins with medical management and follows the medical management algorithm. If this proves ineffective, interventional modalities need to be considered. In the presence of neurovascular compression, surgical techniques are indicated with the type based on age and the presence or absence of comorbidities. If surgery is refused or not indicated because of comorbidities, percutaneous interventions should be offered. Neuromodulation is commonly reserved for cases refractory to the aforementioned therapies. In the absence of neurovascular compression, the treatment is similar although microvascular decompression is seldom considered.

For secondary TN, initial treatment is based on the cause of the TN. Medical management follows for trauma, herpes, and multiples sclerosis. As with idiopathic TN, interventional therapies are considered when medical management is not effective. For tumors, debulking can be effective in alleviating the pain, with radiotherapy and medical management considered if surgery is contraindicated.

Acute TN exacerbations are treated following the acute exacerbation algorithm.

M. Day (✉) · B. Ashworth
Department of Anesthesiology, Texas Tech University Health Sciences Center, Lubbock, TX, USA
e-mail: miles.day@ttuhsc.edu; ben.ashworth@ttuhsc.edu

A. Abd-Elsayed
Department of Anesthesiology, University of Wisconsin School of Medicine and Public Health, Madison, WI, USA
e-mail: abdelsayed@wisc.edu

A. Abd-Elsayed (ed.), *Trigeminal Nerve Pain*,
https://doi.org/10.1007/978-3-030-60687-9_22

Table 22.1 Trigeminal neuralgia algorithm

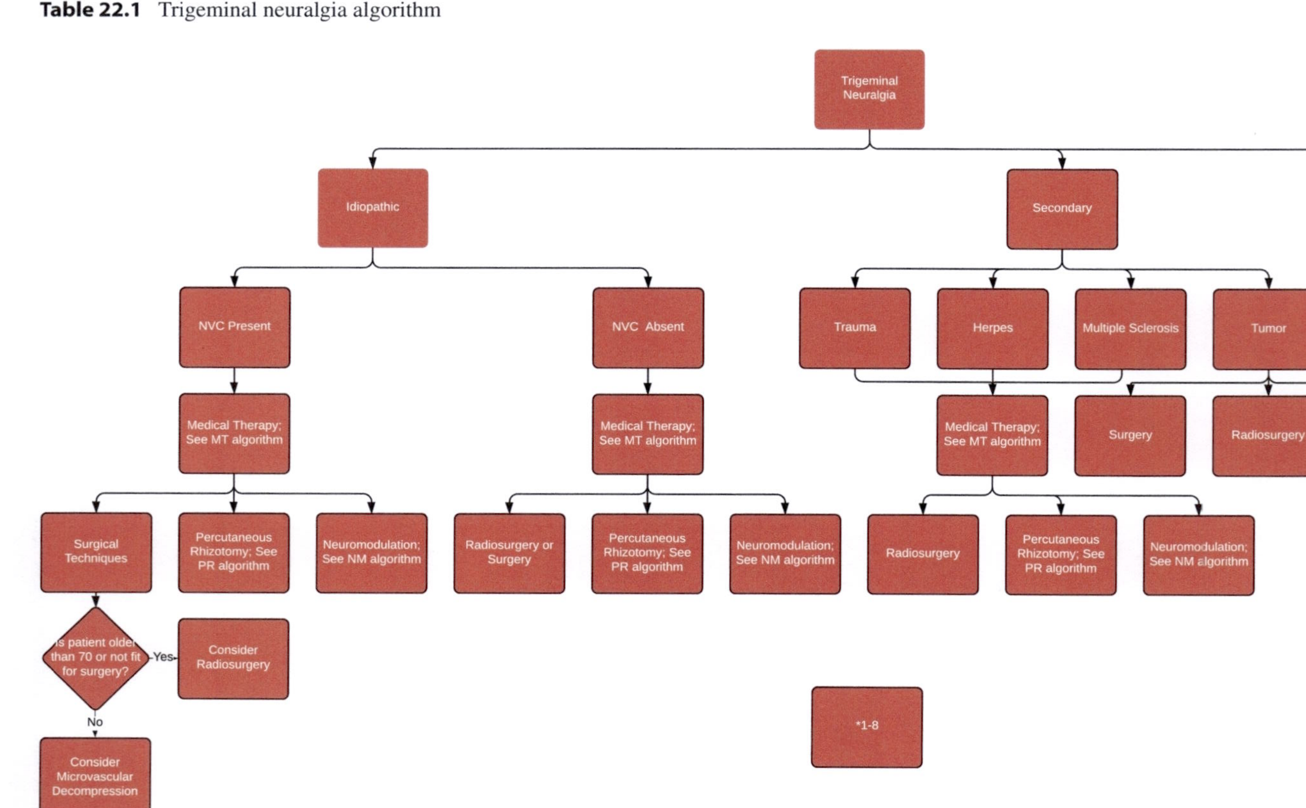

Trigeminal Neuropathic Pain

Trigeminal neuropathic pain is different from TN in that it stems from an unintentional or intentional injury to the trigeminal system, i.e., nucleus, ganglion, or the peripheral branches (Table 22.2) [9, 10]. Causes of unintentional injuries include stroke and trauma. Intentional trigeminal injuries caused by the treatments for TN can cause deafferentation pain and anesthesia dolorosa that oftentimes are worse than the initial TN pain. Regardless of the type of injury, therapy begins with

Table 22.2 Trigeminal neuropathic pain algorithm

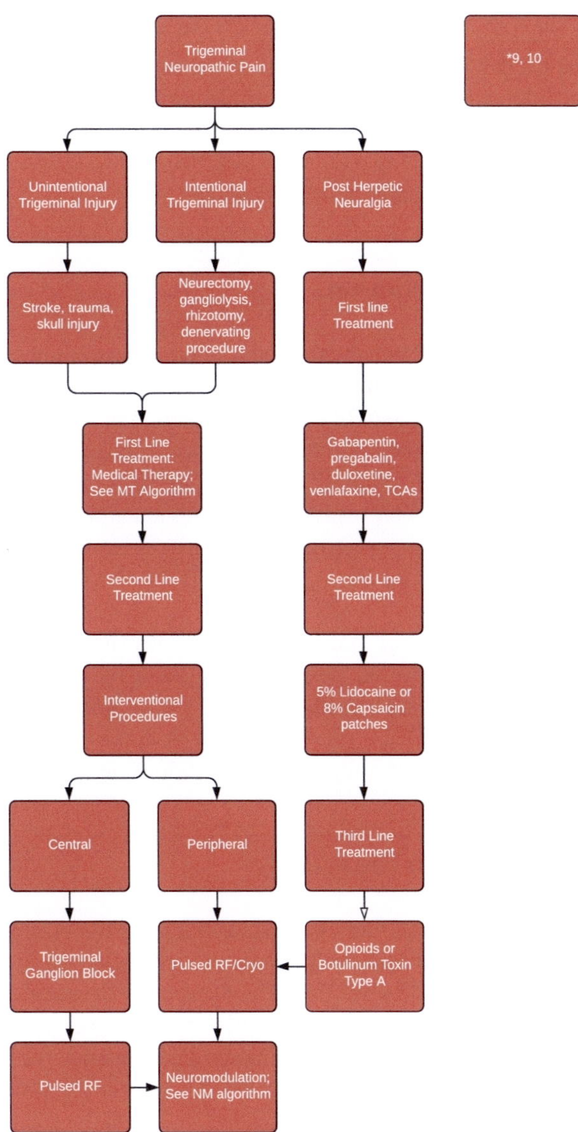

medical management followed by interventional treatments if initial treatment is not effective. Interventional procedures target the peripheral branches or the central components (trigeminal ganglion and nucleus caudalis). The primary author's training suggests not performing conventional RF on a previously injured ganglion or peripheral nerve. Neuromodulation is reserved for refractory cases.

Medical Therapy for Trigeminal Neuralgia

The algorithm for the treatment of TN and trigeminal neuropathic pain begins with medical management (Table 22.3) [2, 5, 6]. Progression down the algorithm is based on the degree of responsiveness of the patient to the medication and/or the presence of intolerable side effects. Multiple options are available at each level of therapy. Effectiveness should be evaluated at regular intervals to ensure appropriate therapy. Some therapies may require regular blood draws to monitor potential abnormalities, i.e., hyponatremia with oxcarbazepine.

Acute Exacerbations

Patients with TN may experience acute exacerbations of their underlying disease that require prompt treatment. This algorithm begins with an evaluation for mucosal trigger points (Table 22.4) [4]. If present, the initial option is intranasal 8% lidocaine. Other concentrations can be used if 8% is not available. The primary author has used aerosolized local anesthetics for the acute treatment of migraine headaches and patients can be instructed on how to safely perform this technique at home. Based on the response, trigger point injections with local anesthetic are next in line. This is followed by Botox injections if the previous two steps do not achieve long-lasting relief.

In the absence of mucosal trigger points, subcutaneous (SQ) sumatriptan is first-line therapy. If the SQ formulation is ineffective or not available, the nasal and oral formulations can be used. If any of these formulations are effective, the patient should be provided a prescription for at-home use. A fourth option is intravenous magnesium, followed by intravenous lidocaine and finally intravenous phenytoin.

Percutaneous Rhizotomy

After a successful diagnostic block, the practitioner must decide on the appropriate procedure for providing long-term relief (Table 22.5) [3]. Several techniques are available to accomplish this. The decision is based on the training of the practitioner, available equipment, available medications, and risk: benefit ratio. Previous chapters have covered the techniques and evidence for these procedures.

Table 22.3 Medical therapy algorithm

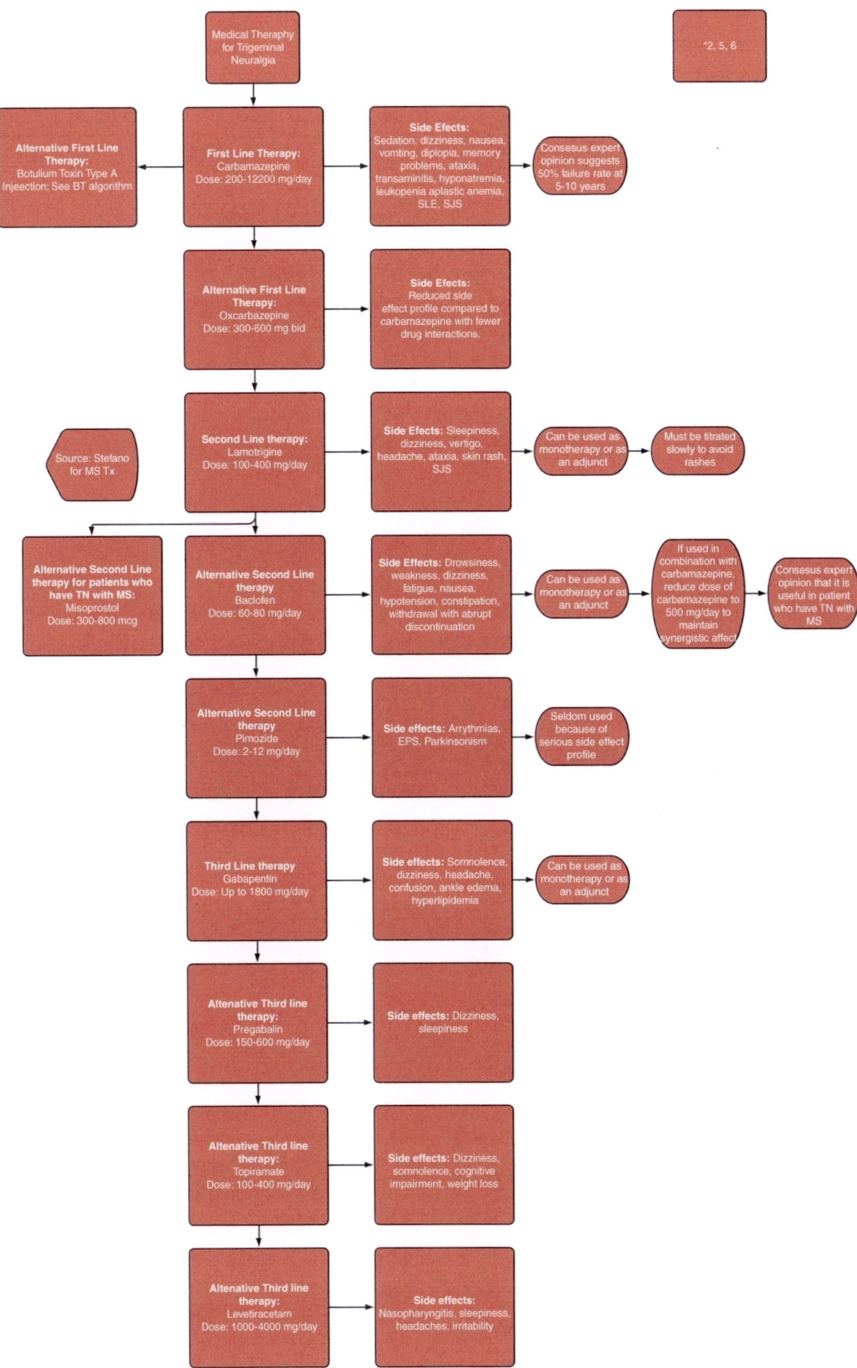

Table 22.4 Acute exacerbation algorithm

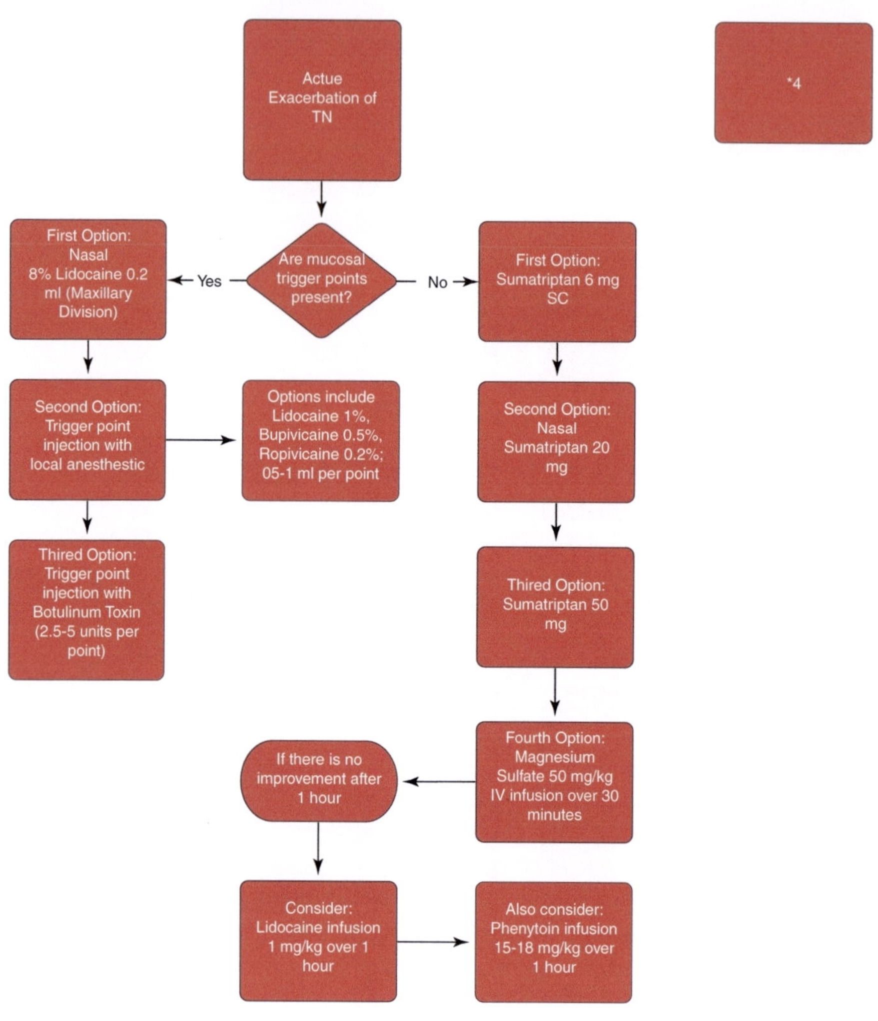

Botulinum Toxin Type A

The use of botulinum toxin type A (BoNT-A) for TN has emerged over recent years as a minimally invasive treatment. As with other algorithms, there must be diminishing efficacy or a failure of medical therapy before initiating (Table 22.6) [5, 7]. The initial dose is 2.5 U/cm^2. If successful, this dose can be used for further treatments. If there is no or an incomplete effect after 4 weeks, a booster dose of 2.5 U/cm^2 is given. If effective, a dose of 5 U/cm^2 can be used for future

Table 22.5   Percutaneous rhizotomy algorithm

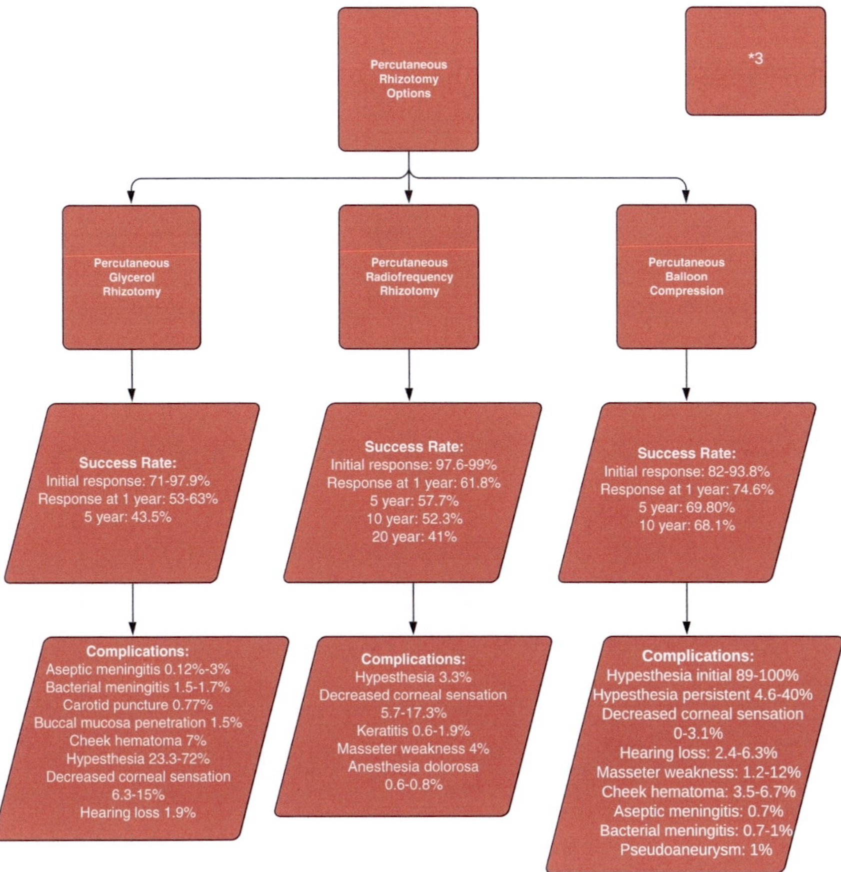

treatments. If the booster dose fails, other invasive modalities should be considered.

Neuromodulation

When conservative and less invasive therapies, i.e., botulinum toxin and rhizotomies, have failed for TN and trigeminal neuropathic pain, neuromodulation is an option that may provide relief (Table 22.7) [1, 8]. Targets include the peripheral nerve branches and central structures. In the periphery, transcutaneous electrical nerve stimulation and subcutaneous implantation of electrodes in the trigeminal nerve distributions have been used. Centrally, the motor cortex, thalamus, Gasserian ganglion, and nucleus caudalis have been targeted for lead placement.

Table 22.6 Botulinum toxin type A algorithm

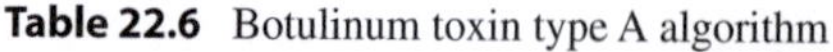

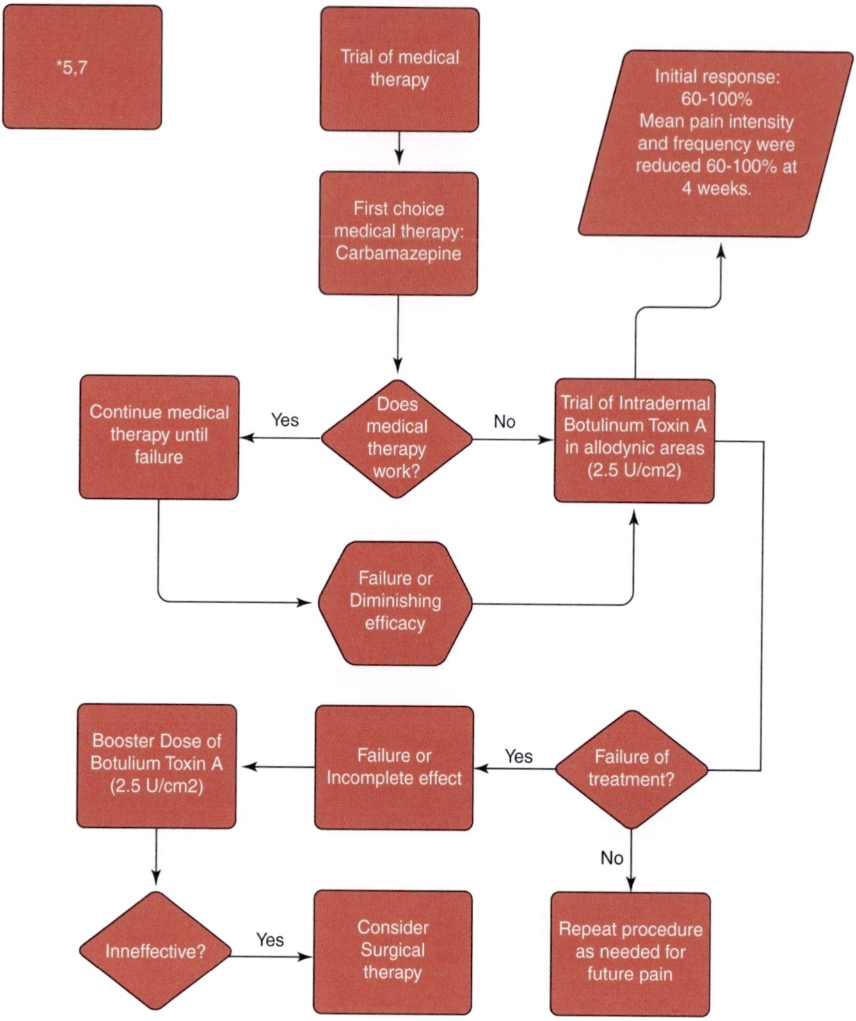

Headache Disorders that Can Mimic TN

There many headaches disorders that can mimic TN including migraine headaches (Table 22.8) [11–14] and the trigeminal autonomic cephalgias: cluster headaches (Table 22.9) [15–17], paroxysmal hemicranias (Table 22.10) [15, 17], short-lasting unilateral neuralgiform headache attacks with conjunctival injection and tearing (SUNCT) (Table 22.11) [16–18], short-lasting unilateral neuralgiform headache attacks with cranial autonomic symptoms (SUNA), hemicrania continua

Table 22.7 Neuromodulation algorithm

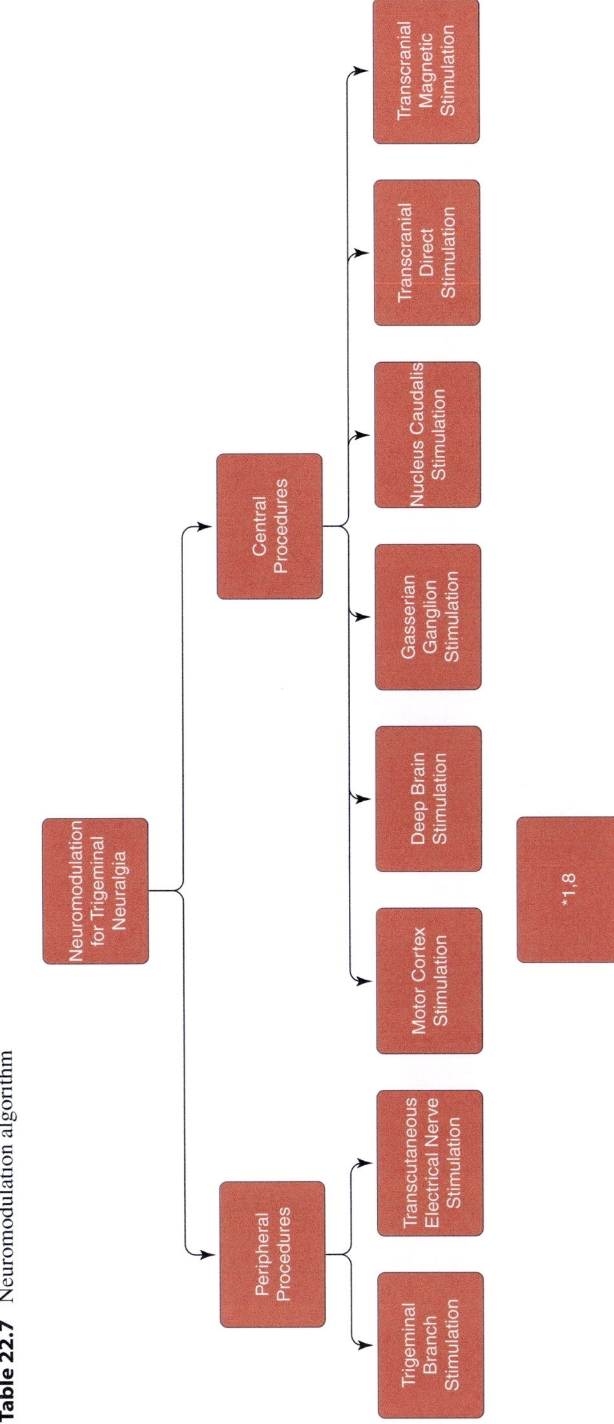

Table 22.8 Migraine headache algorithm

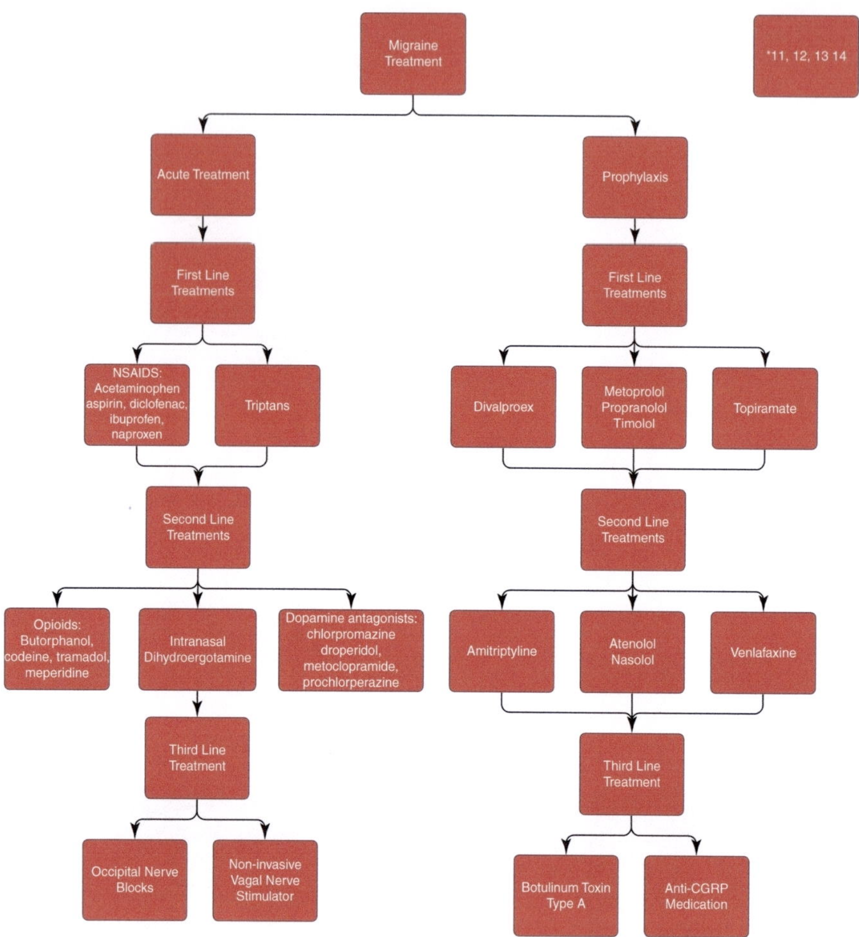

(Table 22.12) [15, 17], and persistent idiopathic facial pain (PIFP) (Table 22.13) [19]. Treatment algorithms begin with medication management and in some cases may include minimally invasive procedures. Medical management for PIFP consists of previously mentioned neuropathic pain medications.

In conclusion, an algorithmic approach to treating trigeminal neuralgia and trigeminal-related diagnosis is important in ensuring that all avenues of treatment are considered as the pain practitioner embarks on treating this life-altering malady. Each step should be reassessed before proceeding to the next. Appropriate referrals should be made once the practitioner has reached their limits.

Table 22.9 Cluster headache algorithm

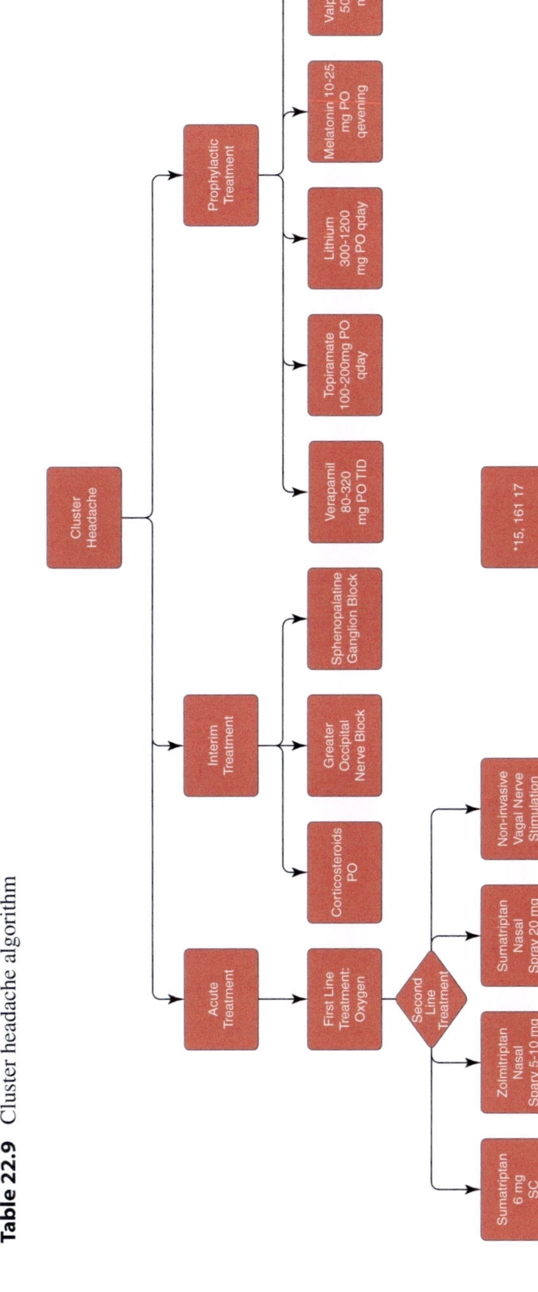

Table 22.10 Paroxysmal hemicrania algorithm

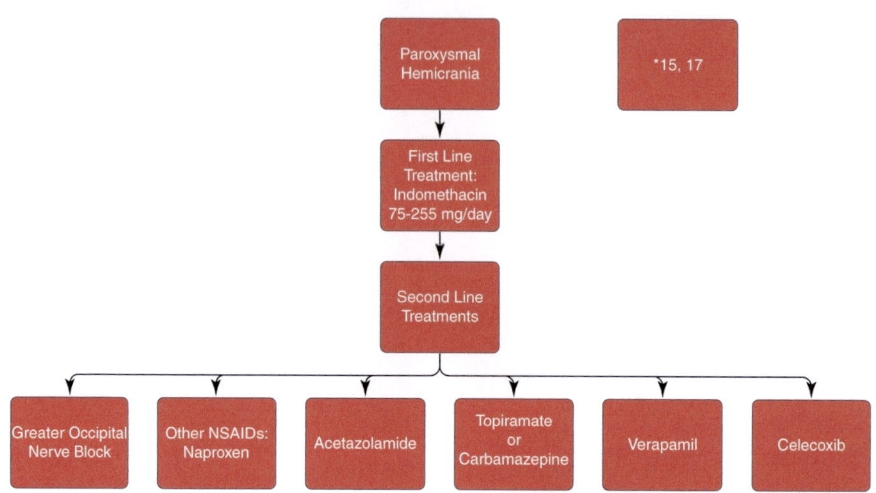

Table 22.11 SUNCT/SUNA algorithm

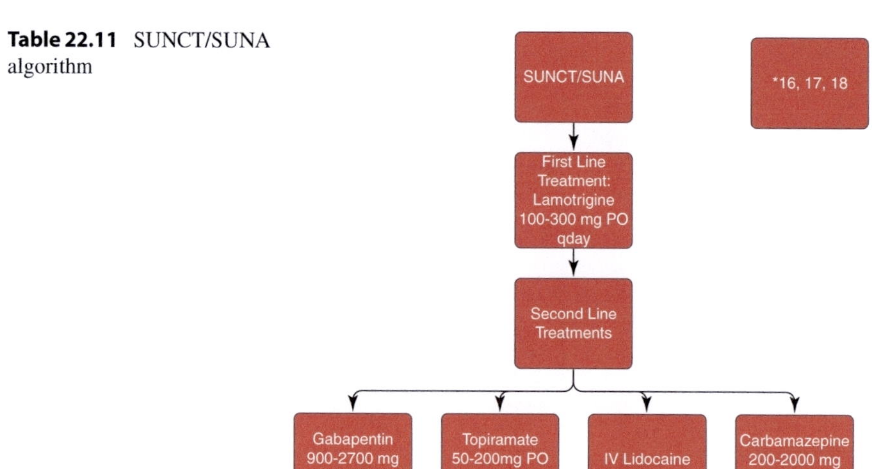

Table 22.12 Hemicrania continua algorithm

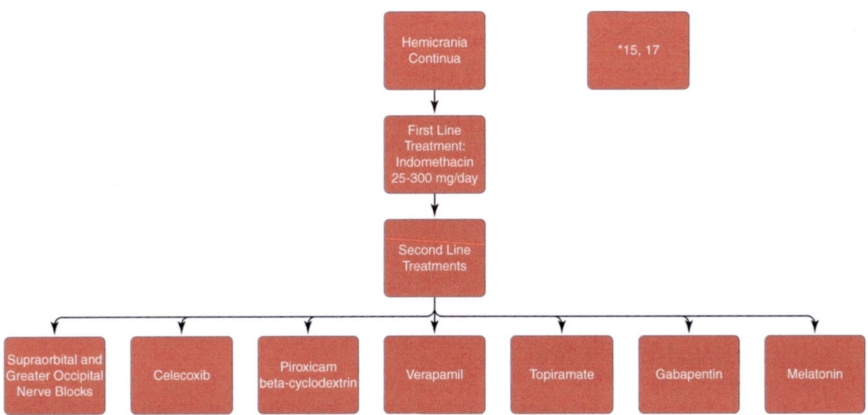

Table 22.13 Persistent idiopathic facial pain algorithm

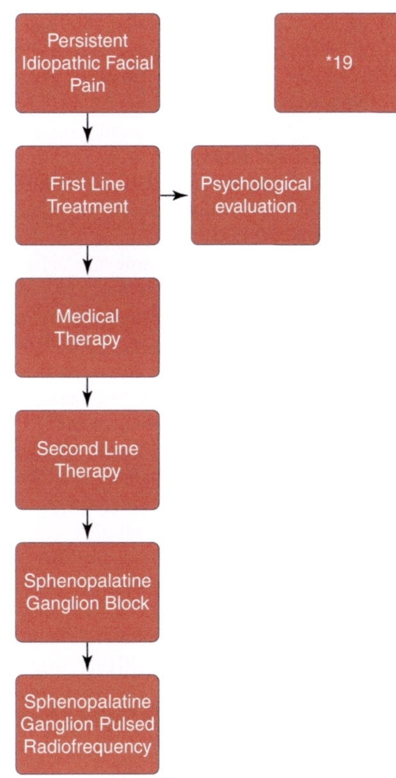

References

1. Spina A, Mortini P, Alemanno F, Houdayer E, Iannaccone S. Trigeminal neuralgia: toward a multimodal approach. World Neurosurg. 2017;103:220–30. https://doi.org/10.1016/j.wneu.2017.03.126.
2. Bendtsen L, Zakrzewska JM, Abbott J, et al. European Academy of Neurology guideline on trigeminal neuralgia. Eur J Neurol. 2019;26(6):831–49. https://doi.org/10.1111/ene.13950.
3. Bick SKB, Eskandar EN. Surgical treatment of trigeminal neuralgia. Neurosurg Clin. 2017;28(3):429–38.
4. Moore D, Chong MS, Shetty A, Zakrzewska JM. A systematic review of rescue analgesic strategies in acute exacerbations of primary trigeminal neuralgia. Br J Anaesth. 2019;123(2):e385–96. https://doi.org/10.1016/j.bja.2019.05.026.
5. Al-Quliti KW. Update on neuropathic pain treatment for trigeminal neuralgia. The pharmacological and surgical options. Neurosciences (Riyadh). 2015;20(2):107–14. https://doi.org/10.17712/nsj.2015.2.20140501.
6. Zakrzewska JM, Linskey ME. Trigeminal neuralgia. BMJ Clin Evid. 2014;2014:1207.
7. Guardiani E, Sadoughi B, Blitzer A, Sirois D. A new treatment paradigm for trigeminal neuralgia using Botulinum toxin type A. Laryngoscope. 2014;124(2):413–7. https://doi.org/10.1002/lary.24286.
8. Weber K. Neuromodulation and devices in trigeminal neuralgia. Headache. 2017;57(10):1648–53. https://doi.org/10.1111/head.13166.
9. Eller JL, Raslan AM, Burchiel KJ. Trigeminal neuralgia: definition and classification. Neurosurg Focus. 2005;18(5):1–3.
10. Schutzer-Weissmann J, Farquhar-Smith P. Post-herpetic neuralgia—a review of current management and future directions. Expert Opin Pharmacother. 2017;18(16):1739–50. https://doi.org/10.1080/14656566.2017.1392508.
11. Mayans L, Walling A. Acute migraine headache: treatment strategies. Am Fam Physician. 2018;97(4):243–51.
12. Ha H, Gonzalez A. Migraine headache prophylaxis. Am Fam Physician. 2019;99(1):17–24.
13. Tassorelli C, Grazzi L, de Tommaso M, et al. Noninvasive vagus nerve stimulation as acute therapy for migraine: the randomized PRESTO study. Neurology. 2018;91(4):e364–73. https://doi.org/10.1212/WNL.0000000000005857.
14. Silberstein SD, Calhoun AH, Lipton RB, et al. Chronic migraine headache prevention with noninvasive vagus nerve stimulation: the EVENT study. Neurology. 2016;87(5):529–38. https://doi.org/10.1212/WNL.0000000000002918.
15. Wei DY, Khalil M, Goadsby PJ. Managing cluster headache. Pract Neurol. 2019;19(6):521–8. https://doi.org/10.1136/practneurol-2018-002124.
16. Benoliel R. Trigeminal autonomic cephalgias. Br J Pain. 2012;6(3):106–23. https://doi.org/10.1177/2049463712456355.
17. Costa A, Antonaci F, Ramusino MC, Nappi G. The neuropharmacology of cluster headache and other trigeminal autonomic cephalalgias. Curr Neuropharmacol. 2015;13(3):304–23. https://doi.org/10.2174/1570159x13666150309233556.
18. Miller S, Matharu M. Trigeminal autonomic cephalalgias: beyond the conventional treatments. Curr Pain Headache Rep. 2014;18(8):438. https://doi.org/10.1007/s11916-014-0438-z.
19. Huygen F, Kallewaard JW, van Tulder M, et al. Evidence-based interventional pain medicine according to clinical diagnoses: update 2018. Pain Pract. 2019;19(6):664–75. https://doi.org/10.1111/papr.12786.

Index

© The Author(s), under exclusive license to Springer Nature
Switzerland AG 2021
A. Abd-Elsayed (ed.), *Trigeminal Nerve Pain*,
https://doi.org/10.1007/978-3-030-60687-9